Handbook of Neuroanesthesia

Fourth Edition

W9-COP-829

Editors

Philippa Newfield, MD
Attending Anesthesiologist
Department of Anesthesiology
California Pacific Medical Center
San Francisco, California

James E. Cottrell, MD
Chairman
Department of Anesthesiology
State University of New York
Downstate Medical Center
Brooklyn, New York

Foreword by

Stephen Onesti, MD
Professor and Chairman
Department of Neurosurgery
State University of New York
Downstate Medical Center
Brooklyn, New York

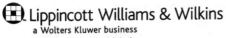

Lippincott Williams & Wilkins
a Wolters Kluwer business
Philadelphia · Baltimore · New York · London
Buenos Aires · Hong Kong · Sydney · Tokyo

Acquisitions Editor: Brian Brown
Managing Editor: Nicole Dernoski
Developmental Editor: Maria McAvey
Project Manager: Alicia Jackson
Senior Manufacturing Manager: Benjamin Rivera
Marketing Manager: Angela Panetta
Design Coordinator: Terry Mallon
Production Service: Laserwords Private Limited, Chennai, India
Printer: RR Donnelley-Crawfordsville

© 2007 by **LIPPINCOTT WILLIAMS & WILKINS, a Wolters Kluwer business**
530 Walnut Street
Philadelphia, PA 19106 USA
LWW.com

3rd edition, © 1999 by Lippincott Williams & Wilkins
2nd edition, © 1991 by Little Brown

Cover Illustration by Frank D. Fasano, MAMS, BFA

Printed in the USA

Library of Congress Cataloging-in-Publication Data
Handbook of neuroanesthesia / editors, Philippa Newfield, James E. Cottrell ; foreword by Stephen Onesti.—4th ed.
  p. ; cm.
Includes bibliographical references and index.
ISBN-13: 978-0-7817-6245-8
ISBN-10: 0-7817-6245-6
  1. Anesthesia in neurology—Handbooks, manuals, etc. 2. Nervous system—Surgery—Complications—Handbooks, manuals, etc. I. Newfield, Philippa. II. Cottrell, James E.
  [DNLM: 1. Anesthesia—Handbooks. 2. Neurosurgical Procedures—Handbooks.
WO 231 H2367 2007]
RD87.3.N47H36 2007
617.9′6748—dc22

                                                                        2006020370

Care has been taken to confirm the accuracy of the information presented and to describe generally accepted practices. However, the authors, editors, and publisher are not responsible for errors or omissions or for any consequences from application of the information in this book and make no warranty, expressed or implied, with respect to the currency, completeness, or accuracy of the contents of the publication. Application of this information in a particular situation remains the professional responsibility of the practitioner.

The authors, editors, and publisher have exerted every effort to ensure that drug selection and dosage set forth in this text are in accordance with current recommendations and practice at the time of publication. However, in view of ongoing research, changes in government regulations, and the constant flow of information relating to drug therapy and drug reactions, the reader is urged to check the package insert for each drug for any change in indications and dosage and for added warnings and precautions. This is particularly important when the recommended agent is a new or infrequently employed drug.

Some drugs and medical devices presented in this publication have Food and Drug Administration (FDA) clearance for limited use in restricted research settings. It is the responsibility of the health care provider to ascertain the FDA status of each drug or device planned for use in their clinical practice.

To purchase additional copies of this book, call our customer service department at (800) 638-3030 or fax orders to (301) 223-2320. International customers should call (301) 223-2300.

Visit Lippincott Williams & Wilkins on the Internet: at LWW.com. Lippincott Williams & Wilkins customer service representatives are available from 8:30 am to 6 pm, EST.

                                                        10 9 8 7 6 5 4 3 2 1

To our neuroanesthesiology fellows who have contributed to improving the quality of care for patients undergoing neurosurgery and neurosurgical critical care procedures through their active involvement in both the clinical and research aspects of our specialty:

Anthony Abadia, MD
Elisabeth Abramowicz, MD
David Acosta, MD
Edwarda Amadeu, MD
Pedro Amorim, MD
Waseem Ashraf, MD
Audrée A. Bendo, MD
Jean Boening, MD
Jean G. Charchaflieh, MD
Lynette Charity, MD
Dennis Dimaculangan, MD
Elie Fried, MD
Lilya Garber, MD
Bhagwandas Gupta, MD
Pavel Illner, MD
Michael Kittay, MD
Brad Litwak, MD
Gina Matei, MD
Michael Mendeszoon, MD
Myrna I. Morales, MD
James K. Ohn, MD
Janet Pittman, MD
Lesly Pompy, MD
Andrew Robustelli, MD
Hector Torres, MD

Contents

I. General Considerations

II. Anesthetic Management

III. Postanesthesia Care Unit & Intensive Care

†Deceased

Contributors List

Steven J. Allen *Chief Executive Officer, Columbus Children's Hospital, Columbus, Ohio*

Miguel F. Arango, MD *Assistant Professor, Department of Anesthesia & Perioperative Medicine, The University of Western Ontario, Anesthesia Consultant, Department of Anesthesia & Perioperative Medicine, London Health Sciences Centre, London, Ontario*

Audrée A. Bendo, MD *Professor, State University of New York, College of Medicine, Vice Chair for Education and Program Director, Department of Anesthesiology, Downstate Medical Center, Brooklyn, New York*

Nicolas J. Bruder, MD *Professor, Department of Anesthesiology and Intensive Care, CHU Timone, Chief, Department of Neuroanesthesiology and Neuro-Intensive Care, CHU Timone, Marseille, France*

Jean G. Charchaflieh, MD, MPH *Associate Professor, Department of Clinical Anesthesiology, State University of New York, College of Medicine, Co-Director Medical / Surgical Intensive Care Unit and Program Director, Critical Care Fellowship Program, Department of Anesthesiology, Downstate Medical Center, Brooklyn, New York*

Daniel J. Cole, MD *Professor, Department of Anesthesiology, Mayo Clinic College of Medicine, Scottsdale, Chair, Department of Anesthesiology, Mayo Clinic Hospital, Phoenix, Arizona*

James E. Cottrell, MD, FRCA *Distinguished Service Professor, State University of New York, College of Medicine, Chairman, Department of Anesthesiology, Downstate Medical Center, Brooklyn, New York*

Gregory Crosby, MD, SM *Associate Professor, Harvard Medical School, Department of Anesthesiology, Brigham & Women's Hospital, Boston, Massachusetts*

Deborah J. Culley, MD *Assistant Professor, Department of Anesthesiology, Harvard Medical School, Assistant Professor, Department of Anesthesiology, Perioperative and Pain Medicine, Brigham and Women's Hospital, Boston, Massachusetts*

Timothy R. Deer, MD, DABPM, FIPP *President and CEO, The Centre for Pain Relief and Clinical Professor of Anesthesiology, West Virginia University School of Medicine, Charleston, West Virginia*

Karen B. Domino, MD, MPH   *Professor, Department of Anesthesiology and Neurological Surgery (Adjunct), University of Washington School of Medicine, Associate Chief of Anesthesiology, Department of Anesthesiology, University of Washington Medical Center, Seattle, Washington*

Lawrence H. Feld, MD   *Attending Anesthesiologist, Vice-Chairman, Department of Anesthesiology, Director of Pediatric Anesthesiology, California Pacific Medical Center, San Francisco, California*

Elie Fried, MD   *Clinical Associate Professor, Department of Anesthesiology, State University of New York, College of Medicine, Downstate Medical Center, Brooklyn, New York*

Adrian W. Gelb, MD   *Professor, Department of Anesthesia and Perioperative Care, University of California San Francisco, San Francisco, California*

Joseph P. Giffin[†]

Rukaiya K. A. Hamid, MBBS, FFARCS, MD   *Department of Pediatric and Adult Anesthesiology, Cedars Sinai Medical Center, Los Angeles, California*

Ian A. Herrick, MD   *Associate Professor, Department of Anesthesia and Perioperative Medicine, and Department of Medicine, Division of Clinical Pharmacology, University of Western Ontario, Chief of Staff, London Health Sciences Centre, London, Ontario, Canada*

Rosemary Hickey, MD   *Professor, Department of Anesthesiology, University of Texas Health Science Center at San Antonio, San Antonio, Texas*

Shailendra Joshi, MD   *Assistant Professor, Department of Anesthesiology, Columbia University, Assistant Attending Anesthesiologist, Department of Anesthesiology, New York Presbyterian Hospital, New York, New York*

Ira S. Kass, PhD   *Professor, Departments of Anesthesiology and Pharmacology, State University of New York, College of Medicine, Downstate Medical Center, Brooklyn, New York*

M. Sean Kincaid, MD   *Acting Assistant Professor, Department of Anesthesiology, University of Washington, Attending in Anesthesia and Critical Care Medicine, Department of Anesthesiology, Harborview Medical Center, Seattle, Washington*

[†]Deceased

Arthur M. Lam, MD   *Professor, Departments of Anesthesiology and Neurological Surgery, University of Washington, Anesthesiologist-in-Chief, Department of Anesthesiology, Harborview Medical Center, Seattle, Washington*

Melissa A. Laxton, MD   *Assistant Professor, Department of Anesthesiology, Wake Forest University School of Medicine, Staff Anesthesiologist, Department of Anesthesiology, Wake Forest University Baptist Medical Center, Winston-Salem, North Carolina*

Linda Liu, MD   *Associate Professor, Department of Anesthesia and Perioperative Care, University of California San Francisco, San Francisco, California*

Sundeep Mangla, MD   *Visiting Associate Professor, State University of New York, College of Medicine, Director of Interventional Neuroradiology, Director of Radiology Research, Departments of Radiology, Neurosurgery and Neurology, Downstate Medical Center, Brooklyn, New York*

Pirjo Hellen Manninen, MD, FRCPC   *Associate Professor, Department of Anesthesia, University of Toronto, Director of Neuroanesthesia, Department of Anesthesia, Toronto Western Hospital, University Health Network, Toronto, Ontario, Canada*

Seth Manoach, MD   *Assistant Professor, Department of Emergency Medicine, State University of New York, College of Medicine, Attending Emergency Physician, Department of Emergency Medicine, Kings County Hospital Center/Downstate Medical Center, Brooklyn, New York*

M. Jane Matjasko, MD   *Professor Emeritus, University of Maryland, Baltimore, Maryland*

Myrna I. Morales, MD   *Clinical Assistant Instructor, Department of Anesthesiology, State University of New York, College of Medicine, Downstate Medical Center, Brooklyn, New York*

Philippa Newfield, MD   *Assistant Clinical Professor, Department of Anesthesia and Neurosurgery, University of California San Francisco, Attending Anesthesiologist, Department of Anesthesiology, California Pacific Medical Center, San Francisco, California*

Stephen Onesti, MD   *Professor and Chairman, Department of Neurosurgery, State University of New York, Downstate Medical Center, College of Medicine, Brooklyn, New York*

C. Lee Parmley, MD *Professor of Anesthesiology, Department of Anesthesiology, Vanderbilt University Medical Center, Director, Division of Critical Care, Department of Anesthesiology, Vanderbilt University Medical Center, Nashville, Tennessee*

Patricia H. Petrozza, MD *Department of Anesthesiology, Wake Forest University School of Medicine, Wake Forest University Baptist Medical Center, Winston-Salem, North Carolina*

Janet Pittman, MD *Attending Anesthesiologist, Department of Anesthesiology, Lutheran Medical Center, Brooklyn, New York*

Patrick A. Ravussin, MD *Professor, Département d'anesthésiologie et de réanimation, Centre Hospitalier Universitaire Vaudois, LAUSANNE, Switzerland, Head, Département d'anesthésiologie et de réanimation, Réseau Santé Valais, CHCVs, site de Sion, SION, Switzerland*

Irene Rozet, MD *Assistant Professor, Department of Anesthesiology, University of Washington, Attending Anesthesiologist, Department of Anesthesiology, Harborview Medical Center, Seattle, Washington*

Takefumi Sakabe, MD *Professor and Chairman, Department of Anesthesiology, Yamaguchi University school of Medicine, Chief, Department of Anesthesiology, Yamaguchi University Hospital, Ube,Yamaguchi, Japan*

David L. Schreibman, MD *Assistant Professor, Department of Anesthesiology, University of Maryland, Director, Neuroanesthesiology, Department of Anesthesiology, University of Maryland Hospital, Baltimore, Maryland*

Jee Jian See, MBBS, MMed *Clinical Teacher, Clinical Research Centre, Yong Loo Lin School of Medicine, National University of Singapore, Consultant, Department of Anesthesiology, Tan Tock Seng Hospital, Singapore*

Gary R. Stier, MD *Associate Professor, Department of Anesthesiology, Loma Linda University School of Medicine, Medical Director-Surgical Trauma ICU, Department of Anesthesiology, Loma Linda University Medical Center, Loma Linda, California*

John M. Taylor, MD *Assistant Clinical Professor, Department of Anesthesia and Perioperative Care, University of California San Francisco, San Francisco, California*

Concezione Tommasino, MD *Associate Professor, Institute of Anesthesiology and Intensive Care, University of Milano, Head of Unit, Department of Anesthesia and Intensive Care San Paolo Hospital, Milano, Italy*

Lela D. Weems, MD   *Clincal Assistant Professor, State University of New York, College of Medicine, Downstate Medical Center, Director, Department of Obstetric Anesthesiology, Long Island College Hospital, Brooklyn, New York*

Deborah M. Whelan, MD   *Department of Anesthesiology, Wake Forest University School of Medicine, Wake Forest University Baptist Medical Center, Winston-Salem, North Carolina*

David J. Wlody, MD   *Clinical Associate Professor, Department of Anesthesiology, State University of New York, College of Medicine, Chairman, Department of Anesthesiology, Long Island College Hospital, Vice Chair for Clinical Affairs, Department of Anesthesiology, Downstate Medical Center, Brooklyn, New York*

Samrat H. Worah, MD   *Clinical Assistant Professor, Department of Anesthesiology, State University of New York-Downstate Medical Center, Attending Anesthesiologist, Department of Anesthesiology, University Hospital of Brooklyn, Brooklyn, New York*

William L. Young, MD   *Professor and Vice Chair, Department of Anesthesia and Perioperative Care, University of California San Francisco, San Francisco, California*

Foreword

It is a distinct honor for me to write the Foreword to the 4th edition of the *Handbook of Neuroanesthesia*. I have had the pleasure of working with one of the editors, James E. Cottrell, at SUNY Downstate Medical Center since 2003. As a neurosurgeon, I have been delighted to work and collaborate with a person who has a deep understanding and love of the human brain and of the practice of neuroanesthesia. Dr. Cottrell has been a mentor, role model, and friend, and his help to the Department of Neurosurgery at Downstate has been invaluable.

The field of neuroanesthesia has advanced dramatically since I first set foot in a neurosurgical operating room more than 20 years ago. Advances in neurologic and physiologic monitoring, pharmacology, and regional anesthetic techniques have created an exceptionally high standard of care that would have been unimaginable a generation ago. The dramatic growth of neurovascular surgery and interventional neuroradiology, skull base surgery, epilepsy and functional neurosurgery, and complex spine surgery would not have been possible without modern neuroanesthetic techniques. As a result, we as neurosurgeons can now offer significantly better care to our patients.

This deceptively small manual has played an outsized role in the education and training of anesthesiologists in the principles of neuroanesthesia since it was first published in 1983. It is a comprehensive guide to the basic science of neuroanesthesia, to the principles of intraoperative management, and to the pre- and postoperative care of the neurosurgical patient. It is essential reading for all anesthesiology residents and fellows. It is also an efficient resource for attending anesthesiologists who need a compact reference that can easily be consulted. In addition, neurointensivists and neurologists will find that it has much to offer in the care of patients in the intensive care unit. Finally, both resident and attending neurosurgeons would benefit greatly by having a thorough knowledge of what is available inside. This will not only make us better neurosurgeons but will also help us understand the issues confronting our neuroanesthesia colleagues in the care of our patients.

Stephen Onesti, MD

Preface

Harvey Cushing, the renowned neurosurgeon, made a number of contributions to anesthesia, setting the stage for the close association between neurosurgeons and neuroanesthesiologists that we have enjoyed ever since. As student "etherizers" at Harvard Medical School in 1894, Cushing and his friend E. Amory Codman developed the first anesthesia record by taking a temperature–pulse–respiration sheet from the ward to the operating room on which to record the patient's intraoperative pulse and respiration. The perhaps apocryphal story is told that Cushing and Codman started a competition as to who could give the best anesthesia. The stakes were dinner and the criterion was the patient's postoperative condition. A perfect anesthetic was one after which the patient was sufficiently conscious when returned to the ward to follow commands and did not vomit subsequently. Cushing also used cocaine as a local anesthetic for shoulder, hip, and hernia operations in 1898 and brought the pneumatic measurement of blood pressure, developed by Scipione Riva-Rocci in Italy, back to Boston in 1902. His excellent record of intracranial operations without significant infection has been attributed to his preferential use of local anesthetic and his dressing the operative site and changing the dressing daily—himself.

It is in this spirit of cooperation, consultation, and collaboration among neuroanesthesiologists, neurosurgeons, neurointensivists, neuropathologists, neuroradiologists, and neurologists that the fourth edition of the *Handbook of Neuroanesthesia* is offered as a concise and easily accessible compendium of neuroanesthetic and neurosurgical critical care. The chapters have been updated to reflect new techniques and practices for awake craniotomy, diagnostic and interventional neuroradiology, management of acute and chronic pain, monitoring modalities, and management of head injury and subarachnoid hemorrhage, among other areas. Suggested readings are included for further exploration of the contents of each chapter.

The advances in neuroanesthesia and neurocritical care of the past several years can be attributed to the intellectual curiosity, creativity, energy, and determination of the physicians who have worked to improve the care of neurosurgical patients. We acknowledge the anesthesiologists who have devoted their careers to advancing the safe and enlightened practice of neuroanesthesia through teaching, research, and clinical care, especially those who have so generously contributed to this volume.

We also express our tremendous appreciation to Anne Minaidis who has shepherded this edition—and the previous three—through the entire process from conceptualization through writing and editing to publication. She has single-handedly functioned as "Mission Control," the liaison among the many editors, authors, and managers involved in this project.

We thank her for seeing the fourth edition through to completion with her organizational skills and characteristic good humor, efficiency, tact, and grace.

Philippa Newfield MD
James E. Cottrell MD

General Considerations

1

Physiology and Metabolism of the Brain and Spinal Cord

Ira S. Kass

I. **Brain and spinal cord physiology.** To understand the effects of anesthesia and surgery on the nervous system, one needs to know basic cellular neurophysiology as well as organ-level physiologic function. This section briefly describes the basic principles of neurophysiology.
   A. **Cellular neurophysiology.** The basic properties of neuronal excitability are due to a change in the membrane potential so that a threshold is reached and the neuron fires an action potential. This propagates to the axon terminal and releases a neurotransmitter that influences the membrane potential of a second neuron.
      1. Membrane potentials are voltages measured across the cell membrane due to an unequal distribution of ions across that membrane. A combination of the equilibrium potential for a particular ion and the membrane's conductance (permeability) for that ion determines its contribution to the membrane potential.
         a. The equilibrium potential (E) for an ion can be calculated using the Nernst equation if the intra- (for potassium, K_i) and extracellular (K_0) concentrations of that ion are known. For an ion with a single positive charge, the equation simplifies to $E_K = -61 \log[K_i/K_0]$ at $37°C$. Under normal conditions in the nervous system, the equilibrium potential for potassium (K) is approximately -90 mV and for sodium (Na) $+45$ mV.
            (1) The relative conductance of the neuronal membrane to different ions determines the membrane potential. This conductance (g) for the different ions varies with conditions, input to the specific neuron, and time. The membrane potential of a neuron at any point in time can be described by the following equation:

$$E_m = \frac{g_K(E_K) + g_{Na}(E_{Na}) + g_x(E_x)}{g_K + g_{Na} + g_x}$$

where g_x is the conductance for ion x and E_x is the equilibrium potential for that ion. The resting membrane potential for a neuron is approximately -70 mV, which

3

is closer to the E_K (-90 mV) than the E_{Na} ($+45$ mV) because g_K is much greater than g_{Na} in resting (unexcited) neurons.

(2) There are concentration-dependent and electrical field-dependent forces acting on ions; the sum of these forces determines whether the net movement of a particular ion will be into or out of that neuron. This is referred to as the electrochemical gradient for that ion.

2. Action potentials are regenerative changes in a neuron's membrane potential due to excitation of the neuron so that its membrane potential depolarizes past a certain threshold. During an action potential, a rapid initial increase in the g_{Na} is followed by a return to baseline and a slower increase in the g_K. These conductance changes lead to a short and rapid depolarization followed by a repolarization. This is sometimes followed by a hyperpolarization after the action potential (Figure 1-1).

   a. The Na conductance changes are due to the opening of a protein channel in the membrane that is selectively permeable to Na ions. This channel has one activation and one inactivation gate, both of which must be in the open configuration if the channel is to allow Na through it. The rapid opening and closing of this channel are in part responsible for the brief duration of the action potential.

   b. At rest, more K than Na channels are open. With the action potential, more Na channels open so that the g_{Na} is greater than the g_K and the neurons depolarize. The depolarization causes a slow opening of K channels, increasing g_K and leading to a repolarization ($g_K > g_{Na}$). In the period after the action potential, when the Na channels have become inactivated, the increased g_K can actually cause a hyperpolarization below the resting potential; this so-called afterhyperpolarization is frequently found in neurons.

3. Synaptic transmission is the process by which one neuron (presynaptic neuron) influences the membrane potential and thereby the action potential generation in a second neuron (postsynaptic neuron). The axon terminals of a neuron contain vesicles with neurotransmitter molecules in them. When a terminal is depolarized, voltage-sensitive calcium (Ca) channels open, increasing the Ca concentration in the terminal. This Ca increase causes the vesicles to release a neurotransmitter into the synaptic cleft. The transmitter diffuses across the synapse and binds to a specific receptor on the postsynaptic neuron. Its effect on the

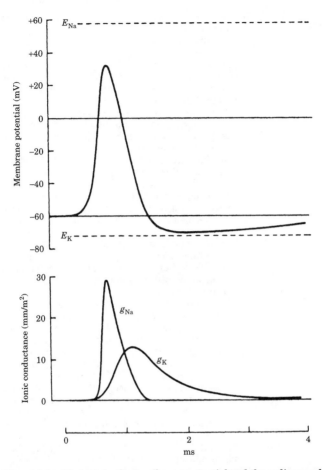

Figure 1-1. Changes in the membrane potential and the sodium and potassium conductances (g_{Na} and g_K) during an action potential. E_{Na} and E_K are the sodium and potassium equilibrium potentials. (In: Aidley DJ. *The Physiology of Excitable Cells.* Cambridge: Cambridge University Press, 1989:65, as redrawn from Hodgkin Al, Huxley AT. A quantitative description of membrane and excitation in nerve current and its application to conduction. *J Physiol* 1952;117: 500–544.)

postsynaptic neuron depends on ion channels that are opened or biochemical processes that are altered by the activation of that receptor.

a. Ionotropic receptor activation opens membrane channels for certain ions that can either hyperpolarize or depolarize the postsynaptic neuron, making it less or more likely to fire an action potential.

b. Metabotropic receptors can activate second messengers that alter neuronal biochemical parameters. This can effect long-term changes in a neuron's activity.

4. Glutamate is a major excitatory neurotransmitter in the central nervous system (CNS). Its activation depolarizes neurons, increasing the number of action potentials generated.

a. There are three major ionotropic glutamate receptors: alpha-amino-3-hydroxy-5-methyl-4-isoxazole propionic acid (AMPA), kainate, and N-methyl-D-aspartic acid (NMDA). The AMPA and kainate receptors are attached to ion channels that allow Na and K to pass through them; a small number of AMPA receptors are also permeable to Ca. The NMDA channels activated when neurons are already depolarized are permeable to Na, K, and Ca. Activation of NMDA channels has been associated with long-term changes in neuronal activity that may be cellular correlates of learning and memory. Overactivation of glutamate receptors has been associated with neuronal injury from epilepsy, trauma, and ischemia.

b. Metabotropic receptors are also activated by glutamate. These receptors act via guanosine 5'-triphosphate (GTP)–binding proteins (G proteins) to affect ion channels or second-messenger pathways (e.g., cyclic 3', 5'-adenosine monophosphate [cAMP], inositol 1,4,5-trisphosphate [IP_3]), which in turn can alter ionic conductance, cell Ca levels, and a host of other biochemical changes. The effect of metabotropic receptor activation is longer in duration than that of inotropic receptor activation.

5. Gamma-aminobutyric acid (GABA) and glycine are major inhibitory neurotransmitters in the CNS. Their activation hyperpolarizes neurons, decreasing the number of action potentials generated. Inhibition is important for the brain and spinal cord to function. When inhibition is substantially reduced, seizures can occur and lead to complete loss of function and permanent brain damage.

a. GABA is a major inhibitory transmitter in the brain and spinal cord. The $GABA_A$ receptor contains a chloride channel that is opened when GABA binds. This activity is augmented by benzodiazepines, volatile anesthetics, and barbiturates. The $GABA_B$ receptor acts via a second messenger to open K channels.

b. Glycine is a major inhibitory transmitter in the spinal cord. Strychnine blocks the action of glycine.

6. Active transport maintains the ionic concentrations required for neuronal function. There is a constant leak of ions down their electrochemical gradients. If not corrected, this leak leads to a loss of these ion gradients. Ion pumps use energy to maintain the ion concentrations necessary for neuronal viability. During ischemia, a decrease in energy production and a loss of ion gradients occurs (Figure 1-2).

a. Adenosine 5'-triphosphate (ATP) is a source of energy for many ion pumps. The Na–K ATPase pump maintains high intracellular K concentrations and low intracellular Na concentrations. The pump compensates for the leak of these ions in inactive neurons and the large changes in these ions during the action potential. If this pump is blocked, neurons quickly lose their ability to function. ATPase

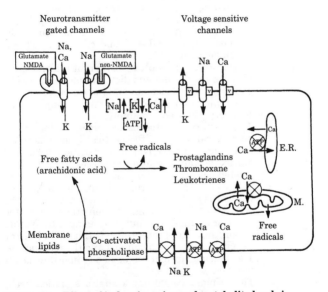

Figure 1-2. Effect of ischemia on ion and metabolite levels in neurons. For clarity, ion channels are shown on the top membrane and ion pumps on the bottom membrane; their actual location can be on any membrane surface. Circles indicate energy-driven pumps; an x through the circle indicates that this pump is blocked or has reduced activity during ischemia. V indicates a voltage-dependent channel. NMDA, *N*-methyl-D-aspartic acid; ATP, adenosine triphosphate. (From: Bendo AA, Kass IS, Hartung J, et al., Anesthesia for neurosurgery. In: Barash PG, Cullen BF, Stoelting RK, eds. *Clinical Anesthesia*, 4th ed. Philadelphia, PA: Lippincott Williams & Wilkins, 2001:743–790.)

pumps in the plasma membrane and the endoplasmic reticulum maintain low cytosolic Ca concentrations in neurons.

b. The Na gradient is a source of energy for ion pumps and amino acid transporters. These active transporters couple the energy of Na as it goes down its electrochemical gradient with the pumping of other ions and metabolites up their gradients. To maintain appropriate cellular levels of Ca and hydrogen (H), Na–Ca and Na–H exchangers are important transporters. The transport of glutamate and other amino acids from the extracellular to the intracellular compartment also uses the energy of the Na gradient. The gradient is maintained by the Na–K ATPase pump; thus, the ultimate energy for this ion exchanger comes from ATP used to power the Na–K pump.

c. When energy fails due to hypoxia or ischemia, the pumps can no longer maintain the gradients, intra- and extracellular ion concentrations change and the neurons depolarize, leading to a rapid and complete membrane depolarization and eventual cell death. This is illustrated in Figure 1-2.

B. **Regional neurophysiology.** Different regions of the brain subserve different and distinct functions. We can provide only a very brief summary of them; for details, refer to *Principles of Neural Science* by Kandel et al. See Figure 1-3 for neuroanatomy.

1. The primary somatosensory cortex located on the postcentral gyrus is the cortical locus where somatic sensations converge. Association areas that aid in the interpretation of these sensations are located posterior to this gyrus.

2. The primary motor cortex is located on the precentral gyrus and has output to motor neurons in the spinal cord. Premotor association areas are located anterior to this gyrus and receive input from other important motor centers of the brain including the cerebellum, the basal ganglia, and the red nucleus. The reticular formation also has important motor functions.

3. The primary visual and visual association areas are located in the occipital lobe.

4. The primary auditory and auditory association areas are located in the temporal lobe.

5. Wernicke's area is located on the angular gyrus in the dominant hemisphere. It is a multimodal association area. Lesions in this area are devastating and can lead to the loss of comprehension of written and spoken words.

6. The frontal association areas are important for controlling personality and directing intellectual activity through sequential steps toward a goal.

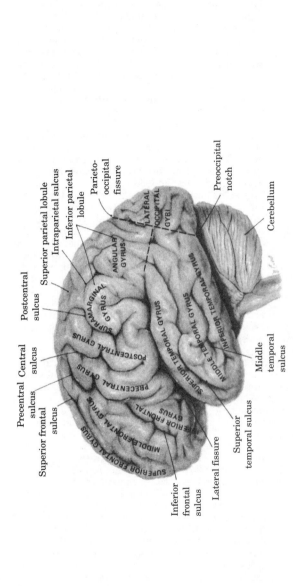

Figure 1-3. Lateral view of the cerebral cortex. (In: Gilman S, Newman SW. *Manter and Gatz's Essentials of Clinical Neuroanatomy and Neurophysiology* 8th ed. Philadelphia, PA: FA Davis Co, 1992:7.)

7. The limbic areas of the brain, not shown in Figure 1-3, are located medially. Limbic system structures include the hypothalamus, the amygdala, the hippocampus, and the limbic cortex. These areas are associated with feelings of reward and punishment, emotional behavior, learning, and memory. The hippocampus is essential for the transformation of short-term to long-term memory. The hypothalamus controls many bodily vegetative functions (cardiovascular, temperature, and water regulation).

8. The brain stem contains the reticular activating system, which is responsible for maintaining alertness. The vasomotor areas located in the brain stem are important for circulatory control. Lesions in the brain stem can lead to coma.

9. The spinal cord is important as a pathway for information between the body and the brain as well as for the generation of certain reflexes. Input to the spinal cord comes via the dorsal root to the dorsal horn; output from motor neurons, which are located in the ventral horn, is via the ventral root. Input to the brain via the spinal cord can be modified before transmission to the brain via ascending tracts. Indeed, descending pathways can reduce pain input at the spinal level. These pathways are activated by periaqueductal and periventricular gray regions of the brain.

II. Brain and spinal cord metabolism

A. Energy utilization by neurons in the brain and spinal cord.

Neurons have a high metabolic rate and use more energy than other cells. Although the brain accounts for 2% of total body weight, it uses 20% of the body's total oxygen consumption. Most energy-requiring processes in cells use either ATP directly or energy stores indirectly derived from ATP such as ion gradients.

1. Ion pumping accounts for a large part of a neuron's energy requirement. The Na–K pump alone accounts for 25% to 40% of a neuron's ATP utilization. Calcium and the transport of other cations (e.g., H) or anions (Cl or HCO_3) also account for significant energy utilization. Some pumping of Ca and H is coupled with Na for an energy source and depletes the Na gradient; thus, Ca and H are indirectly coupled to ATP utilization via the Na–K pump. Energy is required to pump ions from the cytosol to intracellular organelles and to pump molecules across the plasmalemma.

2. Transport of amino acids and other essential small molecules across the cell membranes requires energy. Glutamate and many other neurotransmitters are removed from the extracellular space by active pumps that require energy. Reduced activity

of the glutamate pump can lead to excessive excitability and neuronal damage.

3. Neuronal structure and function require the synthesis of proteins, lipids, and carbohydrates. These substances are continually being formed, modified, and degraded and require ATP for their synthesis.

4. The transport of substances within cells also requires energy. Most synthesis takes place in the cell body, and an energy-dependent transport system distributes these substances to the parts of the neuron that require them. The enormity of the task is apparent when one considers the length of the axons and dendrites of a typical neuron; diffusion is not sufficient, and active transport is required.

B. **Energy synthesis by neurons in the brain and spinal cord**

1. Efficient ATP production from glucose requires oxygen (Figure 1-4).

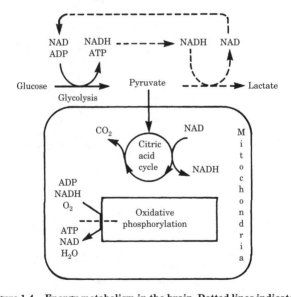

Figure 1-4. Energy metabolism in the brain. Dotted lines indicate reactions that occur during ischemia. The dotted line across the oxidative phosphorylation reaction indicates that this reaction is blocked during ischemia. NAD, nicotinamide adenine dinucleotide; ADP, adenosine diphosphate; NADH, nicotinamide adenine dinucleotide, reduced form; ATP, adenosine triphosphate. (From: Bendo AA, Kass IS, Hartung J, et al. Anesthesia for neurosurgery. In: Barash PG, Cullen BF, Stoelting RK, eds. *Clinical Anesthesia*, 4th ed. Philadelphia, PA: Lippincott Williams & Wilkins, 2001:743–790.)

a. The major portion of energy is generated by glycolysis (breakdown of glucose), the citric acid cycle (a pathway that generates nicotinamide adenine dinucleotide, reduced form [NADH], from nicotinamide adenine dinucleotide [NAD]), and oxidative phosphorylation (coupling of the regeneration of NAD from NADH to the production of ATP). The mitochondria and oxygen are critical for the efficient production of ATP from glucose. The yield of 1 glucose is a maximum of 38 ATP molecules

$$C_6H_{12}O_6 + 6O_2 + 38ADP + 38P_i \rightarrow 6CO_2$$
$$+ 6H_2O + 38ATP$$

(1) In an actual neuron, other synthesis pathways use some of the energy and biochemical intermediates so that the average yield per glucose is between 30 to 35 ATP molecules.

b. In the absence of oxygen, the mitochondria cannot convert NADH to NAD and lose much of the energy of glucose oxidation. Each molecule of glucose yields only 2 ATP molecules. This is insufficient to meet the energy demands of the brain. Glucose $+ 2ADP + 2P_i + 2NAD \rightarrow$ 2pyruvate $+ 2ATP + 2NADH \rightarrow$ 2lactate $+$ 2H $+ 2NAD$. The last step is required to regenerate the NAD from NADH; no energy is obtained from this step in the absence of oxygen. The H ion generated can lead to neuronal damage under certain circumstances.

(1) High blood glucose before hypoxia or ischemia has been shown clinically and in animals to increase damage. The excess H ion production could partially explain this.

C. **Emergency sources of energy during metabolic stress**

1. There are two immediate sources of ATP when energy production does not meet the cell's demand for energy.

a. The enzyme adenylate kinase can convert adenosine diphosphate (ADP) to ATP.

$$ADP + ADP \leftrightarrows ATP + AMP$$

When energy production recovers, this process is reversed.

b. Phosphocreatine (PCr) acts as a store of high-energy phosphate that can be rapidly converted to ATP. Normally there are two to three times more PCr than ATP. Nevertheless, PCr levels fall rapidly during ischemia.

$$PCr + ADP + H \leftrightarrows ATP + Cr$$

2. The mechanism of energy production and its reduced usage during ischemia
   a. In addition to the formation of ATP from 2ADP or PCr, anaerobic glycolysis contributes to ATP maintenance. Anaerobic glycolysis leads to acidosis, which may be damaging to neurons. With ischemia that lasts for more than several minutes, ATP formation from 2ADPs and PCr is exhausted and anaerobic glycolysis continues only so long as glucose is available. Some glucose is produced from the breakdown of glycogen.
   b. Shortly after the onset of ischemia (in about 30 seconds), spontaneous neuronal activity stops and the electroencephalogram (EEG) becomes quiet. This reduces the neuron's metabolic rate and ATP utilization.

D. **The overall metabolic rate for the brain**
   1. The cerebral metabolic rate of awake young adults is 3.5 mL O_2/100 g/minute or 5.5 mg glucose/100 g/minute. This rate is virtually identical in healthy elderly persons. Children have a higher metabolic rate, i.e., 5.2 mL O_2/100 g/minute. The reason for the higher metabolic rate in children is unknown, but it may represent continuing growth and development of the nervous system.

E. **Molecular aspects of neuronal metabolism, survival versus apoptosis**
   1. Many more neurons are formed during mammalian development than the adult organism needs. In many areas of the brain and spinal cord, 50% of the neurons die as the animal matures.
      a. The target cells of a neuron—those cells a neuron innervates—secrete trophic factors (e.g., nerve growth factor and brain-derived neurotrophic factor) in limited quantities. If the neuron receives enough of these trophic factors, it survives; if not, it dies. Because trophic factors are limited, an average 50% of the neurons do not receive enough trophic factors and die.
      b. Neurons also receive trophic factors from nontarget sources such as glia; this also promotes survival. The combination of trophic factors from all sources determines whether a neuron will survive or die.
      c. The trophic factors work by binding to external receptors on membrane-spanning proteins. When their receptor is bound by a trophic factor, these proteins activate intracellular signals, which in some cases phosphorylate other intracellular proteins and alter cellular processes leading to neuronal survival (Figure 1-5).
         One example of such binding is the tyrosine receptor kinase (trk): it binds nerve growth

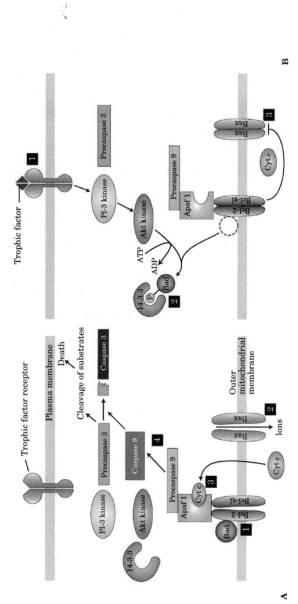

Figure 1-5. Trophic factors and apoptosis. A: Absence of trophic factor: caspase activation. B: Presence of trophic factor: inhibition of caspase activation. ATP, adenosine triphosphate; ADP, adenosine diphosphate. (From: Lodish H, Berk A, Matsudaira P, et al, eds. *Molecular Cell Biology*, 5th ed. New York: W.H. Freeman & Co, 2004:929 as adapted from Pettmann B, Henderson CE. Neuronal cell death. *Neuron* 1998;20:633.)

factor, brain-derived neurotrophic factor, or other neurotrophins, dimerizes (combines two identical molecules), and then becomes active. It adds a phosphate group onto the amino acid tyrosine of certain proteins. This addition alters the activity of these proteins and inhibits cell death pathways.

  d. If a cell does not receive enough trophic factor, certain proteins are not phosphorylated and a programmed cell death pathway is activated. This process is called *apoptosis* and causes cells to die in a way that does not cause inflammation. In the absence of trophic factor–induced phosphorylation, a molecule called *apoptosis activating factor 1* (Apaf-1) is activated, leading to the proteolysis of inactive procaspases to active caspases, which in turn splits other proteins and signals the cell to undergo programmed cell death (apoptosis).

  2. During and after ischemia, hypoxia, or other injury, neurons can die by one of at least two pathways, necrosis or apoptosis.

    a. Necrosis is caused by severe injury that causes neurons to swell and burst apart. In addition to causing the death of that neuron, inflammation and further cell death occur in that region of the brain.

    b. If the injury is less severe and the neuron can recover its ability to make ATP, the neuron can activate the apoptosis pathway and die in a manner similar to the death of excess neurons during development. The advantage of this apoptosis is that the neuron does not break apart and the neurons around it are preserved, resulting in less overall brain damage.

      (1) Apoptosis is triggered by ion flux into the mitochondria through an ion channel formed from the binding of two bax protein molecules together. The ion flux leads to the release of cytochrome c, which binds to Apaf-1, activates it, and initiates the caspase cascade of apoptosis (Figure 1-5).

III. Cerebral and spinal cord blood flow

  A. **Rate of cerebral blood flow (CBF).** CBF rates are largely determined by the cerebral metabolic rate for oxygen consumption; there is exquisite coupling of blood flow and metabolism on a regional basis. The global blood flow to the brain remains fairly stable for a given physiologic state (e.g., awake adult). Anesthetics and hypothermia tend to decrease metabolism throughout the brain and thereby reduce global CBF.

    1. The global CBF in adults is approximately 50 mL/100 g/minute. This global measure is composed of flow from two very different regions: the gray matter, which is where neuronal cell bodies and synapses are located and has a blood flow of 75 mL/100 g/minute, and the white matter, which consists mainly of fiber tracts and has a blood flow of 20 mL/100 g/minute. The higher blood flow to gray matter is primarily due to its greater metabolic rate.

2. The global CBF of children is approximately 95 mL/100 g/minute, which is higher than that of adults. In contrast, infants have a slightly lower CBF than adults (40 mL/100 g/minute).

3. Spinal cord blood flow has been less extensively studied; the gray matter has a rate of 60 mL/100 g/minute and the white matter a rate of 20 mL/100 g/minute.

B. Regulation of CBF

1. Regional flow−metabolism coupling depends on the buildup of metabolites that cause local dilatation of the microvessels.

   a. The precise mechanism of this coupling is unknown. It may be due to the buildup of K or H in the extracellular fluid surrounding the arterioles. Other agents that may mediate flow−metabolism coupling include nitric oxide (NO), calcium, adenosine, and eicosanoids such as thromboxane and prostaglandin. A combination of these factors likely contributes to coupling.

2. NO is a vasodilator that is released locally by the vascular endothelial cells. This vasodilatation is important for vascular regulation throughout the body, but the precise role of NO in the control of CBF remains to be determined. It is likely to be an important regulator of local CBF, perhaps by affecting arterioles upstream of the microvessels dilated by metabolic factors.

3. Carbon dioxide (CO_2) enhances vasodilatation and increases CBF. CO_2 is hydrated with the help of carbonic anhydrase leading to an acidification. This reduction in pH is thought to cause the vasodilatation. When CO_2 is halved from 40 to 20 mm Hg, the CBF is reduced by approximately half (Figure 1-6).

   a. Hyperventilation leads to a reduction in CO_2, an increase in pH, and thereby a reduction in CBF. If hyperventilation is maintained over a period of 6 to 8 hours, the pH returns to normal due to bicarbonate transport and CBF returns to its prehyperventilation levels. Thus, hyperventilation is useful for only short periods of time.

      (1) If hyperventilation is discontinued abruptly, the increase in CO_2 to the normal level, in the presence of reduced HCO_3, leads to acidosis and an above

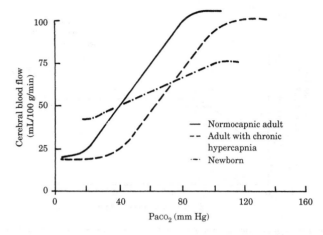

Figure 1-6.   Relationship between cerebral blood flow and arterial carbon dioxide tension (Pa_{CO_2}) in the normocapnic adult, the hypercapnic adult, and the newborn.

normal increase in CBF. This can be a critical problem when hyperventilation is used to reduce intracranial pressure (ICP).

    (2) It is possible that extreme hyperventilation to levels below 20 mm Hg can lead to ischemia due to vasoconstriction; thus, hyperventilation below 30 mm Hg is not recommended clinically.

4. Autoregulation allows CBF to remain constant if the cerebral perfusion pressure (CPP) varies between 50 and 150 mm Hg. Signs of cerebral ischemia are seen below 50 mm Hg; above 150 mm Hg, disruption of the blood-brain barrier (BBB) and cerebral edema may occur. The adjustment of flow to abrupt changes in pressure requires 30 to 180 seconds (Figure 1-7).

    a. The mechanism of autoregulation is not completely understood but is likely to be a combination of effects including myogenic and metabolic factors.

        (1) Myogenic activity of the vessel wall musculature occurs in response to increased distending pressure. In isolated vessels, when the vessel wall is stretched, as it would be by increased blood pressure, the smooth muscle contracts, causing a vasoconstriction that reduces flow. This balances out the increase in blood flow due to the increased pressure, resulting in little net change in blood flow.

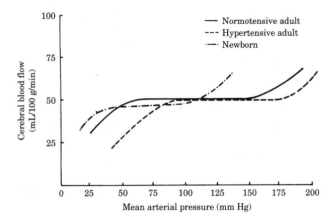

Figure 1-7. Autoregulatory curve of the cerebral vasculature in the normotensive adult, the hypertensive adult, and the newborn.

(2) The metabolic theory states that reduced pressure leads to reduced flow and the buildup of metabolites. This buildup in metabolites and the decrease in local pH lead to a local vasodilatation and thereby an increase in blood flow back to normal.

(3) Autoregulation can be impaired by hypoxia, ischemia, hypercapnia, trauma, and certain anesthetic agents.

(4) Patients who are chronically hypertensive or have a high sympathetic tone have a shift in the autoregulatory curve to the right. They may demonstrate signs of ischemia due to reduced blood flow at pressures above the lower limit for normotensive individuals.

5. The partial pressure of oxygen (Pao_2) has little effect on global CBF until it falls below 50 mm Hg. At this point, a dramatic increase in blood flow with further reductions in Pao_2 occurs. Since the oxygen-carrying capacity of blood is high, a critical reduction in the oxygen content of the blood might not occur until the Pao_2 falls below a threshold of 50 mm Hg (Figure 1-8).

6. Neurogenic factors including adrenergic, cholinergic, and serotonergic systems also influence CBF. Their greatest influence is on larger blood vessels.

7. The hematocrit alters blood viscosity and thereby can affect blood flow. A low hematocrit can increase blood flow by decreasing blood viscosity.

8. Hypothermia decreases neuronal metabolism and thereby reduces CBF; hyperthermia has the opposite effect.

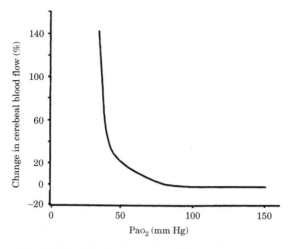

Figure 1-8. Relationship between cerebral blood flow and Pa_{O_2}, arterial oxygen tension.

9. The metabolic rate of neurons surrounding the microvasculature regulates regional blood flow. If the activity of these neurons increases, their metabolic rate increases, and the blood flow to that region increases to meet the demand for oxygen and glucose. This property has been exploited using positron emission tomography to functionally map brain activity.

IV. **Cerebrospinal fluid (CSF) and the blood-brain barrier**

A. **CSF formation** CSF is formed in the choroid plexus of the cerebral ventricles (70%) and across the pial and ependymal surfaces (30%) at a rate of 0.4 mL/minute. The total volume of CSF is between 100 and 150 mL.

1. CSF is an ultrafiltrate of plasma whose final composition is modified by active (mainly Na) and passive (most importantly glucose) transport of ions and other metabolites (Table 1-1). Proteins and other hydrophilic molecules are poorly permeable and excluded from the CSF. The capillary endothelium in the choroid plexus is freely permeable to substances. The epithelial cells of the choroid plexus contain tight junctions and are the site of the blood–CSF barrier.

a. CSF formation is reduced by (a) decreased choroidal blood flow and capillary hydrostatic pressure, (b) hypothermia, (c) increased serum osmolarity, and (d) increased ICP.

2. CSF flows through the ventricles and out to the subarachnoid space of the brain and the spinal

Table 1-1. Composition of cerebrospinal fluid and serum in humans

Component	CSF	Serum
Sodium (mEq/L)	141	140
Potassium (mEq/L)	2.9	4.6
Calcium (mEq/L)	2.5	5.0
Magnesium (mEq/L)	2.4	1.7
Chloride (mEq/L)	124	101
Bicarbonate (mEq/L)	21	23
Glucose (mg/100 mL)	61	92
Protein (mg/100 mL)	28	7000
pH	7.31	7.41
Osmolality (mosmol/kg H_2O)	289	289

Adapted with permission from Artru AA. Cerebrospinal fluid. In: Cottrell JE, Smith DS, eds. *Anesthesia and Neurosurgery.* St. Louis: Mosby, 1994:95.

cord. It is reabsorbed into venous blood via the arachnoid villi. If reabsorption is impeded, CSF builds up and ICP increases.
  B. **Blood-brain barrier.** The BBB isolates the brain from substances in the plasma and is important for normal brain function.
    1. The site of the BBB is the capillary endothelial cells. They are connected to each other via tight junctions that exclude the passage of substances between them. Any substance that crosses into the brain from the blood must cross the capillary epithelial cell. The tight junctions and therefore the BBB are not present in the choroid plexus and certain other small areas of the brain (e.g., restricted areas of the hypothalamus).
    2. Water, gases, and lipophilic substances are freely permeable to the BBB. Proteins and polar (hydrophilic) substances are poorly permeable to the BBB and cross this barrier only if there is a specific transport system for them. Glucose, ions, and certain amino acids are transported across the BBB. Because glucose is passively transported to and metabolized in the CNS, its concentration in the brain is usually 60% of its plasma level. This transport is saturable, so that large changes in glucose concentrations require time to equilibrate (Table 1-1).
V. **Intracranial components and volume**
  A. ICP is determined by the volume of the various intracranial components. Normal ICP is approximately 10 mm Hg. Because the cranium has a fixed volume, an increased volume of any intracranial component must be compensated for by a decrease in the volume

of another component. Otherwise, the pressure in the cranium will increase.

1. There are three major intracranial components.
   a. Brain tissue represents 80% to 85% of the intracranial volume and is composed of a cellular component that includes the neurons and glia, and an extracellular component consisting of the interstitial fluid.
   b. The CSF volume accounts for 7% to 10% of the intracranial volume.
   c. The cerebral blood volume accounts for 5% to 8% of the intracranial volume and includes the blood in the vascular space.
2. There is an elastance or compliance to the components in the cranium such that a small increase in the volume of one component does not cause an increase in pressure. Once this compliance is exhausted, small increases in volume lead to large increases in ICP (Figure 1-9).
3. Increases in cranial volume can be caused by:
   a. Increases in CSF volume due to blockage of the circulation or absorption of CSF.
   b. Increased cerebral blood volume due to vasodilatation (intravascular) or hematoma (extravascular).
   c. Increased brain tissue volume due to a tumor or edema.

B. **Brain edema.** Brain edema is classified as cytotoxic or vasogenic and can increase ICP.
   1. Cytotoxic edema is due to swelling of the neuronal and/or glial cellular component and is frequently the result of cerebral ischemia or trauma.
   2. Vasogenic edema is caused by a breakdown of the BBB. The resultant extra-vascularization of

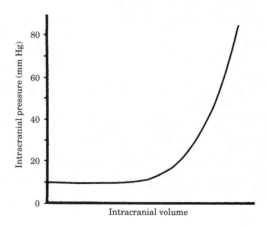

Figure 1-9.   Idealized intracranial pressure–volume curve.

protein increases interstitial water due to an increase in osmotic equivalents in the extravascular space.

C. **ICP pathophysiology.** An increase in ICP can have severe pathophysiologic consequences.

1. CPP can be calculated by subtracting ICP from mean arterial pressure (MAP) (i.e., CPP = MAP − ICP).

a. As ICP increases, CPP decreases. This leads to cerebral ischemia. Normally cerebral ischemia leads to the Cushing reflex, which increases MAP. However, this can compensate only up to a certain point beyond which CPP will fall further, leading to severe ischemia, coma, and death if ICP is uncontrolled.

b. Increased ICP can also cause herniation of the brain, which can lead to rapid neurologic deterioration and death.

SUGGESTED READINGS

Artru AA. Cerebrospinal fluid. In: Cottrell JE, Smith DS, eds. *Anesthesia and Neurosurgery*, 4th ed. St. Louis, MO: Mosby, 2001:83−100.

Bendo AA, Kass IS, Hartung J, et al. Anesthesia for neurosurgery. In: Barash PG, Cullen BF, Stoelting RK, eds. *Clinical Anesthesia*, 4th ed. Philadelphia, PA: Lippincott−Raven Publishers, 2001:743−790.

Dugan LL, Kim-Han JS. Hypoxic-ischemic brain injury and oxidative stress. In: Siegel G, Albers RW, Brady S, et al, eds. *Basic Neurochemistry: Molecular, Cellular and Medical Aspects*, 7th ed. New York, NY: Academic Press an imprint of Elsevier, 2006:559−574.

Fitch W. Brain metabolism. In: Cottrell JE, Smith DS, eds. *Anesthesia and Neurosurgery*, 4th ed. St. Louis, MO: Mosby, 2001:1−18.

Joshi S, Young WL, Ornstein E. Cerebral and spinal cord blood flow. In: Cottrell JE, Smith DS, eds. *Anesthesia and Neurosurgery*, 4th ed. St. Louis, MO: Mosby, 2001:19−68.

Kandel ER, Schwartz JH, Jessell TM, eds. Part II Cell and molecular biology of the neuron. Part III Elementary interactions between neurons: synaptic transmission. In *Principles of Neural Science*, 4th ed. New York, NY: McGraw-Hill, 2000:67−309.

Lodish H, Berk A, Matsudaira P, et al, eds. *Molecular Cell Biology*, 5th ed. New York, NY: W. H. Freeman and Co, 2004, Signaling pathways that control gene activity, 571−610; Cell birth, lineage and death, 899−934.

McKenna MC, Gruetter R, Sonnewald U. Energy metabolism of the brain. In: Siegel G, Albers RW, Brady S, et al, eds. *Basic Neurochemistry: Molecular, Cellular and Medical Aspects*, 7th ed. New York, NY: Academic Press, an imprint of Elsevier, 2006:531−558.

Patel PM, Drummond JC. Cerebral physiology and the effects of anesthetics and techniques. In: Miller RD, ed. *Anesthesia*, 6th ed. Philadelphia, PA: Elsevier Science, 2005:813−858.

Effects of Anesthesia on Cerebral and Spinal Cord Physiology

Rosemary Hickey

The anesthetic management of neurosurgical patients is based on the knowledge of the selected drug's influence on the central nervous system (CNS) physiology. The specific anesthetic regimen is a combination of drugs that favorably affects cerebral hemodynamics, cerebral metabolism, and intracranial pressure (ICP) to provide good operating conditions and to enhance the probability of a quality outcome. Most anesthetic drugs have been studied in this regard and, as new drugs are developed, their effects on cerebral physiology will be elucidated. The effects of anesthetic drugs on cerebrospinal fluid (CSF) volume (as determined by the rate of formation and the resistance to reabsorption) have also been determined.

Few studies have addressed the effects of anesthetic drugs on spinal cord physiology. This could be in part because noninvasive methods of measuring various aspects of spinal cord physiology in the human are not available so that most of the data have been derived from animal studies. Although it has been assumed that the effects of anesthetics on the spinal cord mimic their effects in the brain (and this is likely to be qualitatively correct), to make true comparisons, investigators must examine both brain and spinal cord parameters simultaneously.

I. **Intravenous drugs**
   A. **Barbiturates**
      1. **Effect on cerebral blood flow (CBF) and cerebral oxygen consumption** (Table 2-1). Barbiturates were the first anesthetics to be examined for their cerebral vascular effects. Thiopental decreases CBF and cerebral metabolic rate for oxygen consumption (CMR_{O_2}) in a parallel fashion up to the point of isoelectricity on the electroencephalogram (EEG). The changes in CBF are thought to be secondary to the changes in CMR_{O_2} (a coupled decrease in flow and metabolism). The component of CMR_{O_2} that is affected is related to electrical brain function; there is minimal effect on the component of CMR_{O_2} associated with cellular homeostasis. At the point at which an isoelectric EEG occurs after the administration of thiopental, an approximately 50% decrease in CMR_{O_2} occurs with no cerebral metabolic evidence of toxicity. If barbiturates are used clinically for the purpose of cerebral protection, the endpoint of EEG burst suppression is

Table 2-1. Effects of anesthetic agents on cerebral blood flow, cerebral metabolic rate for oxygen consumption, and intracranial pressure

Anesthetic	CBF	CMRO$_2$	ICP
Thiopental	Decrease	Decrease	Decrease
Etomidate	Decrease	Decrease	Decrease
Propofol	Decrease	Decrease	Decrease
Fentanyl	0/Decrease	0/Decrease	0/Decrease
Alfentanil	0/Decrease/ increase	0/Decrease	0/Decrease/ increase
Sufentanil	0/Decrease/ increase	0/Decrease	0/Decrease/ increase
Ketamine	Increase	0/Increase	Increase
Midazolam	Decrease	Decrease	0/Decrease
Nitrous oxide	Increase	0/Increase	Increase
Isoflurane	Increase	Decrease	Increase
Desflurane	Increase	Decrease	Increase
Sevoflurane	Increase	Decrease	Increase

CBF, cerebral blood flow; CMRO$_2$, cerebral metabolic rate for oxygen consumption; ICP, intracranial pressure.

often used to provide near-maximal metabolic suppression. The reduction in mean arterial pressure (MAP) associated with the high doses of thiopental needed to provide EEG burst suppression may require concomitant use of a vasopressor to maintain cerebral perfusion pressure (CPP), the difference between MAP and ICP. Methohexital differs from other barbiturates in regard to epileptiform activity in that it may induce seizures in patients who have epilepsy and thus increase CMRO$_2$ and CBF.

2. **Effect on autoregulation and CO$_2$ reactivity.** Thiopental, even in high doses, does not appear to abolish cerebral autoregulation or CO$_2$ reactivity.

3. **Effect on CSF dynamics** (Table 2-2). Low doses of thiopental cause no change in the rate of CSF formation (V_f) and either no change or an increase in the resistance to reabsorption of CSF (R_a). This would predict no change or an increase in ICP. High doses of thiopental cause a decrease in V_f and either no change or a decrease in R_a with a predicted decrease in ICP.

4. **Effect on ICP.** As a result of the reduction in both CBF and cerebral blood volume (CBV), barbiturates lower ICP. Barbiturates are used clinically for this purpose and may even be effective when other methods for reducing ICP have failed.

5. **Effect on spinal cord blood flow (SCBF) and metabolism.** Barbiturates produce a significant

Table 2-2. Effects of intravenous drugs on rate of cerebrospinal fluid formation, resistance to reabsorption of cerebrospinal fluid, and the predicted effect on intracranial pressure

Intravenous drug	V_f	R_a	Predicted ICP effect
Thiopental			
Low dose	0	+, 0*	+, 0*
High dose	−	0, −*	−
Etomidate			
Low dose	0	0	0
High dose	−	0, −*	−
Propofol	0	0	0
Ketamine	0	+	+
Midazolam			
Low dose	0	+, 0*	+, 0*
High dose	−	0, +*	−, ?*

V_f, rate of CSF formation; R_a, resistance to CSF reabsorption; ICP, intracranial pressure; 0, no change; +, increase; −, decrease; *, effect dependent on dose; ?, uncertain.
Adapted from Artru AA. CSF dynamics, cerebral edema, and intracranial pressure. In: Albin MS, ed. *Textbook of Neuroanesthesia with Neurosurgical and Neuroscience Perspectives.* New York: McGraw-Hill, 1997:61.

reduction in SCBF. Autoregulation of SCBF remains intact under barbiturate anesthesia (as demonstrated with thiopental) with an autoregulatory range of approximately 60 to 120 mm Hg. Pentobarbital has been shown to decrease local utilization of glucose in the spinal cord, although the magnitude of this effect is smaller than that seen in the brain.

B. Etomidate

  1. **Effect on CBF and $CMRo_2$.** Etomidate, like the barbiturates, reduces CBF and $CMRo_2$. An isoelectric EEG can be induced with etomidate, and, as with thiopental, there is no evidence of cerebral toxicity as reflected by normal brain metabolites. In addition, no further reduction in $CMRo_2$ occurs when additional doses are given after EEG burst suppression is achieved. Myoclonus produced by the drug has the disadvantage of being misinterpreted as seizure activity in neurosurgical patients. Prolonged use of etomidate may suppress the adrenocortical response to stress. However, this may not be an issue in patients who have intracranial tumors because they are already receiving steroids frequently. Less cardiovascular depression with etomidate as compared to thiopental makes this drug advantageous for the induction of

anesthesia in trauma patients and older neurosurgical patients who have multiple medical problems.

2. **Effect on autoregulation and CO_2 response.** Reactivity to CO_2 is maintained with the administration of etomidate. The effect of etomidate on autoregulation has not been evaluated.

3. **Effect on CSF dynamics.** Low-dose etomidate causes no change in V_f and R_a with no predicted effect on ICP. High-dose etomidate causes a decrease in V_f and either no change or a decrease in R_a with a predicted decrease in ICP.

4. **Effect on ICP.** Etomidate has been shown to reduce ICP without decreasing CPP and is clinically useful in neurosurgical patients for this purpose.

C. **Propofol**

1. **Effect on CBF and CMR_{O_2}.** Propofol produces dose-related reductions in both CBF and CMR_{O_2}. In neurosurgical patients who are hypovolemic, the reduction in MAP might be substantial when they receive large bolus doses of propofol. Either the intravascular volume of these patients should be restored before the administration of propofol or an alternative induction drug should be used. A continuous infusion of propofol may be used intraoperatively as part of a total intravenous technique. The combination of an infusion of propofol and a narcotic (such as remifentanil) is particularly useful when the monitoring of evoked potentials precludes the use of other than low concentrations of inhalational drugs. Propofol is also useful for sedation during awake craniotomies and as a substitute for an inhalational drug at the end of a general anesthetic to shorten the wake-up time.

2. **Effect on autoregulation and CO_2 response.** Autoregulation and CO_2 response are preserved during the administration of propofol.

3. **Effect on CSF dynamics.** Propofol causes no change in V_f or R_a with no predicted effect on ICP.

4. **Effect on ICP.** Propofol reduces ICP. Because it also reduces MAP, its effect on CPP must be carefully monitored. Nonetheless, propofol's ICP-lowering effect makes it useful in the intensive care unit (ICU) for the sedation of patients in whom elevated ICP is a concern. Propofol has the advantage of allowing prompt awakening which is advantageous in patients whose neurologic status needs to be evaluated serially. In the operating room, moderately deep sedation with propofol does not increase ICP in comparison to no sedation in patients undergoing stereotactic biopsy for brain tumors. During craniotomy for resection of brain tumors, ICP has been shown to be lower in patients who receive propofol-fentanyl in comparison to

patients anesthetized with isoflurane-fentanyl or sevoflurane-fentanyl. The antinausea effect of propofol is also advantageous in neurosurgical patients because many of them receive moderate to large doses of narcotics, which are associated with a high incidence of nausea and vomiting. This can be particularly deleterious because nausea-induced retching and vomiting might increase ICP. Careful attention to sterile technique is essential when using propofol as an infusion because the solubilizing agent in which propofol is prepared provides an excellent medium for bacterial growth.

5. **Effect on spinal cord metabolism.** Propofol decreases local spinal cord metabolism in both the gray and white matter, as expressed by local reductions in glucose utilization.

D. **Narcotics**

1. **Effect on CBF and CMR_{O_2}.** The effects of narcotics on CBF are difficult to characterize accurately because of conflicting experimental reports. It appears, however, that low doses of narcotics have little effect on CBF and CMR_{O_2} whereas higher doses progressively decrease both CBF and CMR_{O_2}.

   The baseline anesthetic state also plays a role. If a cerebral vasodilator is used to achieve the control anesthetic state to which a narcotic is added, a decrease in CBF and CMR_{O_2} occurs. If either an anesthetic possessing cerebral vasoconstricting properties or no anesthetic is used as the control, narcotics have little effect on CBF. The observed reductions in CBF and CMR_{O_2} parallel progressive slowing of the EEG. However, burst suppression and an isoelectric EEG are never achieved. High doses of narcotics have been shown to produce seizures in laboratory animals but rarely in humans. Seizures have been reported with high-dose fentanyl. Normeperidine, a metabolite of meperidine, is a known convulsant.

2. **Effect on autoregulation and CO_2 reactivity.** Cerebral autoregulation and CO_2 reactivity are maintained with narcotics.

3. **Effect on CSF dynamics** (Table 2-3). At low doses, fentanyl, alfentanil, and sufentanil cause no change of V_f and a decrease in R_a with a predicted decrease in ICP. At high doses, fentanyl decreases V_f and causes either no change or an increase in R_a with either a predicted decrease or an uncertain effect on ICP. At high doses, alfentanil causes no change in V_f and R_a with no predicted effect on ICP. High doses of sufentanil cause no change of V_f and either no change or an increase in R_a, predicting either no change or an increase in ICP.

Table 2-3.   Effects of narcotics on rate of cerebrospinal fluid formation, resistance to reabsorption of cerebrospinal fluid, and the predicted effect on intracranial pressure

Narcotic	V_f	R_a	Predicted ICP effect
Fentanyl, alfentanil, and sufentanil (low dose)	0	−	−
Fentanyl (high dose)	−	0, +*	−, ?*
Alfentanil (high dose)	0	0	0
Sufentanil (high dose)	0	+, 0*	+, 0*

V_f, rate of CSF formation; R_a, resistance to CSF reabsorption; ICP, intracranial pressure; 0, no change; −, decrease; +, increase; *, effect dependent on dose; ?, uncertain.
Adapted from Artru AA. CSF dynamics, cerebral edema, and intracranial pressure. In: Albin MS, ed. *Textbook of Neuroanesthesia with Neurosurgical and Neuroscience Perspectives.* New York: McGraw-Hill, 1997:61.

4. **Effect on ICP.** Under most conditions, narcotics produce either no change or a slight decrease in ICP. Narcotics can, however, increase ICP under certain study conditions. For example, the bolus administration of sufentanil has been shown to produce transient but pronounced increases in ICP in patients who have severe head injury. Likewise, the bolus administration of sufentanil and alfentanil has been shown to produce increases in cerebrospinal fluid pressure (CSFP) in patients who have supratentorial tumors. The autoregulation-induced vasodilatation of cerebral vessels from the decrease in MAP may explain the changes in CSFP. Thus, when narcotics are administered to the neurosurgical patient, they should be given in a manner that does not cause a sudden reduction in MAP. The narcotic antagonist naloxone, when carefully titrated, has little effect on CBF and ICP. When used in large doses to reverse narcotic effects, however, the administration of naloxone may be associated with hypertension, cardiac arrhythmias, and intracranial hemorrhage.

E. **Ketamine**

1. **Effect on CBF and CMR_{O_2}.** Ketamine produces an increase in CBF and CMR_{O_2}. The mechanism of the increase in CBF may be several-fold: respiratory depression with mild hypercapnia in spontaneously ventilating subjects, regional neuroexcitation with a concomitant increase in

cerebral metabolism, and direct cerebral vasodilatation as demonstrated by an increase in CBF during normocapnia and in the absence of changes in cerebral metabolism. Although seizures have been reported in epilepsy patients receiving ketamine, generally no epileptiform activity is seen on EEG analysis.

2. **Effect on autoregulation and CO_2 reactivity.** Cerebral autoregulation and CO_2 reactivity are maintained with ketamine.

3. **Effect on CSF dynamics.** Ketamine increases R_a and causes no change in V_f, which would predict an increase in ICP.

4. **Effect on ICP.** During spontaneous ventilation, ketamine produces an increase in Pa_{CO_2} and ICP, in both the presence and absence of preexisting intracranial hypertension. Increases in ICP might also occur in the presence of normoventilation. Interestingly, ketamine is a noncompetitive N-methyl-D-aspartate antagonist. In one animal model of incomplete cerebral ischemia, ketamine was shown to reduce cerebral infarct size. In the clinical arena, however, ketamine is still avoided in most neurosurgical patients, particularly those who have mass lesions and the potential for increased ICP.

F. **Benzodiazepines**

1. **Effect on CBF and CMR_{O_2}.** Benzodiazepines, including diazepam, midazolam, and lorazepam, produce small decreases in CBF and CMR_{O_2} in both small and large doses. A ceiling effect on these parameters is seen, which may represent saturation of receptor-specific binding sites. As with the barbiturates, some of the CBF-lowering effect of benzodiazepines is thought to be secondary to a reduction in CMR_{O_2}. Electroencephalographic effects include a shift from alpha to low-voltage beta and then theta waves, although an isoelectric EEG is not produced. Benzodiazepines are known *anticonvulsants* and are used clinically for this purpose.

2. **Effect on cerebral autoregulation and CO_2 reactivity.** CBF autoregulation and CO_2 reactivity are maintained with benzodiazepines.

3. **Effect on CSF dynamics.** Midazolam causes no change in V_f at low doses and a decrease in V_f at high doses. R_a is either not changed or increased. The predicted effect on ICP from these changes in CSF dynamics is uncertain.

4. **Effect on ICP.** ICP effects are small with benzodiazepines, which cause either no change or a slight reduction in ICP. Midazolam is commonly used as a premedication in neuroanesthesia, with small intravenous doses titrated to the patient's response, and as an anesthetic adjuvant. Large doses are generally avoided, however, because of

the potential for prolonged sedation. Flumazenil is a receptor-specific benzodiazepine antagonist that can increase CBF and ICP when used in large doses to reverse midazolam sedation. Seizures can also be precipitated by the administration of large doses of flumazenil.

II. Inhalational drugs

A. Nitrous oxide (N_2O)

1. **Effect on CBF and $CMRo_2$.** Although many clinicians once thought N_2O to be devoid of cerebrovascular effects, it is now known that it can cause large increases in CBF. The effects of N_2O vary depending on the presence or absence of other anesthetics. When administered alone or with minimal background anesthesia, N_2O increases CBF. In contrast, when it is administered with certain intravenous anesthetics (barbiturates, narcotics), its effects on CBF may be attenuated. When the effects of a 1 minimum alveolar concentration (MAC) anesthetic produced by a volatile drug alone are compared to the effects of a 1 MAC anesthetic provided by the combination of 0.5 MAC volatile drug and 0.5 MAC N_2O, CBF is higher in the presence of N_2O. $CMRo_2$ may be unchanged or increased with N_2O. Although brain activity on EEG might be increased with N_2O, it does not cause seizures.

2. **Effect on CO_2 reactivity.** CO_2 reactivity is preserved during the use of N_2O.

3. **Effect on CSF dynamics** (Table 2-4). Either the addition to or the withdrawal of N_2O from the inhalational drugs halothane and enflurane causes no change in either V_f or R_a with no predicted effect on ICP.

Table 2-4.   Effects of inhaled agents on rate of cerebrospinal fluid formation, resistance to reabsorption of cerebrospinal fluid, and the predicted effect on intracranial pressure

Inhaled agent	V_f	R_a	Predicted ICP effect
Nitrous oxide	0	0	0
Isoflurane			
Low dose	0	0, +[*]	0, +[*]
High dose	0	−	−
Desflurane	0, +[a]	0	0, +[a]
Sevoflurane	−	+	?

V_f, rate of CSF formation; R_a, resistance to CSF reabsorption; ICP, intracranial pressure; 0, no change; −, decrease; +, increase; *, effect dependent on dose; ?, uncertain.

[a]Effect occurs only during hypocapnia combined with increased CSF pressure. Adapted from Artru AA. CSF dynamics, cerebral edema, and intracranial pressure. In: Albin MS, ed. *Textbook of Neuroanesthesia with Neurosurgical and Neuroscience Perspectives*. New York: McGraw-Hill, 1997:61.

4. **Effect on ICP.** N_2O can increase ICP in patients who have mass lesions. The ICP response can be attenuated if either intracranial compliance is improved first or drugs that decrease CBV such as barbiturates are administered concomitantly. N_2O is known to diffuse rapidly into and expand closed air-filled spaces. Pneumocephalus produced by a recent craniotomy contraindicates the use of N_2O for the repeat procedure. If a venous air embolism (VAE) occurs, N_2O can increase the size of the air bubble and worsen the consequences of the air embolism. N_2O should be discontinued if a VAE occurs. Some clinicians avoid the use of N_2O altogether in procedures in which the likelihood of VAE is high, such as a posterior fossa craniectomy performed with the patient in the sitting position.

5. **Effect on spinal cord metabolism.** N_2O increases the spinal cord's utilization of glucose, which is quantitatively similar to that effect produced in the brain (approximately 25%).

B. **Isoflurane**

1. **Effect on CBF and $CMRo_2$.** Isoflurane is a cerebrovasodilatator that increases CBF. Although it is one of the least potent cerebrovasodilatators, it is the most potent depressant of $CMRo_2$. The techniques of CBF measurement may influence the interpretation of CBF studies with the different inhalational drugs. For example, cortical blood flow is higher with halothane than isoflurane. By contrast, the increase in CBF seen with isoflurane is higher in the subcortical areas. Therefore, if a technique of CBF measurement that selectively looks at cortical flow (radioactive xenon techniques, transcranial Doppler, venous outflow) is used, halothane might demonstrate a greater effect on CBF than isoflurane. If whole-brain blood flow is measured (microspheres, positron emission tomography [PET], autoradiography), the effects might appear more similar among the different volatile anesthetics.

Isoflurane is unique among the inhalational drugs in that it has the capacity to induce an isoelectric EEG at a concentration that is clinically relevant because it is tolerated hemodynamically. This occurs at approximately 2 MAC. The reduction in $CMRo_2$ plateaus at the point at which an isoelectric EEG is reached. A normal cerebral energy state is also present at this point.

2. **Effect on cerebral autoregulation and CO_2 reactivity.** Cerebral autoregulation is impaired with isoflurane in a dose-related manner. CO_2 reactivity is maintained with isoflurane. The achievement of hypocapnia may restore cerebral autoregulation impaired by isoflurane.

3. **Effect on CSF dynamics.** At low concentrations, isoflurane causes no change in V_f and either no change or an increase in R_a with either no change or an increase in ICP predicted. At high concentrations, isoflurane causes no change in V_f and a decrease in R_a, predicting a decrease in ICP.

4. **Effect on ICP.** Isoflurane has the potential to increase ICP. However, it may not be necessary to induce hypocapnia before introducing isoflurane. The simultaneous introduction of hyperventilation and isoflurane may be sufficient to prevent an increase in ICP.

5. **Effect on SCBF and metabolism.** At both 1 and 2 MAC concentrations, isoflurane produces an increase in SCBF and an attenuation of autoregulation. The changes seen at 2 MAC are greater for the spinal cord than for either the cortex or the subcortex.

C. **Desflurane**
1. **Effect on CBF and CMRo$_2$.** The effects of desflurane on CBF and CMRo$_2$ appear to be very similar to those of isoflurane. The use of desflurane is associated with a dose-related decrease in CMRo$_2$ (although slightly less than with isoflurane) and, if the blood pressure is maintained, an increase in CBF. At 2 MAC, EEG burst suppression can occur, but it may revert with the passage of time. Desflurane has a low blood-gas partition coefficient (0.4), which provides rapid titration of anesthetic depth and prompt emergence.

2. **Effect on cerebral autoregulation and CO$_2$ reactivity.** Cerebral autoregulation is impaired with concentrations of desflurane in excess of 1 MAC. The CO$_2$ reactivity is maintained at desflurane concentrations of between 0.5 and 1.5 MAC.

3. **Effect on CSF dynamics.** Desflurane causes no change in either V_f or R_a under conditions of normocapnia and either normal or increased CSF pressure and hypocapnia and normal CSF pressure. This would predict no effect on ICP. With hypocapnia and increased CSF pressure, however, desflurane increases V_f with a predicted increase in ICP.

4. **Effect on ICP.** Like isoflurane, desflurane can produce an increase in ICP from general cerebrovascular dilatation. When hypocapnia is maintained, however, the effect on ICP is minimized. Altered CSF dynamics such as an increase in V_f (as noted previously) may play a role in desflurane's ability to decrease intracranial compliance.

D. **Sevoflurane**
1. **Effect on CBF and CMRo$_2$.** Sevoflurane's effects on CBF and CMRo$_2$ are similar to those of isoflurane. CBF increases with sevoflurane secondary to cerebral vasodilatation. CMRo$_2$ decreases and

EEG burst suppression can be achieved with a clinically relevant concentration of approximately 2 MAC (similar to isoflurane). Anesthesia with high concentrations of sevoflurane has not provided any evidence of cerebral toxicity. Sevoflurane's relatively low blood-gas partition coefficient (0.6) provides for rapid induction and emergence. Unlike desflurane, sevoflurane is not irritating to the airway and can be used for inhalational induction. Inhalational inductions are avoided, however, in most neurosurgical patients because of the volatile drugs' potential for producing vasodilatation with a subsequent increase in CBF, CBV, and ICP and the potential for uncal, tentorial, or transforaminal herniation. Approximately 2% of the absorbed sevoflurane is metabolized with inorganic fluoride produced as one of the metabolites. Compound A, a degradation product from the interaction of sevoflurane with CO_2 absorbents, can also be produced. There is no agreement on the clinical significance of the levels of fluoride and Compound A so generated, but they are unlikely to be associated with renal injury in humans.

2.   **Effect on cerebral autoregulation and CO_2 reactivity.** Cerebral autoregulation and CO_2 reactivity are preserved during the administration of low concentrations of sevoflurane.

3.   **Effect on CSF dynamics.** Sevoflurane decreases V_f and increases R_a. The predicted effect on ICP is uncertain.

4.   **Effect on ICP.** The effect of sevoflurane on ICP is similar to isoflurane. A minimal change in ICP occurs in patients who have normal intracranial compliance. Caution should be exercised, however, when this drug is given to patients who have large mass lesions and reduced intracranial compliance because of the potential for cerebrovasodilatation and an increase in CBF, CBV, and ICP.

III.   **Muscle relaxants.** Muscle relaxants do not cross the blood-brain barrier. Any cerebral effects are thus secondary to histamine release, systemic hemodynamic changes, actions of metabolites, and altered cerebral afferent input.

A.   **Nondepolarizing muscle relaxants**

1.   **Short-acting drugs.** Mivacurium is a short-acting relaxant that is metabolized by plasma cholinesterase (at about 88% of the rate of succinylcholine) and undergoes ester hydrolysis in the liver. It is commonly given by infusion because of its rapid metabolism. When large doses of mivacurium are given rapidly, some histamine release can occur. Therefore, bolus doses should be given slowly over a period of 30 to 60 seconds to avoid histamine release and the potential for an increase in CBF and ICP.

2. **Intermediate-acting drugs.** Atracurium causes histamine release when given in large bolus doses. It is metabolized by ester hydrolysis and Hoffmann elimination and has an advantage in that with renal or liver dysfunction, atracurium does not alter its metabolism. Laudanosine, a metabolite of the Hoffmann elimination of atracurium, has been shown to cause seizures in laboratory animals although this has not been noted at the level obtained clinically. The newer analog of atracurium, *cis*-atracurium, does not cause histamine release and is not associated with the formation of toxic metabolites.

   Vecuronium has the advantage of maintaining stable hemodynamics even when given in large doses. One possible exception is that bradycardia may occur when vecuronium is combined with large doses of narcotics for induction of anesthesia, leaving the vagotonic effect of the narcotic unopposed. Vecuronium does not alter ICP or CSF dynamics with no change in V_f or R_a. Its stable hemodynamics and lack of cerebral effects have made vecuronium a popular choice in neuroanesthesia.

   Rocuronium is a nondepolarizing muscle relaxant that has a relatively stable hemodynamic profile (weakly vagolytic) and is excreted unchanged by the biliary system and the kidneys. Unlike vecuronium, it is not associated with the production of active metabolites. The rapid onset of rocuronium makes it an excellent choice for intubation in the neurosurgical patient who is at risk for succinylcholine side effects but in whom rapid onset of action is desirable.

3. **Long-acting drugs.** Pancuronium decreases the MAC of volatile anesthetics, secondary to the decrease in cerebral input from paralyzed muscle spindles. Large doses of pancuronium may cause hypertension and tachycardia, which could increase CBF and ICP. These effects may not occur when pancuronium is combined with narcotics for induction or when it is given in smaller doses for maintenance of relaxation.

   Doxacurium, a long-acting muscle relaxant, is devoid of significant cardiovascular side effects and has not been shown to have any adverse cerebral effects. It is eliminated unchanged in the kidney and bile. Doxacurium's lack of side effects and long duration of action make this relaxant useful for very lengthy neurosurgical procedures.

B. **Depolarizing muscle relaxants.** Succinylcholine can cause an increase in CBF that is associated with an increase in ICP. This is secondary to increases in muscle spindle activity, which increase cerebral afferent input. These effects can be blocked by prior paralysis or pretreatment with a nondepolarizing muscle relaxant. The changes in ICP are modest and transient, however, and may be outweighed by the benefit of rapid and reliable onset of muscle relaxation in instances in which rapid control of the airway is necessary. Succinylcholine produces no change in either V_f or R_a and no predicted effect on ICP. Of greater concern than succinylcholine's effect on ICP in the neurosurgical patient is the exaggerated release of potassium that occurs with certain neurologic injuries such as closed head trauma, cerebrovascular accidents, hemiparesis, spinal cord trauma, and neuromuscular disorders.

SUGGESTED READINGS

Artru AA. CSF dynamics, cerebral edema, and intracranial pressure. In: Albin MS, ed. *Textbook of Neuroanesthesia with Neurosurgical and Neuroscience Perspectives*. New York, NY: McGraw-Hill, 1997:61–115.

Girard F, Moumdjiian R, Boudreault D, et al. The effect of propofol sedation on the intracranial pressure of patients with an intracranial space-occupying lesion. *Anesth Analg* 2004;99:573–577.

Kaye A, Lucera IJ, Heavner J, et al. The comparative effects of desflurane and isoflurane on lumbar cerebrospinal fluid pressure in patients undergoing craniotomy for supratentorial tumors. *Anesth Analg* 2004;98:1127–1132.

Klimscha W, Ullrich R, Nasel C, et al. High dose remifentanil does not impair cerebrovascular carbon dioxide reactivity in healthy male volunteers. *Anesthesiology* 2003;99:834–840.

Marx W, Shah N, Long C, et al. Sufentanil, alfentanil, and fentanyl: impact on cerebrospinal fluid pressure in patients with brain tumors. *J Neurosurg Anesthesiol* 1989;1:3–7.

McCulloch TJ, Boesel TW, Lam AM. The effect of hypocapnia on the autoregulation of cerebral blood flow during administration of isoflurane. *Anesth Analg* 2005;100:1463–1467.

Petersen KD, Landsfeldt U, Cold GE, et al. Intracranial pressure and cerebral hemodynamics in patients with cerebral tumors: a randomized prospective study of patients subjected to craniotomy in propofol-fentanyl, isoflurane-fentanyl, or sevoflurane-fentanyl anesthesia. *Anesthesiology* 2003;98:329–336.

Pinaud M, Lelausque J-N, Chetanneau A, et al. Effects of propofol on cerebral hemodynamics and metabolism in patients with brain trauma. *Anesthesiology* 1990;73:404–409.

Warner DS, Hindman BJ, Todd MM, et al. Intracranial pressure and hemodynamic effects of remifentanil versus alfentanil in patients undergoing supratentorial craniotomy. *Anesth Analg* 1996;83:348–353.

Young WL. Effects of desflurane on the central nervous system. *Anesth Analg* 1992;75:S32–S37.

Neurophysiologic Monitoring

M. Sean Kincaid and Arthur M. Lam

Patients with neurologic disease undergoing surgical procedures have increased risk of ischemic/hypoxic damage to the central nervous system (CNS). This risk may be related to hemodynamic/embolic events associated with a non-neurosurgical operation (e.g., patients with significant carotid stenosis undergoing cardiopulmonary bypass [CPB] procedures) or the risk may be inherent in the neurosurgical procedure itself (e.g., temporary clipping of feeding artery during cerebral aneurysm surgery). Intraoperative neurophysiologic monitoring may improve patient outcome by (a) allowing early diagnosis of ischemia/hypoxia before irreversible damage occurs and (b) enabling surgeons to provide optimal operative treatment as indicated by the monitoring parameter.

Although not universally adopted, neurophysiologic monitoring has become routine for some surgical procedures in many centers.

Broadly speaking, the brain can be monitored in terms of (a) function, (b) blood flow, and (c) metabolism (Tables 3-1 to 3-3).

I. **Monitoring of function**
   A. **Electroencephalography.** Summation of the excitatory postsynaptic potential generated by the pyramidal cells of the cerebral cortex gives rise to the electrical activity of the brain, which can be recorded as an electroencephalogram (EEG). The EEG comprises many underlying components with different frequencies and harmonics. The component waves are typically classified according to the respective frequencies (Table 3-4). This electrical activity is volume conducted and can be recorded from the scalp and forehead, using surface or needle electrodes.
      1. **Recording techniques.** Because the scalp has no electrically neutral area, EEG is typically recorded using a montage (electrode arrangement) with bipolar recording. Thus, both electrodes are active, and the polarity of the signal recorded depends on the arbitrary designation of recording versus referential electrode. Other electrical activities generated in the body such as electromyographic and electrocardiographic potentials are minimized but not eliminated using common-mode rejection which rejects the electrical signals that are measured in both recording sites (common) in comparison to a third "ground electrode." The number of channels used and the placement of electrodes determine the specificity of the EEG as a monitor of the occurrence of regional ischemia. The gold

Table 3-1. Monitoring of function

Electroencephalogram
  Raw electroencephalogram
  Computerized processed
    Compressed spectral array
    Density spectral array
    Aperiodic analysis
  Bispectral Analysis
Evoked potentials
  Sensory evoked potentials:
    Somatosensory EP
    Brain stem auditory EP
    Visual EP
  Motor evoked potentials
    Transcranial magnetic MEP
    Transcranial electric MEP
    Direct spinal cord stimulation
Electromyography
  Cranial nerve functions (V, VII, IX, X, XI, XII)

EP, evoked potential; MEP, motor evoked potential.

standard for raw EEG recording is 16-channel recording (eight channels for each hemisphere) with electrodes placed according to the International 10–20 System (Figure 3-1). With the exception of monitoring in carotid endarterectomy (CEA) in some centers, 16-channel EEG recording is seldom performed intraoperatively because of its relative complexity and the inaccessibility of recording sites in intracranial surgical procedures.

To simplify recording and interpretation of EEG, most EEG machines designed for intraoperative

Table 3-2. Monitoring of flow/pressure

Cerebral blood flow
  Nitrous oxide wash-in
  Radioactive xenon clearance
  Laser Doppler blood flow
  Transcranial Doppler
Intracranial pressure
  Intraventricular catheter
  Fiberoptic intraparenchymal catheter
  Subarachnoid bolt
  Epidural catheter

Table 3-3. Monitoring of metabolism

Invasive monitor

Intracerebral P_{O_2} electrode (Paratrend, Licox)

Noninvasive monitor

Transcranial cerebral oximetry (near-infrared spectroscopy)

Jugular venous oximetry

monitoring use two- to four-channel recording with computer processing to simplify the output. Although different vendors use different algorithms, the basic premise is to filter out the high frequency activity (likely to be artifacts or interference), typically at 30 Hz. The raw EEG is then separated into its component waves using Fast Fourier Transform and then they are grouped together according to the frequency spectrum. Thus, raw EEG recorded in a time domain is displayed in a frequency domain. The resultant power (square of the amplitude of the EEG wave) spectrum can be displayed in a number of ways, the most common ones being compressed spectral array or density spectral array with either the peaks and valleys or the density of the gray scale representing the power of the spectrum. Aperiodic analysis is another method of EEG processing that tracks each wave and plots it as a "telephone pole" with its height representing the amplitude or power of the wave.

2. **Interpretation of EEG**
   a. The EEG is a random activity reflecting the state of arousal and metabolic activity. The generation of electrical activity is an energy-requiring process that depends on an adequate

Table 3-4. Electroencephalogram

Beta	13–30 Hz	High frequency, low amplitude, dominant during awake state
Alpha	9–12 Hz	Medium frequency, higher amplitude seen in occipital cortex with eyes closed while awake
Theta	4–8 Hz	Low frequency, not predominant in any condition
Delta	0–4 Hz	Very low frequency, low to high amplitude signifies depressed functions, consistent with deep coma (cause can be anesthesia, metabolic, or hypoxia)

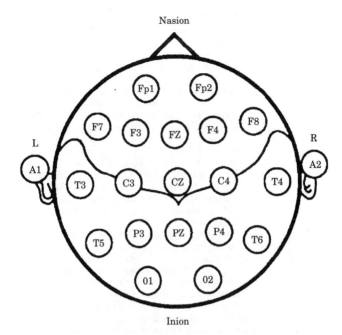

Figure 3-1. The International 10–20 System for placement of EEG electrodes. It is based on dividing each head circumference (anteroposterior from nasion to inion over the vertex, coronal from tragus of one ear to the other) into two halves and then subdividing each half (50%) into 10%, 20%, 20% sectors. Fp, frontal pole; F, frontal; C, central; P, parietal; T, temporal; A, ear lobe; M, mastoid (not shown). Odd number subscripts denote the left hemisphere, and even numbers denote the right hemisphere.

supply of substrates including oxygen and glucose. Thus, significant reductions of blood flow, oxygen, or glucose all lead to depression of EEG activity. Gradual reduction of cerebral blood flow (CBF) can be correlated with characteristic changes in EEG and constitutes the most frequent underlying indication for EEG monitoring.

b. Awake EEG is dominated by beta activity with high-frequency and low-amplitude waves. With the onset of ischemia/hypoxia, initially a transient increase in beta activity occurs, followed by development of slow waves (theta and delta) with large amplitude, disappearance of beta activity, and eventually the occurrence of delta waves with low amplitude. The ischemic changes can progress to suppression of electrical activity with an occasional burst of activity (burst suppression) and finally to complete electrical silence with flat EEG, signaling the onset of irreversible damage. Thus, the sudden development of delta waves coincident with a surgical maneuver such as cross-clamping of the common carotid artery would warn the anesthesiologist and the surgeon that the patient is at risk of cerebral injury. In the region of the ischemic penumbra where blood flow is inadequate to generate electrical activity but sufficient to maintain neuronal viability for a period of time, EEG has poor predictive power for brain damage. Thus, EEG is sensitive to the occurrence of ischemia but lacks specificity as a diagnostic test for irreversible damage. In general, the quicker the onset of the ischemic EEG changes, the higher the probability for irreversible damage.

3. **Confounding factors.** The observed changes in EEG with ischemia/hypoxia are not unique, and similar changes occur with anesthetic-induced metabolic depression, albeit in a reversible manner. Most intravenous (with the exception of ketamine) and inhalation anesthetics cause a dose-dependent depression of EEG and virtually all of them can produce a burst-suppression pattern on EEG. Similarly, hypothermia decreases cerebral metabolism and causes slowing of the EEG. EEG changes, therefore, should always be interpreted in concert with other physiologic variables, not in isolation.

4. **Indications for EEG monitoring**
   a. All surgical procedures that potentially place the brain at risk are theoretically amenable to EEG monitoring. In practice, EEG monitoring is often difficult to perform during intracranial procedures because of the lack of access to scalp recording. The use of needle electrodes may ameliorate this problem. CEA, which places the ipsilateral hemisphere at risk during cross-clamping of the common carotid artery, is the most frequent indication for EEG monitoring. When EEG changes indicate that CBF is inadequate, the placement of an intraluminal shunt restores blood flow.
   b. Some anesthesiologists and surgeons utilize anesthesia-induced metabolic suppression to provide cerebral protection during risky procedures. EEG monitoring in these circumstances allows optimal metabolic suppression with anesthesia administered by titration to achieve burst suppression. The main indications for EEG monitoring are listed in Table 3-5.

Table 3-5.   Indications for electroencephalogram monitoring

1. Carotid endarterectomy
2. Cerebral aneurysm surgery when temporary clipping is used
3. Cardiopulmonary bypass procedures
4. Extracranial-intracranial bypass procedures
5. Deliberate metabolic suppression for cerebral protection

        c. Although uncommon in the anesthetized patient, occult seizures occur frequently in patients with head injury in the intensive care unit (ICU). These seizures, which may worsen the outcome, may be detectable only with continuous EEG monitoring. Although treatment of these seizures is likely beneficial, it is yet to be determined whether continuous EEG monitoring in the ICU will improve outcome in a cost-effective manner.

    5. Bispectral analysis. The bispectral index is a derived EEG parameter designed not to detect ischemia but to monitor the degree of hypnosis. Based on both power spectrum analysis and phase change or coherence of the different frequencies, the value is normalized to a range of 0 to 100. A value between 40 and 60 is considered adequate hypnosis to prevent possible recall, whereas a value above 80 is consistent with impending emergence from anesthesia. Strictly speaking, this is not a parameter used to preserve the integrity of the CNS but is derived from the raw EEG and, as such, it is potentially influenced by the occurrence of ischemia that results in changes in the EEG. The frontal location of electrode placement, however, renders the bispectral index less sensitive to development of regional ischemia.

B. Evoked potential monitoring

    1. Sensory evoked potentials (SEPs). SEP is a time-locked, event-related, pathway-specific electroencephalographic activity generated in response to a specific stimulus such as electrical stimuli applied to the median nerve. The typical peaks and troughs are described by their polarity and latency (Figure 3-2). For example, the cortical negative peak that typically occurs 20 msec after stimulation of the median nerve is called $N20$. Alternatively, it is numbered according to the sequence in which it is generated; thus, the first positive wave that occurs following posterior tibial nerve stimulation is called $P1$. The amplitude of evoked potential waves is small relative to conventional

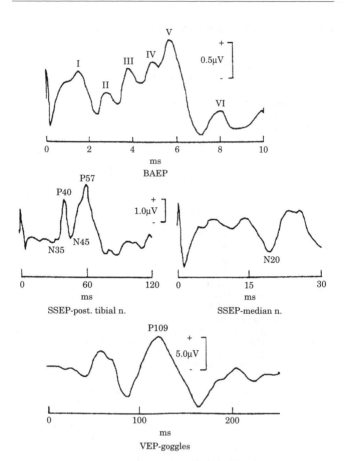

Figure 3-2. Common modalities of sensory evoked responses. BAEP, brain stem auditory evoked potential; SSEP-median n, somatosensory evoked potential with median nerve stimulation; SSEP-post tibial n, somatosensory evoked potential with posterior tibial nerve stimulation; VEP-goggles, visual evoked potential in response to stimulation with light-emitted diode goggles.
(Reproduced from Lam AM. Monitoring neurologic evoked potentials, *ASA Refresher Course* **1989;17(13):175–192, with permission.)**

EEG and is not easily visualized without computer averaging of repetitive stimuli. SEPs are anatomically pathway specific and theoretically assess only the integrity of the pathway monitored. The contrast between conventional EEG and SEP is summarized in Table 3-6.

a. SEP can be recorded in response to stimulation of any sensory nerve, cranial or peripheral. The common modalities of evoked potentials

Table 3-6.   Difference between sensory evoked potential (SEP) and electroencephalogram (EEG)

SEP	EEG
Event-related	Random
Anatomically pathway specific	Primarily cortical activity
Monitors integrity of the pathway	Monitors only the cortex
Small amplitude	Large amplitude
Requires computer averaging	No averaging required
Resistant to intravenous anesthetics, recordable during inhaled anesthetics	Abolished by high dose intravenous or inhalation anesthetics

used in clinical practice are (a) somatosensory evoked potentials (SSEPs), (b) visual evoked potentials (VEPs), and (c) brain stem auditory evoked potentials (BAEPs). Of these three, VEP is profoundly influenced by inhalation anesthesia, is difficult to perform, and is seldom utilized as an intraoperative monitor. The SSEPs recorded in response to stimulation of the median nerve, ulnar nerve, and posterior tibial nerve monitor the integrity of the respective pathways from the periphery to the cortex. They are a routine monitor for surgical procedures on the spinal column with potential risk to the spinal cord such as scoliosis surgery.

SEPs are also used during CEA and cerebral aneurysm surgery with the theoretical advantage over EEG that even subcortical ischemia can be detected. Indications for different SEP-monitoring modalities are summarized in Table 3-7.

Table 3-7.   Indications for sensory evoked potential (SEP) monitoring

SSEP monitoring

 Spinal column surgery

 Carotid endarterectomy

 Cerebral aneurysm surgery

BAEP monitoring

 Acoustic neuroma

 Vertebral-basilar aneurysms

 Other posterior fossa procedures

SSEP, somatosensory evoked potential; BAEP, brain stem auditory evoked potential.

    b.   BAEPs include a series of seven short-latency peaks generated in response to stimulation of the auditory (VIII) nerve, typically with repetitive clicks delivered to the ears with a head phone or ear-inserted transducers. A specific neurogenerator produces each peak, numbered with a Roman numeral. Examination of the change in latency interval between various peaks can localize the specific site of the injury. Monitoring BAEPs during acoustic neuroma surgery, when feasible, has been shown to help preserve the integrity of the auditory nerve. Although the neurogenerators are specific to the VIII nerve, BAEP monitoring has also been used to reflect the general well-being of the brain stem in posterior fossa procedures.

2. **Interpretation of evoked potentials.** As with EEG, ischemia/hypoxia leads to depression of conduction with resultant decrease in amplitude and increase in latency of the specific peaks. For SSEPs, 50% reduction in amplitude from baseline in response to a specific surgical maneuver is generally accepted to be a significant change warranting alteration of surgical strategy to avert potential damage. Some centers also consider a 10% increase in latency of SSEP signals to be significant. For BAEP, an increase in latency of more than 1 msec, particularly in wave V, is considered to be clinically significant. In addition, a 50% decline in amplitude is a concern, and a loss of wave V is strongly predictive of postoperative hearing loss.

3. **Confounding factors.** As with EEG, anesthetic agents influence cortical evoked potentials. Unlike EEG, SSEPs resist the influence of intravenous agents. Although the amplitude may be slightly reduced and the latency increased, cortical SSEPs can be recorded even during deep barbiturate-induced coma with isoelectric EEG. In contrast, inhalation anesthetics cause a dose-related decrease in amplitude and increase in latency. With high doses, SSEP can become unrecordable. Nitrous oxide also has a profound depressant effect on the amplitude of SSEP, particularly when used in combination with an inhalation anesthetic. Therefore, the combination of inhalation anesthetic and nitrous oxide is avoided. Intraoperative recording of SSEP is best accomplished using an intravenous anesthetic technique or low-dose inhalation anesthetic (<1 minimum alveolar concentration [MAC]). Opioids have negligible effects on SSEP. Ketamine and etomidate have a paradoxical effect of augmenting the amplitude of SSEP and could make monitoring possible in patients with otherwise unrecordable SSEP. BAEP, unlike cortical SSEP, resists the influence of anesthetic agents and can be recorded even during high-dose inhalation anesthetics. For surgical procedures on the spinal column, evoked potentials can also be recorded directly from the epidural space; these potentials are robust and can be recorded regardless of anesthetic agents used. As with EEG, hypothermia also decreases amplitude and increases latency.

4. **Motor evoked potentials.** Because SSEP monitors only the integrity of the sensory pathway, it is theoretically possible to miss an injury specifically affecting the motor pathway but sparing the sensory tracts. Thus, motor evoked potential (MEP) recording was introduced into clinical practice to complement SSEP recording. The MEP is basically an electromyographic potential recorded over muscles in the hand or foot in response to depolarization of the motor cortex (Figure 3-3). Depolarization can be achieved using transcranial magnetic or electrical stimulation.

Unfortunately, anesthetic agents profoundly influence both modalities, rendering the transcranial magnetic stimulation essentially unrecordable during anesthesia and the electrical stimulation recordable only during total intravenous anesthesia. The use of a train-of-four stimuli has augmented MEP and makes it easier to record under general anesthesia. In contrast to SSEP, the relatively large voltage of MEP abrogates the need

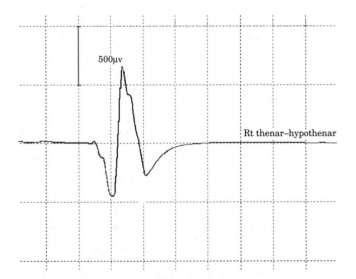

Figure 3-3.   **Motor evoked potential from stimulation of left cranium.**

for averaging and provides almost instant feedback. In many centers, MEP monitoring is used in addition to SSEP during operations on the spinal column. MEPs cannot be recorded in the presence of neuromuscular blockade.

5. **Spontaneous electromyography.** Although not technically an evoked potential, spontaneous electromyography (EMG) is frequently recorded during surgical procedures of both the cervical spine and lumbar spine. Irritation of peripheral nerves, such as spinal nerve roots, invokes immediate motor activity in muscles that should otherwise be silent under general anesthesia. Spontaneous EMG is particularly useful when the surgeon is working around nerve roots and needs immediate feedback regarding injury or irritation to them.

C. **Monitoring cranial nerve functions.** Operations in the posterior fossa and the lower brain stem are associated with potential injury to the cranial nerves. Monitoring the electromyographic potential of the cranial nerves with motor components (V, VII, IX, X, XI, XII) can preserve the integrity of these cranial nerves. Two types of potentials can be recorded: spontaneous and evoked activity. Measuring spontaneous activity can detect injury potential, signifying accidental surgical trespass. Evoking the nerve with electrical stimulation facilitates identification and thus preservation of the cranial nerve. Although EMG theoretically can be recorded during partial neuromuscular blockade, it is best not to administer any muscle relaxants during cranial nerve monitoring.

II. **Monitoring of CBF and intracranial pressure (ICP)**

A. **Absolute CBF.** Most methods of CBF measurement are not applicable to intraoperative monitoring. Nitrous oxide wash-in is the classic method of measuring global hemispheric CBF, but it necessitates cannulation of the jugular bulb and clinically is cumbersome to use. Radioactive xenon clearance is a method that allows noninvasive measurement of regional CBF. Although some centers use it clinically to determine adequacy of hemispheric CBF during CEA, it is primarily a research tool.

B. **Relative CBF.** Other tools used for real-time evaluation of relative changes in CBF include laser Doppler flowmetry (LDF) and transcranial Doppler (TCD) sonography.

1. **LDF.** This tool is a parenchymal or surface Doppler probe that measures tissue local CBF in a quantitative manner. However, the flow can be expressed only in a relative manner in arbitrary units. Because the volume of tissue monitored is limited to 1 mm, its clinical use, both in the operating room (OR) and the ICU, remains limited. Its insertion also requires a burr hole. Its incorporation

into the intracranial monitor may increase its functionality.

2. **TCD sonography.** This procedure allows measurement of CBF velocity in the major vessels of the Circle of Willis noninvasively and continuously. For intraoperative purposes, velocity in the middle cerebral artery (V_{mca}) is measured transtemporally over the zygomatic arch. Although it does not derive the absolute CBF, it can measure relative changes in CBF in a quantitative manner. The waveform profile also provides a qualitative assessment of ICP/cerebral perfusion pressure (CPP). In addition, the occurrence of air or particulate emboli can be detected. TCD can be used to determine cerebral autoregulation and carbon dioxide (CO_2) reactivity.

   a. **Physiological principles of TCD**

      (1) **The diameter of the basal cerebral arteries is constant.** Flow velocity is proportional to CBF only when the diameter of the insonated vessel and the angle of insonation remain constant. There is considerable evidence to suggest that the basal cerebral arteries, as conductance vessels, do not dilate or constrict as the vascular resistance changes. Angiographic and CO_2 reactivity studies confirm that changes in CO_2 tension and blood pressure have negligible influence on the diameter of the proximal basal arteries. Intravenous and inhaled anesthetic agents do not constrict or dilate the middle cerebral artery (MCA) appreciably. Probably the only clinically important situation in which the basal cerebral vessels vasoconstrict is when vasospasm occurs as a complication of a subarachnoid hemorrhage. Vasospasm renders the relationship between CBF velocity and CBF invalid; as the vessel constricts, the flow velocity increases but the CBF actually decreases. This increase in flow velocity with constriction of the basal cerebral artery represents one of the most important and established uses of the TCD. Once angiography confirms the diagnosis of vasospasm, TCD can track the patient's response to therapy and the time course of resolution of the vasospasm.

      (2) **Changes in CBF velocity reflect relative changes in CBF.** Although correlation between absolute flow velocity and CBF in any given population is poor, good correlation exists between relative changes in flow velocity and CBF.

b. Clinical applications of intraoperative TCD monitoring

(1) Carotid endarterectomy

(a) Detection of ischemia. TCD monitoring during CEA can detect cerebral ischemia during cross-clamping of the carotid artery and allows selective shunting. The correlation between changes in flow velocity and in EEG appears to be excellent in many studies. A decrease in V_{mca} of more than 60% compared to preclamped baseline suggests inadequate CBF and the need for an intraluminal shunt. TCD can also detect malfunctioning shunts due to kinking or thrombosis.

(b) Detection of microemboli. Microemboli occur frequently during CEA; embolic events may outweigh hemodynamic events as an etiology of perioperative stroke. TCD can detect both air and particulate emboli.

(c) Diagnosis and treatment of postoperative hyperperfusion syndrome. Approximately 1% of patients develop hyperperfusion syndrome following CEA, resulting in cerebral hemorrhage. TCD monitoring allows this diagnosis to be made and treatment to be implemented. Patients who develop the hyperperfusion syndrome show sustained elevation of flow velocities after release of carotid occlusion and often develop headaches. Prompt reduction of blood pressure is effective in normalizing the ipsilateral flow velocity and alleviating symptoms.

(d) Diagnosis and treatment of postoperative intimal flap or thrombosis. Occlusion of the carotid artery postoperatively can occur due to clot formation or the presence of an intimal flap. Sudden development of clinical symptoms in the postanesthesia care unit should prompt an immediate TCD examination. A prompt exploration may prevent an impending stroke.

(2) Cardiac surgery. Stroke as a complication of cardiac surgical procedures occurs in up to 10% of patients. More subtle neurologic and cognitive dysfunction has been reported in 30% to 70% of patients.

Adverse cerebral outcomes are due either to embolic events or hypoperfusion, or both.

(a) **Cerebral emboli during CPB.** There is considerable evidence to suggest that the delivery of micro-emboli (air, platelet aggregate, and thrombus) into the cerebral circulation is responsible for the neuropsychologic deterioration seen after bypass procedures. Patients with the highest emboli counts have been observed to have greater neurologic deterioration. Other studies have shown that the presence of arterial line filters reduces the incidence of emboli detected by TCD. Despite these published findings, TCD monitoring of emboli is still evolving and faces a number of technical challenges.

(b) **Cerebral perfusion during CPB.** Brain injury during CPB may also occur as a result of hypoperfusion. TCD has been used as a noninvasive tool for examining CBF in patients having cardiac surgical procedures performed under CPB. The validity of TCD as a surrogate estimate of CBF during CPB is unclear at present, however.

(3) **Closed head injury.** TCD can be used to assess autoregulation and diagnose hyperemia and vasospasm as well as intracranial circulatory arrest. With elevation of ICP and cessation of CBF (intracranial circulatory arrest), a characteristic oscillating pattern is evident on TCD, with forward flow during systole and backward flow during diastole. In this context, although not widely used intraoperatively, TCD may be useful in monitoring patients with head injuries undergoing non-neurosurgical procedures.

(4) **Diagnosis of brain death.** When the oscillating pattern is persistent and reproducible, the American Academy of Neurology accepts it as a useful adjunct for the confirmation of brain death.

c. **Limitations of TCD as a routine intraoperative monitor**
   (1) Most TCD monitors are designed for diagnostic rather than monitoring purposes. A fixation device is needed to allow

continuous, reliable recording that does not interfere with the surgical procedure.

(2) Although most TCD equipment is fairly easy to operate, skill and training are nevertheless required.

(3) The successful transmission of ultrasound through the skull depends on the thickness of the skull, and the temporal bone thickness varies with gender, race, and age. The failure rate can be anywhere from 5% to 20%, depending on the patient population.

C. **ICP.** Monitoring ICP allows optimization of CPP and possibly prevents herniation. Monitoring methods currently available include ventriculostomy, subarachnoid bolt, epidural sensor, and fiberoptic intraparenchymal monitor; the latter is the most commonly used. The fiberoptic ICP monitors may allow simultaneous measurement of brain temperature, a function that is particularly useful in the ICU where fever exacerbates secondary injury. In addition, some incorporate LDF, partial pressure of arterial oxygen (Pa_{O_2}), partial pressure of arterial carbon dioxide (Pa_{CO_2}), and pH monitoring.

Although its use is fairly common in the management of patients with head injury in the ICU, the ICP monitor is available only as an intraoperative monitor when placed preoperatively by the neurosurgeon.

III. **Monitoring cerebral oxygenation and metabolism**

A. **Invasive monitoring**

1. **Brain tissue oxygenation (P_{O_2}).** In the setting of head injury, where secondary injury from ischemia/hypoxia is of concern, maintaining a reasonable CPP may not be adequate for brain preservation. Significant inter-patient variability exists with respect to the CPP below which brain hypoxia is encountered. In this situation, a tissue P_{O_2} monitor is useful for assessing the balance between oxygen supply and demand.

When a miniature Clarke-type polarographic electrode originally designed for continuous intra-arterial monitoring is used, the tissue P_{O_2} monitor is placed intraparenchymally, typically in conjunction with an ICP monitor. As such, the monitor reveals regional or local, rather than global, oxygen levels. An oxygen tension of 10 mm Hg is considered the threshold for brain hypoxia. This value can be increased either by increasing supply of oxygen (supplemental O_2, raising CPP, treating anemia) or by decreasing demand (propofol or barbiturate therapy). In addition to identifying inadequate cerebral P_{O_2}, this monitor may demonstrate hyperoxia that could occur with absolute or relative cerebral hyperemia such as from loss of cerebral autoregulation.

Some controversy exists regarding whether tissue Po_2 monitors should be placed within a region of normal brain parenchyma or adjacent to the injured brain area.

2. **Jugular bulb venous oximetry monitoring.** In contrast to the *regional* information that the tissue Po_2 monitor provides, the jugular bulb oximeter allows continuous or intermittent estimate of the *global* balance between cerebral oxygen demand and supply. Provided the cerebral metabolic rate for oxygen consumption ($CMRo_2$) remains constant, calculation of the arteriovenous oxygen content allows estimation of the relative CBF. Even if $CMRo_2$ does not stay constant, the arteriovenous oxygen content difference always reflects the balance between the brain's oxygen demand and supply. Because arterial oxygenation is usually 100%, provided that hematocrit remains constant, the jugular venous oxygen saturation ($Sjvo_2$) equally reflects this balance. The physiological principle behind jugular venous oximetry is shown in Figure 3-4. Thus, intraoperative cerebral ischemia from inadequate perfusion pressure or excessive hyperventilation can be diagnosed readily. The influence of jugular venous desaturation on prognosis in patients with a head injury has been documented, and continuous jugular venous oximetry has become a routine monitor in many neurointensive care units. The thermistor-tipped catheter also measures temperature approximating that of the brain. Its major limitations include its global nature and therefore inability to detect focal cerebral ischemia and its invasive nature. Its reliability during CPB is also controversial.

Figure 3-4. Physiologic principles of jugular venous oximetry.

$CMRo_2 = CBF \times AVDo_2$

$AVDo_2 = CMRo_2 \div CBF$

$AVDo_2$ = arterial O_2content(Cao_2) $-$ jugular venous O_2

content($Cjvo_2$)

$= (Hgb \times 1.39 \times Sao_2 + 0.003 \times Pao_2) - (Hgb \times 1.39$

$\times Sjvo_2 + 0.003 \times Pjvo_2)$

$= Hgb \times 1.39(Sao_2 - Sjvo_2) + 0.003(Pao_2 - Pjvo_2)$

$= Hgb \times 1.39(Sao_2 - Sjvo_2)$(ignoring the amount

of dissolved O_2)

Since, under most circumstances, $Sao_2 = 1$, thus $AVDo_2 \propto 1 - Sjvo_2$ where $AVDo_2$ = arteriovenous O_2 content, $Sjvo_2$ = jugular venous O_2 saturation, $Pjvo_2$ = jugular venous O_2 tension, Sao_2 = arterial O_2 saturation, Pao_2 = arterial O_2 tension. Therefore, a change in $Sjvo_2$ will reflect corresponding change in $AVDo_2$ provided hemoglobin saturation stays constant.

a. **Interpretation of $Sjvo_2$ values.** The normal arterio-jugular difference for O_2 ($AVDO_2$) value is 2.8 mcmol/mL or 6.3 vol% of oxygen. (Range 2.2 to 3.3 mcmol/mL, or 5 vol% to 7.5 vol%), and $Sjvo_2$ is between 60% and 70%. When oxygen delivery is higher than oxygen demand, as in hyperemia, $AVDo_2$ decreases and $Sjvo_2$ increases. During periods of global cerebral ischemia, $AVDo_2$ widens and $Sjvo_2$ decreases.

(1) **Increased values.** An $Sjvo_2$ value of more than 90% indicates absolute or relative hyperemia. This can occur as a result of a reduced metabolic need (e.g., a comatose or brain-dead patient) or from excessive flow (e.g., severe hypercapnia). Patients with cerebral arteriovenous malformations have a direct arterial shunt into the venous circulation and thus have abnormally increased $Sjvo_2$ values. Extracranial contamination, either from the facial vein or from rapid withdrawal in blood sampling (intermittent measurement), also results in an elevated value.

(2) **Normal values.** Although a normal balance between flow and metabolism results in a normal $Sjvo_2$, it does not exclude the presence of focal ischemia. Because the blood in the jugular veins drains all areas of the brain, a discrete area of ischemia or infarction might not influence the overall level of saturation.

(3) **Decreased values.** On the other hand, $Sjvo_2$ is sensitive to global cerebral ischemia. A value of <50% reflects increased O_2 extraction and indicates a potential risk of ischemic injury. This may be due to increased metabolic demand, as in fever or seizure, not matched by an equivalent increase in flow, or due to an absolute reduction in flow. A significant decrease in O_2-carrying capacity due to a decrease in hematocrit also leads to desaturation. Ischemia may also alter $CMRo_2$ measurements and affect the interpretation of $Sjvo_2$. As ischemia progresses to infarction, oxygen consumption decreases and $Sjvo_2$ normalizes.

3. **Microdialysis catheters.** A small catheter, typically inserted in conjunction with an ICP or tissue Po_2 monitor, allows sampling of small molecules in the interstitial fluid. The catheter, 0.6 mm in diameter, has a 10-mm dialysis membrane. Artificial cerebrospinal fluid (CSF) circulates through the catheter, allowing equilibration with the extracellular fluid and subsequent analysis of its chemical

composition. This monitor's value is in determining the metabolic state of the brain and assessing the local cellular integrity. Three markers are thought to be valuable for these purposes. An increasing lactate/pyruvate ratio is sensitive to the onset of ischemia. High levels of glycerol suggest inadequate energy to maintain cellular integrity and the resultant membrane breakdown. Finally, excitatory amino acids, such as glutamate, are both a marker for neuronal injury and a factor in its exacerbation.

Currently, the microdialysis catheter is primarily used in two situations: (a) extensive subarachnoid hemorrhage where subsequent vasospasm is likely and (b) traumatic brain injury (TBI) of sufficient severity to warrant ICP/CPP monitoring. In either situation, a significant risk exists for the development of secondary injury due to cerebral ischemia.

Location of the microdialysis catheter is important because it provides information regarding only a small surrounding region of brain. With subarachnoid hemorrhage, the catheter should be placed in the region of the brain perfused by the vessel most likely at risk for vasospasm. Placement in TBI depends on the nature of the injury. With diffuse injury, the recommendation is to place the catheter in the right frontal region. A focal contusion warrants one catheter in the pericontusional area but not within the contusion and a second catheter in the normal brain.

B. **Noninvasive monitoring.** Near-infrared spectroscopy (NIRS) or transcranial oximetry measures cerebral regional oxygen saturation by measuring near-infrared light reflected off the chromophobes in the brain, the most important of which are oxyhemoglobin, deoxyhemoglobin, and cytochrome A3. NIRS has been studied in a variety of clinical settings including CEA and hypothermic circulatory arrest. Its major limitations include the intersubject variability, the variable length of the optical path, the potential contamination from extracranial blood, and most important, the lack of a definable threshold. Because of the thin scalp and skull in the neonate and infant, NIRS holds promise in this patient population but remains an investigative tool in its present form.

SUGGESTED READINGS

Bellander BM, Cantais E, Enblad P, et al. Consensus meeting on microdialysis in neurointensive care. *Intensive Care Med* 2004;30: 2166–2169.

Lam AM. Do evoked potentials have any value in anesthesia? *Anesthesiol Clin North America* 1992;10:657–682.

Lam AM, Mayberg TS. Jugular venous oximetry. *Anesthesiol Clin North America* 1997;15:533–549.

MacLennan N, Lam AM. Intraoperative neurological monitoring with transcranial Doppler ultrasonography. *Seminars in Anesthesiol* 1997;16:56–68.

Minahan RE. Intraoperative neuromonitoring. *Neurologist* 2002;8: 209–226.

Rampil I. What every neuroanesthesiologist should know about electroencephalograms and computerized monitors. *Anesthesiol Clin North America* 1992;10:683–718.

Rosow C, Manberg PJ. Bispectral index monitoring. *Ann Anesth Pharmacol* 1998;2:89–107.

Sloan MA, Alexandrov AV, Tegeler CH, et al. Assessment: Transcranial Doppler ultrasonography Report of the Therapeutics and Technology Assessment Subcommittee of the American Academy of Neurology. *Neurology* 2004;62:1468–1481.

Vespa PM. Multimodality monitoring and telemonitoring in neurocritical care: from microdialysis to robotic telepresence. *Curr Opin Crit Care* 2005;11:133–138.

Cerebral Protection and Resuscitation

Myrna I. Morales, Janet Pittman,
and James E. Cottrell

I. **Cerebral protection and resuscitation**
   A. **Cerebral protection.** Cerebral protection is the preemptive use of therapeutic interventions to improve neurologic outcome in patients who will be at risk for cerebral ischemia. The primary objective is **prevention** of the deleterious effects of ischemia.
   B. **Resuscitation.** Resuscitation refers to therapeutic interventions initiated after an ischemic event. The goal is treatment of ischemia and attenuation of neuronal injury.

II. **The ischemic brain**
   A. **Cerebral ischemia.** Cerebral ischemia is defined as perfusion insufficient to provide the supply of oxygen and nutrients needed for maintenance of **neuronal metabolic integrity (40% to 45% of total cerebral metabolic rate for oxygen consumption [CMR_{O_2}]) and function (55% to 60% of CMR_{O_2}).** It is assumed that a hierarchy of ischemic damage exists in which neuronal function is abolished before cellular integrity is lost.
      1. **Cellular integrity.** The brain utilizes **glucose** as its primary substrate for energy production. In the nonfasting state, glucose is metabolized via oxidative phosphorylation to adenosine triphosphate (ATP), which is needed for cellular activities such as homeostasis, protein synthesis, removal of carbon dioxide (CO_2), mitochondrial activity, and maintenance of ionic gradients and cell membrane stability.
      2. **Neuronal function.** Normal neuronal functional activity consists of the generation and transmission of nerve impulses and is manifest by the presence of normal electroencephalographic (EEG) activity.
   B. **Ischemia.** Ischemia may be **global or focal**, as well as **complete or incomplete**. Complete global ischemia occurs with cardiac arrest; incomplete global ischemia occurs with hypotension or shock. Focal ischemia involves the occlusion of a single vessel and is thus incomplete.
   C. **The ischemic cascade.** The ischemic cascade occurs when inadequate cerebral perfusion leads rapidly to

a cascade of pathophysiologic changes involving a multitude of chemical mediators of neuronal damage.

1. **Decreased availability of oxygen and glucose** results in immediate depletion of ATP, which is required for all active cellular processes. This depletion occurs within 2 to 4 minutes of complete ischemia. Phosphocreatine (PCr) is a source of high energy phosphate that allows the resynthesis of ATP from adenosine diphosphate (ADP). Brain PCr levels are normally three times those of ATP. A decrease in PCr is one of the earliest harbingers of ischemia.

2. **Lactate** levels increase because of anaerobic metabolism of glucose. Lactic acidosis aggravates ischemic damage. Lactic acid reduces ferric to ferrous iron, which in turn promotes free radical formation followed by lipid peroxidation of cell membranes. With incomplete ischemia, the persistence of residual perfusion facilitates increased lactate production in the presence of ongoing anaerobic metabolism and is thought to be the mechanism for increased damage with this type of ischemia. In contrast, complete ischemia results in complete cessation of metabolism.

3. Increased plasma **glucose** is an independent risk factor for aggravation of ischemia. The primary mechanism appears to be increased production of lactate with intracellular acidosis which contributes to neuronal necrosis. Hyperglycemia also prevents the increase in brain adenosine that occurs with ischemia. Adenosine, a purine nucleotide, inhibits excitatory amino acid (EAA) release and promotes cerebrovasodilatation, thus theoretically attenuating ischemic damage. In addition, there is some evidence that insulin has neuroprotective effects independent of its glucose-lowering properties. Hypoglycemia can also exacerbate ischemic brain injury. The persistence of hypoglycemia results in seizure activity and neuronal injury, particularly to the hippocampus.

4. Cerebral ischemia increases release of the **EAA neurotransmitters glutamate** and **aspartate**.

   a. Three receptors for the excitatory neurotransmitters are currently identified.

      (1) **N-methyl-D-aspartate (NMDA)** receptors are located in layers three, five, and six of the cerebral cortex, thalamus, striatum, and Purkinje fibers, the granule cell layers of the cerebellum, and the CA1 region of the hippocampus, which is particularly susceptible to ischemia. NMDA receptors mediate the influx of sodium (Na) and calcium (Ca) through membrane channels. Magnesium and the experimental drug

dizocilipine maleate (MK-801) block the NMDA receptor site in a noncompetitive fashion.

(2) **Quisqualate (alpha-amino-3-hydroxy-5-methyl-4-isoxazole-propionic acid [AMPA])** receptors occur in the deep cortical layers, thalamus, striatum, molecular layer of the cerebellum, and pyramidal cell layer and striatum lucidum of the hippocampus. AMPA receptors mediate the influx of Na.

(3) **Kainate** receptors, located in the striatum lucidum of the hippocampus, also mediate the influx of Na.

Glutamate stimulates all three receptors, but aspartate affects only the NMDA receptor. The presence of glycine is necessary for activation of NMDA receptors by glutamate.

b. Glutamate causes neuronal cell death by two mechanisms: **immediate** and **delayed**. In immediate neurotoxicity, glutamate activates the NMDA receptor, leading to Na, chloride (Cl), and water (H_2O) influx, which results in cellular edema, membrane lysis, and cell death. In delayed neurotoxicity (24 to 72 hours), the activated NMDA receptor promotes a cycle of ischemia initiated by the influx of Ca. This leads to activation of phospholipases, proteases, and eventually free fatty acids (FFAs), formation of arachidonic acid and free radicals, lipid peroxidation, and, ultimately, cell death.

5. Increased **Ca influx** is an early, pivotal event in the ischemic cascade and is caused by several mechanisms.

a. Depletion of ATP results in failure of the energy-requiring sodium/potassium (Na/K) ATPase-dependent ion pumps. Na and Cl influx and K efflux ensue. Influx of H_2O and edema occur secondarily. The resulting membrane depolarization leads to opening of voltage-sensitive Ca channels and Ca influx.

b. Decreased ATP leads to Ca release from endoplasmic reticulum.

c. EAA levels increase during ischemia, leading to stimulation of glutamate receptors and the opening of NMDA-mediated Ca channels.

d. Ca extrusion from the cell is an active process that stops when ATP stores are exhausted.

6. Numerous ischemic effects of Ca form a common pathway leading to neuronal cell destruction. Increased intracellular Ca activates **phospholipase A_1, A_2,** and **C**, which leads to the hydrolysis of membrane phospholipids and the release of FFAs.

Loss of membrane phospholipids also results in mitochondrial and cell membrane destruction.

    a. Arachidonic acid. The major FFA, arachidonic acid, is metabolized to **prostaglandins, leukotrienes**, and **free radicals**. Both prostaglandins (via the cyclooxygenase pathway) and leukotrienes (via lipoxygenase) cause cerebral edema. **Thromboxane A_2**, a prostaglandin derived from arachidonic acid with potent vasoconstrictor and platelet aggregation properties, potentiates ischemia and has been implicated in reperfusion injury (see **VII.E.**).

    b. Free radical formation. Superoxide, peroxide, and **hydroxyl radicals** cause lipid peroxidation within neuronal cell membranes. This alters membrane function and releases toxic by-products (aldehydes, hydrocarbon gases). These by-products cause edema, blood-brain barrier disruption, and inflammation. The superoxide radical itself can create an inflammatory response with vascular plugging.

D. Clinical ischemia

    1. Of all body organs, the brain is the most vulnerable to ischemia. Loss of consciousness occurs within 15 seconds of cardiac arrest. Brain PCr becomes negligible within 1 minute. Glucose and ATP stores are exhausted within 4 to 5 minutes. Critical levels for cerebral blood flow (CBF), cerebral perfusion pressure (CPP, the difference between the mean arterial pressure [MAP] and the intracranial pressure [ICP]), and the partial pressure of arterial oxygen (Pa_{O_2}) have been determined below which cerebral ischemia occurs (Figure 4-1) with characteristic EEG changes.

    2. Critical CBF is 18 to 20 mL /100 g of brain/minute. The **penumbra** is a hypoperfused region that may remain viable depending on timely reperfusion. The EEG becomes isoelectric at a CBF of 15 mL/ 100 g/minute. Metabolic failure occurs at a CBF of 10 mL /100 g/minute.

    3. Critical CPP is 50 mm Hg in the normal individual.

    4. Critical Pa$_{O_2}$ is 30 to 35 mm Hg in healthy awake patients.

E. Reperfusion injury refers to damage that occurs after the restoration of cerebral perfusion. An initial phase of hyperperfusion occurs, followed by a gradual decline in CBF referred to as the *noreflow phenomenon*. Hypoperfusion results from thromboxane-induced vasoconstriction and platelet aggregation, impaired red cell deformability, tissue edema, and the persistence of abnormal Ca levels. In addition, intracellular acidosis, continued EAA,

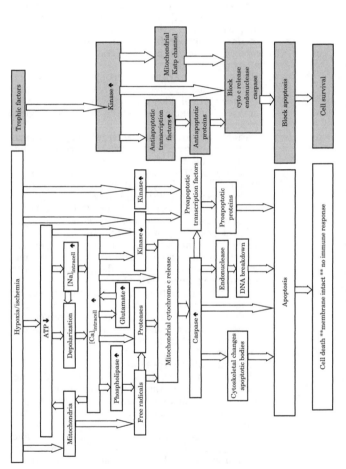

Figure 4-1. ATP, adenosine triphosphate. Brain metabolism and mechanisms of cerebral ischemia. From: Kass IS. In: Schwartz A, Butterworth J, Gross J, eds. Refresher Courses in Anesthesiology. Philadelphia, PA: Lippincott Williams and Wilkins, 2006;34:85–93.

neurotransmitter and catecholamine release, and free radical formation contribute to delayed neuronal damage. This no-reflow phenomenon can last for up to 24 hours.

III. **Clinical cerebral protection**
   A. **Rationale for treatment.** The goal is to maximize the available oxygen by **increasing oxygen supply (delivery)** and **decreasing oxygen demand**. Preservation of CBF and the avoidance of hypoxia and hypoxemia are critical.
   B. **Candidates for cerebral protection.** Candidates for cerebral protection include patients who have the following characteristics:
      1. Patients who have space-occupying lesions such as tumor, abscess, hematoma, hydrocephalus, and chronic cystic fluid collections with or without increased ICP who are scheduled for neurosurgical procedures.
      2. Patients who are scheduled for intracranial vascular procedures, such as cerebral aneurysm coiling/clipping and excision of arteriovenous malformation (AVM) and cavernous angioma, and extracranial vascular procedures including carotid endarterectomy (CEA) and superficial temporal artery to middle cerebral artery (STA-MCA) bypass, which involve temporary vessel occlusion and the possibility of focal ischemia.
      3. Patients who are scheduled for the clipping or coiling of giant or complex basilar artery aneurysms, which may be facilitated by **deep hypothermic circulatory arrest (DHCA)**.
      4. Cardiac bypass patients who typically are at risk from either global ischemia from low-flow states or focal ischemia from multiple small emboli.
      5. Patients who have had a cardiac arrest with circulation reestablished within 2 hours.

IV. **Clinical therapies**
   A. **Nonpharmacologic treatment**
      1. **Hypothermia** decreases both metabolic and functional activities of the brain. Although hypothermia reduces $CMRo_2$ by roughly 7% for each degree Celsius, the mechanism is not uniformly linear. The temperature coefficient (Q_{10}), used to describe the relationship between temperature and $CMRo_2$, is the ratio of two $CMRo_2$ values separated by 10°C. For most biological reactions, the Q_{10} is approximately 2 (a 50% decrease in $CMRo_2$ for every 10°C decrease in temperature). Thus, if the normothermic brain (37°C) can tolerate 5 minutes of complete ischemia, at 27°C the brain should tolerate 10 minutes of ischemia. The actual Q_{10} is 2.2 to 2.4 between 37°C and 27°C, resulting in a reduction of >50% in $CMRo_2$ at 27°C. Between 27°C and 17°C, the Q_{10} is approximately 5. This correlates with the gradual

loss of neuronal function, as demonstrated by an isoelectric EEG (which occurs between 18°C and 21°C) and the ability of the brain to tolerate more prolonged ischemia than would be predicted based on a linear model. Below 17°C, the Q_{10} is 2.2 to 2.4 again.

However, small decreases in temperature have also resulted in significant reductions in the damage from cerebral ischemia. Possible mechanisms of auxiliary hypothermic protection include decreased Ca influx, decreased EAA release, blood-brain barrier preservation, and prevention of lipid peroxidation. Although mild hypothermia (brain temperature of 32°C to 35°C) can be neuroprotective in the animal model, clinical evidence indicates that it is not beneficial during aneurysm surgery.

Correlation between esophageal and brain temperatures should not be assumed. Either tympanic membrane or nasopharyngeal temperature should therefore be measured as a more accurate estimate of brain temperature. Avoidance of hyperthermia is paramount because above-normal temperatures markedly increase $CMRo_2$ and exacerbate ischemic damage.

a. **Deep hypothermic circulatory arrest** to core temperatures of 13°C to 21°C might be indicated for clipping giant or complex basilar artery aneurysms. Peripheral arterial and large-bore intravenous catheters are inserted before induction of anesthesia. After induction, either a central venous or a pulmonary artery catheter, a second arterial catheter for phlebotomy, and a lumbar subarachnoid drain are inserted. Electrophysiologic monitoring of EEG, somatosensory evoked potentials (SSEPs), and brain stem auditory evoked potentials (BAEPs) is begun. The SSEPs persist to 15°C to 18°C and a CBF of 10 to 15 mL/100 g/minute, which is beyond hypothermic EEG isoelectricity (18°C to 20°C).

Cooling at a rate of 0.2°C/minute is performed by using a cooling blanket, infusing cold saline, and decreasing ambient temperature. Barbiturate-induced burst suppression is initiated and maintained intraoperatively. Hemodilution to a hematocrit of 28% to 30% is accomplished by phlebotomy; this blood is reserved in an anticoagulant solution to be reinfused after termination of bypass for replacement of essential clotting factors.

The aneurysm is dissected with meticulous attention to hemostasis before beginning femoral artery–femoral vein bypass. Heparin, 300 to 400 IU/kg, is administered, and the activated clotting time (ACT) is kept between 450 and 480 seconds. Cardiopulmonary bypass is begun when the patient's temperature is 34°C and continued until the desired core temperature is reached. Spontaneous atrial fibrillation may occur below 30°C, and continuous ventricular fibrillation frequently occurs below 28°C. To prevent myocardial ischemic injury, persistent ventricular fibrillation should be terminated by the administration of potassium chloride (KCl), 20 to 60 mEq. Cardioversion with 100 to 250 J may be used to induce asystole in patients resistant to KCl or in anephric patients in whom KCl is contraindicated. MAP should be maintained between 40 to 80 mm Hg during bypass.

Circulatory arrest occurs between 22°C and 18°C. The bypass pump is stopped. The duration of circulatory arrest is limited to aneurysm clip application time. Bypass is resumed and rewarming proceeds at 0.2 to 0.5°C/minute. Spontaneous ventricular fibrillation occurs with rewarming. Cardioversion (200 to 400 J) is required to restore sinus rhythm. Extracorporeal bypass is terminated when the patient's temperature reaches 34°C and normal sinus rhythm and cardiac output are present. Inotropic support may be required. The previously removed whole blood is reinfused to promote normal coagulation. Heparin is reversed with protamine to achieve an ACT of 100 to 150 seconds. Complications of this technique include coagulopathy, postoperative hemorrhage, metabolic acidosis, hyperglycemia, myocardial depression, and dysrhythmias.

2. **Avoidance of hyperglycemia.** The current recommendation is to keep the serum glucose below 150 mg/dL. Serum glucose is monitored frequently, and hypoglycemia (serum glucose below 60 mg/dL) is scrupulously avoided.

3. **Avoidance of hypotension, hypoxia, and hypercapnia.** The surgeon may request induced hypertension to improve CPP during temporary proximal occlusion of the parent vessel before definitive aneurysmal clip-ligation. Induced hypotension can be detrimental in patients at risk for vasospasm.

4. **Hemodilution** to a hematocrit of 32% to 34% increases CBF by decreasing viscosity, thereby improving oxygen delivery.

5. **Normalization of increased ICP** is achieved through moderate hyperventilation (partial pressure of arterial carbon dioxide [Pa_{CO_2}] of

25 to 30 mm Hg), head elevation to 30° in the neutral position, mannitol and/or furosemide diuresis, cerebrospinal fluid (CSF) drainage via ventriculostomy, limited fluid restriction, and barbiturate coma in patients unresponsive to these techniques.

6. **Correction of acidosis and electrolyte imbalance** including Na and K abnormalities should be prompt.

B. **Pharmacologic treatment**

1. **Barbiturates and erythropoietin** remain the only drugs shown to be effective for pharmacologic cerebral protection against ischemic damage in humans.

   a. **Thiopental**, a potent cerebrovasoconstrictor, decreases $CMRo_2$, CBF, cerebral blood volume (CBV), and ICP. CO_2 reactivity is preserved.

      (1) The primary mechanism of protection involves a **reduction in $CMRo_2$** of up to 55% to 60% at which point the EEG becomes isoelectric. Further reduction in $CMRo_2$ confers no additional protection. Thiopental's beneficial effects are thus limited to preservation of neuronal function.

      (2) Thiopental may cause an **inverse steal** phenomenon whereby vasoconstriction in normal tissue improves perfusion of ischemic areas that are unable to vasoconstrict.

      (3) Thiopental is an effective **anticonvulsant**.

      (4) Other possible mechanisms include gamma-aminobutyric acid (GABA) agonism, free radical scavenging, membrane stabilization, NMDA antagonism, Ca channel blockade, and maintenance of protein synthesis.

      (5) Thiopental does not improve outcome in global or complete ischemia after cardiac arrest.

      (6) The thiopental dose in focal ischemia is 3 to 5 mg/kg every 5 to 10 minutes titrated to EEG burst suppression up to a total of 15 to 20 mg/kg. Maintenance of cardiovascular stability could determine the rate of administration.

   b. **Pentobarbital's** cerebral effects are similar to those of thiopental. Pentobarbital is longer acting ($t1/2 = 30$ hours). The current clinical indication for pentobarbital is limited to barbiturate coma in patients who have increased ICP resistant to standard therapy. A loading dose of 3 to 10 mg/kg over 0.5 to 3 hours is given, followed by a maintenance infusion of 0.5 to 3 mg/kg/hour titrated to EEG burst suppression. The currently accepted therapeutic plasma concentration of pentobarbital is 2.5 to 4 mg/dL.

c. **Methohexital,** a short-acting barbiturate, can precipitate seizures in individuals who have epilepsy. Methohexital is useful for the induction of anesthesia for brief procedures in which seizure activity is desired (e.g., electroconvulsive therapy [ECT] and epilepsy surgery).

2. **Other intravenous anesthetics.** Anesthetic drugs that maintain ATP levels by decreasing cerebral metabolism while simultaneously preserving CBF and cardiovascular stability have theoretical potential for cerebral protection.

a. **Etomidate** is a short-acting imidazole compound which, like barbiturates, causes cerebral vasoconstriction. Electroencephalographic burst suppression occurs with higher doses. Most studies have not shown beneficial effects after cerebral ischemia. The administration of induction doses of etomidate has been associated with cerebral desaturation.

(1) Etomidate reduces $CMRo_2$ (by as much as 50%), CBF, and ICP while maintaining cardiovascular stability and CPP. CO_2 reactivity is preserved.

(2) Etomidate can cause **adrenocortical suppression** for up to 24 hours after a single induction dose (inhibition of 11 beta-hydroxylase). This may be of clinical concern when etomidate is used as an infusion, especially in patients who are not concomitantly receiving steroids.

(3) Myoclonic activity has been reported with etomidate, and seizures may occur.

(4) Side effects of etomidate include nausea, vomiting, and pain on injection.

b. **Propofol** (2, 6-diisopropylphenol), a short-acting induction drug also used to maintain anesthesia, has a cerebrovascular profile similar to that of barbiturates. Beneficial effects of propofol after brain ischemia have not been demonstrated.

(1) Propofol decreases $CMRo_2$, ICP, and CBF (via cerebrovasoconstriction). Hemodynamic depression decreases CPP more than with barbiturates.

(2) Burst suppression on EEG occurs with larger doses of propofol.

(3) Propofol may decrease postoperative nausea and vomiting.

c. **Benzodiazepines,** sedative-hypnotic drugs most commonly used as anesthetic adjuncts, stimulate the inhibitory neurotransmitter GABA and decrease CMR_{O_2} and CBF while preserving CO_2 reactivity. ICP may be decreased slightly. Benzodiazepines are potent anticonvulsants. They also produce amnesia and anxiolysis.

(1) **Diazepam** is used as an oral premedicant at a dose of 0.1 to 0.25 mg/kg. Its prolonged $t1/2$ of 21 to 37 hours limits its use in neurosurgical patients in whom prompt emergence and postoperative neurologic assessment are critical. Diazepam remains an effective treatment for status epilepticus.

(2) **Midazolam** has a $t1/2$ of 1 to 4 hours. The intravenous dose of midazolam for premedication is 0.5 to 2.5 mg up to 0.1 mg/kg. Excessive sedation and the possibility of hypoventilation-induced hypercapnia should be avoided in patients at risk for increased ICP. Midazolam in larger doses may have beneficial effects after brain ischemia.

(3) **Lorazepam** is also an effective premedicant in doses of either 0.5 to 4 mg by mouth or 2 to 4 mg intravenously (i.v.) or intramuscularly (i.m.). Like diazepam, its use is limited in neurosurgery by a $t1/2$ of 10 to 20 hours.

d. **Opioids** produce sedation and analgesia and cause a reduction in neurotransmitter release while preserving autoregulation, CO_2 reactivity, and cardiovascular stability. CBF, CMR_{O_2}, and ICP are unchanged or slightly decreased. Delta waves are seen on EEG; burst suppression does not occur.

(1) **Morphine** is a potent analgesic with relatively poor central nervous system (CNS) penetration. Commonly used for postoperative analgesia in neurosurgical patients, morphine can cause hypotension secondary to histamine release.

(2) **Meperidine** may increase the heart rate because of its atropine-like structure and effect. Normeperidine is a metabolite of meperidine that can cause CNS excitation and seizures.

(3) **Fentanyl** is 100 times more potent than morphine. Fentanyl does not cause histamine release, is shorter acting than morphine, and decreases ICP and CBV slightly while maintaining CPP.

(4) **Sufentanil** is more potent than fentanyl and may increase ICP (via vasodilatation) in patients who have severe head

trauma. The use of another opioid should be considered in such instances.

(5) **Remifentanil** is a very short-acting ($t1/2 = 3$ to 10 minutes) esterase-metabolized opioid that compared favorably to fentanyl in reduction of ICP and CBV and maintenance of CPP in a recent clinical trial.

e. **Ca channel-blocking drugs** should theoretically provide cerebral protection by vasodilatation and diminution of the consequences of Ca influx.

(1) **Nimodipine decreases vasospasm** after aneurysmal subarachnoid hemorrhage (SAH). Nimodipine may increase CBF to underperfused areas by redistribution through an inverse steal effect. The dose of nimodipine, presently available only in oral form, is 60 mg every 4 hours for 21 days after SAH. Hypotension may occur with the administration of nimodipine.

(2) **Nicardipine,** available for intravenous administration, has decreased ischemic damage in animal studies, but clinical trials have not shown improved neurologic outcome after ischemia.

f. **Ketamine,** a phencyclidine derivative, produces dissociative anesthesia.

(1) Ketamine markedly increases ICP and CBF (60%) via cerebrovasodilatation. The $CMRo_2$ is unchanged or slightly increased. Autoregulation is abolished.

(2) **Seizures** can occur.

(3) Although it is a noncompetitive NMDA antagonist, ketamine is not recommended for patients who have intracranial pathology.

g. **Local anesthetics** are commonly used as adjuvants in neuroanesthesia.

(1) Lidocaine's clinical effects are determined by the dose. When administered after EEG isoelectricity induced by pentobarbital, lidocaine may decrease $CMRo_2$ by an additional 15% to 20%. At clinically recommended doses (1.5 mg/kg), lidocaine may reduce ischemic damage. Lidocaine also blunts the hemodynamic response to intubation by increasing anesthetic depth. At lower doses, lidocaine possesses anticonvulsant activity and can be used as ancillary therapy for status epilepticus. At toxic doses, lidocaine causes seizures.

C. Potent inhaled anesthetics

1. All potent inhaled anesthetics are cerebrovasodilatators and thereby increase CBF and ICP to different degrees. This effect can be attenuated by prior hyperventilation. The volatile anesthetics also decrease CMR_{O_2} while uncoupling CBF and CMR_{O_2}. Autoregulation is impaired but CO_2 reactivity is preserved.

   a. **Isoflurane** causes the greatest decrease in CMR_{O_2} (40% to 50%) and is the least potent vasodilator. The EEG becomes isoelectric EEG at 2 minimum alveolar concentration (MAC) or 2.4%. Isoflurane has no effect on the production of CSF but does increase CSF resorption. The critical CBF for isoflurane, the lowest of all the volatile agents, is 10 mL/100 g/minute. Thus, the use of isoflurane in patients undergoing CEA may have advantages. Isoflurane may also offer protection after brain ischemia. Studies of isoflurane in animal models of ischemia and hypoxemia have shown some limited protection from isoflurane. Preconditioning with isoflurane seems to confer tolerance to ischemia and some neuroprotection. *In vitro* studies have also shown improved recovery after ischemia and a reduction in cell death through the postischemic activation of ATP-regulated K channels and protein kinases.

   b. The cerebral effects of **sevoflurane** are similar to those of isoflurane; both cause a slight increase in CBF and ICP and a decrease in CMR_{O_2}. Nephrotoxic inorganic fluoride may accumulate when patients receive sevoflurane for prolonged periods of time. Induction and emergence are rapid. Sevoflurane may offer protection after brain ischemia through preconditioning. Preconditioning with sevoflurane and subsequent cerebral protection have been demonstrated during incomplete ischemia *in vitro*. Improved recovery in CA1 pyramidal cells in rats has occurred at clinical concentrations known to be useful in humans.

   c. **Desflurane** is similar to isoflurane in its cerebrovascular profile, but ICP might increase despite normocapnia with desflurane compared to isoflurane. Induction and emergence with desflurane are rapid. Desflurane may also be protective after brain ischemia. Studies after hypoxia and after incomplete cerebral ischemia in rats have shown cerebral protective effects.

2. **Nitrous oxide,** a cerebrovasodilatator, increases CBF, CMR_{O_2}, and ICP. The increase in CBF

is attenuated by barbiturates, opioids, and hypocapnia. Nitrous oxide is 32 times more soluble in blood than nitrogen and is thus capable of diffusing into air-containing body cavities with extreme rapidity. Therefore, nitrous oxide is avoided in the presence of pneumocephalus and in any surgical procedure within 2 weeks of a craniotomy in which nitrous oxide was used. Nitrous oxide is also discontinued immediately if air embolism is suspected and may increase neurologic deficits after brain injury.

D. **Anticonvulsant drugs** are indicated in patients at risk for seizure activity including individuals who have epilepsy, head trauma, or craniotomy, and their administration is continued into the postoperative period. Seizure activity exacerbates the effects of ischemia through activation of anaerobic metabolic pathways. CBF, $CMRO_2$, and intracellular Ca increase during seizures, and EAA neurotransmitters, including glutamate, are released.

1. Once seizure activity occurs, the patient's airway is immediately secured and adequate ventilation is ensured to prevent hypoxemia and hypercapnia.
2. Avoidance of hypotension is essential.
3. Anticonvulsant therapy is administered promptly:
   - **Thiopental,** 25 to 100 mg i.v.
   - **Diazepam,** 2 to 20 mg i.v.
   - **Midazolam,** 1 to 5 mg i.v.
   a. **Fosphenytoin,** 15 to 20 mg phenytoin equivalents (PE)/kg, or **phenytoin**, 15 mg/kg, may be administered to prevent further seizure activity once the acute episode has been terminated. Fosphenytoin, 75 mg, is equivalent to phenytoin, 50 mg, and has the advantage of increased speed of administration (up to 150 mg PE/minute). Phenytoin is limited to 50 mg/minute because it may induce hypotension. The loading dose of fosphenytoin can be given in 5 to 7 minutes, whereas the equivalent dose of phenytoin would require 15 to 20 minutes.

V. **Cerebral preconditioning and neurogenesis.** Models of cerebral ischemia in animals have shown that the induction of endogenous proteins of repair and genes that code for them can set the stage for cerebral preconditioning that may protect the brain during subsequent ischemia. Prodromal transient ischemic attacks (TIAs) may protect the brain during subsequent ischemic strokes. Recent evidence indicates that neurogenesis and diaschisis occur after injury. Diaschisis is a reduction in blood flow and metabolism in an area distant from the site of focal damage. It may represent a process of structural reorganization after injury. Apoptosis, or programmed cell death, may also be part of the process of structural reorganization after injury. Ischemia stimulates neurogenesis and new neurons migrate to the site of tissue injury and contribute to functional recovery. Activated neural stem cells contribute to stroke-induced neurogenesis and the migration of neuroblasts toward the infarct boundary in adult rats. Therapy for stroke in rats with a nitric oxide (NO) donor and human bone marrow stromal cells enhances angiogenesis and neurogenesis subsequent to middle cerebral artery occlusion.

VI. **Cerebral resuscitation.** Patients who require resuscitation from cerebral ischemia include the following:

  A. **Intensive care unit (ICU) patients** who have traumatic but nonoperative brain injury such as **diffuse axonal injury** (DAI) with increased ICP and cerebral edema who may be candidates for barbiturate coma.

  B. Patients who have **Reye's syndrome** and cerebral edema with increased ICP.

  C. Near-drowning victims who have **anoxic encephalopathy,** cerebral edema, and intracranial hypertension who are treated like Reye's syndrome patients.

  D. Patients who have **nonhemorrhagic stroke** who may be candidates for fibrinolytic therapy with tissue plasminogen activator (TPA).

  Anesthesiologists may encounter these patients when they are consulted about the management of cerebral edema and increased ICP or the induction and maintenance of barbiturate coma. These patients may also require sedation, analgesia, and neuromuscular blockade.

VII. **Experimental modalities**

  A. **NMDA receptor antagonists** were developed to prevent neuronal damage from the excessive accumulation of the excitatory neurotransmitter glutamate. The NMDA receptor antagonists have not conferred consistently reproducible neuroprotection in experimental studies and may worsen injury. One of the difficulties has been the development of drugs that effectively penetrate the blood-brain barrier.

    1. **Dizocilpine maleate (MK-801)** is a noncompetitive NMDA receptor antagonist whose beneficial effects in laboratory experiments may be partially attributable to drug-induced hypothermia. Dizocilpine is not approved for use in humans and does not appear to be promising.

    2. **Magnesium,** a noncompetitive NMDA antagonist, binds within the ion channel, preventing ion flux, and may be helpful after brain injury.

    3. **Glycine binding site antagonism** with HA-966 and 7-chlorokynurenic acid is still in the investigational stage but shows promise.

    4. **AMPA receptor antagonism** with 2, 3-dihydroxy-6-nitro-7-sulfamoylbenzo (f)quinazoline **(NBQX)** has proved beneficial when given after the ischemic insult in experimental models.

  B. **Sodium channel-blocking drugs** such as **riluzole** may reduce glutamate release during ischemia.

Lamotrigine, an anticonvulsant with Na channel-blocking activity, is known to reduce glutamate release and ischemic damage. Further studies are warranted.

C. **Tirilazad,** a lipid-soluble 21-aminosteroid, crosses the blood-brain barrier and acts as a lipid antioxidant, inhibiting free radical formation and lipid peroxidation. Studies indicate protection only when tirilazad is administered before an ischemic event.

D. **Free radical scavengers. Superoxide dismutase (SOD), deferoxamine, vitamin E, mannitol,** and **glucocorticoids** all possess free radical scavenging activity. The utility of SOD has been limited by its short $t1/2$ (8 minutes) and poor blood-brain barrier penetration. While glucocorticoids have membrane-stabilizing properties and decrease cerebral edema from brain tumors, they have not been shown to improve outcome in cerebral ischemia. The clinical usefulness of free radical scavengers is still under investigation.

E. **Modification of arachidonic acid synthesis.** Ischemia-induced excess of the vasoconstrictor thromboxane relative to the vasodilator prostacyclin (PGI_2) has led to the development of **thromboxane synthetase inhibitors** and **PGI_2synthetase stimulation** to prevent the formation of excessive thromboxane.

F. **Dexmedetomidine, an alpha$_2$ agonist,** decreases central sympathetic activity by decreasing plasma norepinephrine release. Dexmedetomidine has been found to be neuroprotective in a model of focal ischemia, perhaps because excess catecholamine levels correlate with increased neuronal ischemic damage. Dexmedetomidine also decreases the MAC for halothane and isoflurane and decreases CBF without significantly altering CMR_{O_2}.

G. **NO** is a free radical with complex neuronal activity. Nitric oxide synthase (NOS) catalyzes the formation of NO from the amino acid L-arginine, which itself decreases neuronal damage in experimentally induced focal ischemia. Three forms of NOS have been discovered:

   1. **Neuronal NOS (nNOS)** enhances glutamate release and NMDA-mediated neurotoxicity. Selective nNOS inhibition has been shown to be neuroprotective.

   2. **Immunologic NOS (iNOS)** is not detectable in healthy tissue. Induction of iNOS causes delayed neuronal cell death and can exacerbate glutamate excitotoxicity. Inhibition of iNOS by **aminoguanidine** reduces ischemic damage in experimental models.

   3. Stimulation of **endothelial NOS (eNOS)** by an ischemia-induced increase in intracellular Ca improves CBF by dilatation of cerebral blood vessels and has been shown to reduce ischemic damage in a rodent model.

H. **Erythropoietin (EPO)** is a substance produced in the brain after hypoxic or ischemic insults. Primarily elaborated in the adult mammalian astrocytes in the ischemic penumbra, EPO stimulates neurogenesis, angiogenesis, and production of the proteins of repair, diminishes neuronal excitotoxicity, reduces inflammation, and inhibits neuronal apoptosis. It has been used in humans for cerebral preconditioning in patients after ischemic stroke. EPO may be more effective, however, as a prophylactic protectant when given preoperatively. Nonhematopoietic analogs of EPO, such as asialoEPO, have been developed and are showing equivalent potency as neuroprotectants in the laboratory. These analogs do not increase the hematocrit and thus do not exacerbate the ischemia injury through an increase in blood viscosity.

I. **Other experimental modalities.** Experimental results with preoperative hyperbaric oxygen, normobaric 100% oxygen exposure, electroconvulsive shock, and the potassium channel-opening drug, diazoxide, have shown that all of these modalities can be used to accomplish cerebral preconditioning.

J. **Anesthesia duration and depth.** Minimizing the duration of the time during which the patient is deeply anesthetized may provide cerebral protection by preventing neuronal apoptosis. A growing body of evidence indicates that cumulative deep anesthesia time is an independent predictor of increased postoperative mortality in adult patients.

SUGGESTED READINGS

Amadeu MF, Abramowicz AE, Chambers G, et al. Etomidate does not alter recovery after anoxia of evoked population spikes recorded from the CA1 region of rat hippocampal slices. *Anesthesiology* 1998;88:1274.

Amorim P, Cottrell JE, Kass IS. Effects of small changes in temperature on CA 1 pyramidal cells from rat hippocampal slices during hypoxia: implications about the mechanisms of hypothermic protection against neuronal damage. *Brain Res* 1999;844(1–2): 143–149.

Bendo AA, Kass IS, Hartung J, et al. Anesthesia for neurosurgery. In: Barash PG, et al., eds. *Clinical Anesthesia*, 5th ed. Philadelphia, PA: Lippincott Williams & Wilkins, 2006:746–789.

Cottrell JE. Techniques and drugs for cerebral protection. In: *Annual Meeting Refresher Course Lectures*. American Society of Anesthesiologists. Atlanta, GA, 2005.

Dimaculangan D, Bendo AA, Sims R, et al. Desflurane improves the recovery of the evoked postsynaptic population spike from CA1 pyramidal cells after hypoxia in rat hippocampal slices. *J Neurosurg Anesthesiol* 2006;18:78–82.

Engelhard K, Werner C, Reeker W, et al. Desflurane and isoflurane improve neurological outcome after incomplete cerebral ischemia in rats. *Br J Anaesth* 1999;83:415–421.

Grasso G. Erythropoietin: A new paradigm for neuroprotection. *J Neurosurg Anesthesiol* 2006;18:91.

Guy J, Hindman BJ, Baker KZ, et al. Comparison of remifentanil and fentanyl in patients undergoing craniotomy for supratentorial space-occupying lesions. *Anesthesiology* 1997;86:514–524.

Jevtovic-Todorovic V, Wozniak DF, Benshoff ND, et al. A comparative evaluation of neurotoxic properties of ketamine and nitrous oxide. *Brain Res* 2001;895(1–2):264–267.

Kass IS, Cottrell JE. Pathophysiology of brain injury. In: Cottrell JE, Smith DS, eds. *Anesthesia and Neurosurgery*, 4th ed. St. Louis, MO: Mosby, 2001:69–82.

Lam AM. Anesthetic management of patients with traumatic head injury. In: Lam AM, ed. *Anesthetic Management of Acute Head Injury*. New York, NY: McGraw-Hill, 1995:183.

Lei B, Cottrell JE, Kass IS. Neuroprotective effect of low-dose lidocaine in a rat model of transient focal cerebral ischemia. *Anesthesiology* 2001;95:445–451.

Lei B, Popp S, Capuano-Waters C, et al. Effects of low-dose lidocaine on cytochrome c release and caspase 3 activation after transient focal cerebral ischemia in rats. *Anesthesiology* 2002;96:A800.

Lipton P. Ischemic cell death in brain neurons. *Physiolog Rev* 1999;79(4):1431–1568.

Matei G, Pavlik R, McCadden T, et al. Sevoflurane improves electrophysiological recovery of rat hippocampal slice CA 1 pyramidal neurons after hypoxia. *J Neurosurg Anesthesiol* 2002;14:293–298.

The National Institute of Neurological Disorders and Stroke rt-PA Stroke Study Group. Tissue plasminogen activator for acute ischemic stroke. *N Engl J Med* 1995;333(24):1581–1587.

Raley-Susman KM, Kass IS, Cottrell JE, et al. Sodium influx blockade and hypoxic damage to CA 1 pyramidal neurons in rat hippocampal slices. *J Neurophysiol* 2001;86:2715–2726.

Sullivan B, Leu D, Taylor DM, et al. Isoflurane prevents delayed cell death in an organotypic slice culture model of cerebral ischemia. *Anesthesiology* 2002;96(1):189–195.

Wang T, Raley-Susman KM, Wang J, et al. Thiopental attenuates hypoxic changes of electrophysiology, biochemistry, and morphology in rat hippocampal slice CA 1 pyramidal cells. *Stroke* 1999;30:2400–2407.

Xie Z, Dong Y, Maeda U, et al. The common inhalation anesthetic isoflurane induces apoptosis and increases amyloid β protein levels. *Anesthesiology* 2006;104:988–994.

Zhu H, Cottrell JE, Kass IS. The effect of thiopental and propofol on NMDA- and AMPA-mediated glutamate excitotoxicity. *Anesthesiology* 1997;87:944–951.

Management of Pain in the Neurosurgical Patient

Timothy R. Deer

It has been 30 years since John Bonica, the great anesthesia-based pain educator, expressed concern that pain was not well controlled because of the failure of physicians to apply available knowledge. That thought may hold more credence in the area of neurosurgery than in any other area of postoperative pain treatment. The shortcomings in this arena can be attributed to the common belief of clinicians that pain is minimal after intracranial procedures. Because of this controversial notion, many patients are undertreated in the immediate postoperative period.

A comprehensive look at the issue of postoperative pain in the patient undergoing intracranial surgery led to some clarification of the issue. Dunbar compared those undergoing intracranial surgery to those with select extracranial procedures. In this 200-patient retrospective study, the intracranial group did have significantly less pain than the comparison group ($p<0.05$). A subset of intracranial patients did have significantly more pain than others in the group. Those requiring frontal craniotomies did have an increased need for opioids, and elevated heart rates, blood pressure, and intracranial pressure (ICP). Based on this analysis, a general statement cannot be made about all patients undergoing intracranial procedures.

Other factors, including the need to monitor neurologic and cognitive functions closely, contribute to this problem. This monitoring can be affected adversely if the patient is sedated or obtunded. This conflict of treatment goals can lead to withholding pain medication and techniques. It has also led to the use of less potent opioids and banning morphine from some neurosurgical intensive care units. Recent studies have shown that when morphine and other potent opioids are titrated it does not alter the outcomes or postsurgical monitoring.

Another factor complicates postoperative pain treatment in modern times. The use of new rapidly acting intravenous agents has led to rapid wake-up and recovery and unfortunately to the increased importance of postoperative pain assessment. With the rapid breakdown of these agents, the patient has no opioid level present and may experience significant pain on awakening.

It is critical to realize that the treatment of pain in the neurosurgical patient may influence outcomes in a variety of ways. Studies have shown that pain in the postoperative period can adversely influence ICP. Proper pain control may stabilize hemodynamics and blood pressure as well as lower the ICP. In addition to pain issues, the perioperative period in the intracranial patient is complex in a systemic fashion. Recovery from neurosurgical anesthesia is followed by elevations in body oxygen consumption and serum catecholamine concentrations. Systemic hypertension is often present after neurosurgical procedures and has been linked to intracranial hemorrhage. The cerebral consequences of the recovery period can lead to cerebral hyperemia and increased ICP. Prevention or control of pain is one of the major factors in limiting these adverse systemic effects.

Over the past decade, developments in intravenous opioids, new regional techniques, and local anesthetics have greatly enhanced our abilities to treat this patient group. Preemptive analgesia may lead to the improved stability of the patient throughout the surgical experience. To minimize pain and decrease the stress response and hemodynamic changes, the surgeon and the anesthesiologist must work as a team. The importance of the anesthesiologist in decreasing anxiety, creating a treatment plan, and executing the plan is crucial to a successful surgical experience.

The opportunities to have an effect on the pain pathway are numerous. The pain response has a three-part complex. Pain transduction is the initial impulse. Pain transmission is the transfer of pain information via the C and A delta fibers through the spinothalamic tracts to the thalamus and cortex. Pain modulation is the interpretation of the pain signal. The cortex then processes this pathway into an emotional interpretation. The patient's genetic, social, and cultural backgrounds influence this interpretation. By understanding this complex pain neural network, the opportunity to impact the pain response is great. The method chosen to impact the pain network depends on the surgical procedure and patient comorbidities. The remaining sections of this chapter focus on key points to enhance outcomes, patient satisfaction, and patient safety.

I. **Preoperative assessment**
   A. **Preadmission or presurgical considerations**
      1. **Reducing anxiety.** Recent studies have shown that reducing anxiety preoperatively or in the immediate postoperative period enhances the ease of controlling pain. In the preoperative and postoperative patient groups, the need for medication has been reduced. There was a decrease in pain scales and hypertension. It is important for the anesthesiologist to use part of the preoperative interview to discuss the plan for postoperative pain treatment. Studies have shown that a discussion of the patient's previous experiences, expectations, and fears can be as useful as some anxiolytic medications. Patients should have a chance to ask questions and express concerns prior to the scheduled procedure.
      2. **Pain treatment history.** The prolonged use of oral opioids for chronic pain makes determining the baseline dose of opioids in chronic pain patients somewhat difficult. The tolerance to opioid medication can influence dosing in both the intraoperative anesthetic and postoperative pain course. It is important to realize that the use of

chronic medications is for a stable pain condition and it will be necessary to supplement this baseline dose with additional medication. It is helpful to obtain a history of previous experiences with postoperative pain treatment, complications, and adverse reactions. The anesthesiologists should explain in detail the pain treatment plan; patient reassurance should be a high priority.

3. **Understanding the procedure.** The physician providing the postoperative pain relief should understand the procedure being performed. An understanding of the patient's postsurgical mental status is helpful when the physician chooses a pain treatment plan. Techniques that require an alert patient, such as patient-controlled analgesia, should be offered only to those who are able to comply with instructions. Regional anesthesia is possible if the procedure involves only limited portions of the spine.

4. **Role of coexisting disease.** The patient's nonsurgical disease processes must be considered when tailoring a pain treatment plan. The review of systems is critical in determining what recommendations should be made. The following factors should be considered in a presurgical assessment.

    a. **Neurologic system.** The site of surgery and the perioperative morbidity should be considered. The patient's baseline cognitive function also determines whether a patient-controlled analgesia (PCA) system can be used. PCA can be used in children as young as 5 years but should be instituted with caution and requires the education of both patients and their parents.

    b. **Renal system.** A patient with renal disease is prone to complications from drugs with metabolites removed by the kidneys. Meperidine, for example, breaks down to normeperidine, which can cause seizures in these patients. Meperidine should be used in a limited fashion in any postsurgical patient but the risk is high in those with renal impairment.

    c. **Infectious disease.** Neuroaxial procedures may be contraindicated in the patient with systemic infection or local infection at the site of the proposed procedure. If a patient is bacteremic or has local site infections, regional anesthesia is contraindicated.

    d. **Hematologic system.** The epidural hematoma is a rare but disastrous complication of regional anesthesia. Factors that may contribute to this adverse outcome include abnormalities of the clotting cascade, a history of bleeding during previous surgery, and the use of low molecular weight heparin and other coagulants during the postoperative period. This condition may be evaluated both historically and by laboratory values.

   e. **Cardiovascular system.** As noted in a previous section the physiological response to intracranial surgery includes hypertension, tachycardia, and catecholamine surges. An increase in blood pressure, heart rate and catecholamine results in an increase in cardiac workload and may lead to ischemia in those with perioperative risks. When in doubt, a cardiology consultation may be useful in planning the postoperative pain treatment plan. The other risk of the anesthetic and pain treatment is the issue of patients who are cardiovascularly unstable and require support.

   f. **Gastrointestinal system.** A history of ileus may be a cause for concern for the surgeon in regard to a local anesthetic infusion and use of narcotics. In these cases, it is important to implement a bowel support regimen as a standard part of the program when using intravenous or oral opioids or epidural infusions.

B. **Summary of the preoperative period.** The preoperative period is crucial in the overall success of the neurosurgical pain treatment program. The clinician should develop a mental checklist of assessment points prior to bringing the patient to the operating theater.

II. **The importance of pain treatment**
   A. The patient undergoing neurosurgical intervention may develop many perioperative changes that can affect the overall outcome without attempts at intervention. The stress response, which is somewhat dependent on the complexity and site of surgery, can affect the immunologic response, coagulation, cardiac function, hormonal response, and other systems crucial to the recovery of the neurosurgical patient. The anesthesiologist has several options to blunt the stress response, but these methods are successful only when the appropriate procedure is matched with the right patient.

   B. In some areas of anesthesia, the technique of postoperative pain control has been shown to have a major impact on outcomes and pain reduction. An example of this impact occurs in thoracic surgery. At the current time, no significant studies exist in the neurologic patient, and the significance of postoperative pain is unclear.

III. **The stress response: an overview**
   A. **Changes in other organ systems.** The patient undergoing neurologic surgery is often very sensitive to

subtle changes in other organ systems. The patho-physiologic changes associated with the stress response from surgical trauma can greatly affect the outcome from procedures with high risk of morbidity and mortality.

B. Physiologic effects of the stress response. The stress response includes an initial depressed phase and a subsequent hyperdynamic phase.

1. **The depressed phase.** In the initial portion of the response, the body responds by depressing most physiologic functions. This phase is brief in the surgical patient and might be unidentifiable in some patients.

2. **The hyperdynamic phase.** The portion of the stress response of most concern to the anesthesiologist and most involved in morbidity and mortality in the neurosurgical patient is the period of recovery after surgery. This lasts for a period of time that is directly proportional to the amount of tissue trauma and the patient's pre-existing disease state. A characterization of this response is given below.

   a. **Endocrinologic changes.** Both catabolic and anabolic responses are seen during this phase of response.

      (1) **Catabolic changes** include increases in several hormones: catecholamines, renin, angiotensin II, aldosterone, glucagon, cortisol, tumor necrosis factor, adrenocorticotropic hormone (ACTH), growth hormone, and interleukin (primarily IL-1 and IL-6). These changes lead to hemodynamic instability in some patients and perhaps to changes in cerebral blood flow (CBF) and ICP.

      (2) **Anabolic changes** include decreases in insulin and testosterone. The changes can lead to imbalances in the hormonal axis and impact wound healing and response to tissue trauma.

   b. **Metabolic changes.** The overall impact on the patient outcome by the stress response can be understood by considering the metabolic balance during this tumultuous time.

      (1) The catabolic and anabolic effects noted here create intense changes in the patient's physiologic stability. These changes include shifts in insulin resistance, muscle breakdown, glucose intolerance, fat breakdown, increased tissue oxidation with the creation of free radicals, sodium and water retention, hyperglycemia, increased acute phase proteins, and fluid shifts and third spacing.

(2) The end effect is a change in fluid balance, protein metabolism, fat metabolism, and carbohydrate metabolism.

C. **Body system responses to the stress response**

1. Mechanisms to block the stress response have focused on beta blockade and blockade of other receptors. While these mechanisms are important, the physician should not forget the importance of impacting the pain pathways. Using both techniques enhances the chance of blocking the unstable response. The uninhibited stress response has been shown to increase cardiac workload; increase vascular tension; adversely affect platelet function; decrease fibrinolysis; decrease renal perfusion; decrease the urinary excretion of water, wastes, and electrolytes; decrease hepatic function; increase oxygen consumption; decrease immunocompetence; and decrease the centrally mediated temperature regulation mechanisms.

2. Considering these enormous changes noted in the preceding text in the unbridled stress response, the importance of blunting this response in enhancing outcomes becomes critical. Pain treatment mechanisms utilized in limiting this systemic response are detailed.

IV. **Mechanisms of blunting the stress response to surgery**

A. **General anesthesia.** The use of inhalational anesthetics and total intravenous anesthetic techniques including remifentanil have been responsible for tremendous advances in improving the surgical experience and reducing pain at the time of surgery. Unfortunately, although interrupting pain at the time of surgical insult, most agents have not been shown to substantially block the metabolic and endocrine response to tissue trauma. A few anesthetic agents have shown promise compared to alternatives.

1. **Etomidate.** When given by the intravenous route, etomidate may have some ability to blunt the adrenocortical system's response to stress. This effect is seen by a blunting of the rise in cortisol expected with similar tissue trauma. Etomidate is thought to accomplish this by blocking enzymes in the cortisol synthesis pathway. The clinical benefit of this drug has not been proved in prospective randomized trials. Its long recovery time may also limit its use as a neuroanesthetic agent.

2. **Inhalational agents.** Sevoflurane and isoflurane are both useful drugs in low concentrations in the patient undergoing intracranial surgery. The ability to use these drugs to limit the stress response is minimal because of the effects of higher concentrations in changing CBF, cerebral blood volume, and ICP.

3. **High-dose opioids.** Recent years have shown a dramatic increase in the utilization of high-potency short-acting opioids. Remifentanil, a compound of the 4-anilidopiperidine derivatives, is an ideal drug because of its ultrashort duration of action and metabolic independence of both hepatic and renal functions. The advantages of this drug may be some of the critical issues that lead to poor outcomes in regard to postprocedural pain complaints. The rapid increase in serum levels leads to an initial blunting of the stress response, but as the drug is discontinued, the patient is at risk for hyperalgesia and substantial increases in the stress response. It is critical that longer acting opioids be considered when the intravenous infusions of short-acting opioids are discontinued. Remifentanil, like other intravenous opioids, often leads to a stable hemodynamic course during the surgery.

4. **Propofol.** Propofol has been used to try to limit the wake-up time from general anesthesia and to blunt the initial stress and pain responses. Limited studies provide no evidence that this drug changes the immediate stress response even when a slow reduction of dosage lengthens the wake-up phase until the patient slowly recovers to baseline cognitive function.

B. **Regional anesthesia: neuroaxial.** Regional anesthetic techniques appear to have the greatest ability to block the stress response. The ability to use regional anesthetics in the neurosurgical patient is minimal and acceptable only in a few surgical techniques. Possible opportunities include spinal instrumentation, spinal repair surgeries, plexus operations, and surgery on peripheral nerves. The ability to use these techniques is also limited in surgery of the neuroaxis because it may delay the ability to do neurologic checks postsurgery. While studies have shown epidural or intrathecal analgesia has improved postoperative nitrogen balance, renal function, glucose metabolism, oxygen consumption, coagulation and fibrinolysis, and hepatic and immunologic function, and decreased cardiac workload, it has very little use in the neurosurgical patient.

C. **Peripheral nerve blockade.** Peripheral nerve blocks can blunt the initial response to surgery and may be used as a sole anesthetic. The use of this technique in neurosurgical patients is limited. Common locations for peripheral nerve blockade include the brachial plexus, the cervical plexus, the femoral nerve, and peripheral nerves of the lower extremities. The need to assess nerve function in the immediate postoperative period could limit the technique.

D. Adrenergic blockade. Clonidine has been used in patients with brain trauma and after extensive neurologic surgery to blunt the stress response. The drug has also been shown to blunt the possibilities of vasogenic edema. The use of spinal or epidural alpha-adrenergic blockade has also been shown to reduce the stress response. It is unclear whether the reduction in adrenergic response with epidural or intrathecal clonidine is a direct effect of the alpha-adrenergic blockade or a response to the clonidine-induced analgesia. The use of systemic beta-adrenergic and alpha-adrenergic agents has been shown to stabilize the hemodynamic response and the cerebral circulation.

E. Nonsteroidals. The perioperative use of nonsteroidal anti-inflammatory drugs (NSAIDs) may enhance the ability of other techniques such as regional analgesia and anesthesia in blocking the stress response. The enhancement of regional analgesia and anesthesia is thought to be directly related to the NSAIDs' action at peripheral receptors involved in the tissue trauma cascade. Recent data on dangers of cyclooxygenase 2 inhibition have led to exercise of caution in using this class of drugs in the perioperative period. These drugs have been linked to hypertension, stroke, myocardial infarction, and blood clotting.

F. Intravenous opioids. The use of PCA has led to markedly improved patient satisfaction and improved pain scores. Studies have shown that opioid-induced pain control can improve immunologic function in the patient undergoing neurosurgical procedures, which may lead to improved outcomes.

G. Transcutaneous electrical nerve stimulation (TENS). TENS has been used to treat postoperative pain. Current data do not support its efficacy or any effect on blunting stress response.

H. Psychological counseling. As noted earlier in this chapter, biofeedback, music therapy, relaxation training, and simple conversation have been shown to lessen the stress response to surgery and lessen the overall stress response.

V. Intraoperative and postoperative pain treatment interventions

    A. Preemptive analgesia

        1. Preoperative local anesthetic infiltration of the surgical field. The blunting of the response to incision may be crucial to the overall ability to provide a stable postoperative pain treatment course, lessen amount of anesthetic involved, and blunt the initial stage of the surgical stress response. Combining local anesthetics with general anesthetics can result in lower minimum alveolar concentrations when compared with using general anesthetics alone. Recovery is also superior with this method. The combined use of general and local anesthetic may reduce the afferent barrage of surgery, and preemptive analgesia may lead to decreased postoperative pain and blunt the stress response. Local anesthetic should be considered for the wound field even when general anesthesia is the method of choice for the anesthetic.

2. **Anesthetics and systemic opioids.** There is no evidence that use of high-dose opioids or inhalational agents results in any change in postoperative pain levels or need for pain medications.

3. **Neuroaxial anesthetic techniques.** Recent randomized controlled studies in the Japanese literature show that using epidural anesthesia for spine surgery has a preemptive effect on postoperative pain and leads to less perioperative bleeding. An understanding of these techniques is important to be able to use them properly.

B. **Neuroaxial infusion therapy: epidural.** The use of epidural infusion therapy has increased in recent years as a primary method of acute pain control in patients undergoing surgical procedures involving peripheral nerves. The proper use of an epidural infusion requires a working knowledge of dermatomal anatomy, drug pharmacokinetics, drug synergies, and postoperative follow-up requirements.

1. **Epidural location.** This is important in the dosage requirement and infusion rate required for proper analgesia. Epidural placement should ideally be within two levels of the nerve root of primary focus of the surgical procedure.

2. **Lipophilia.** This is crucial in drug selection for postoperative pain. A lipophilic drug such as fentanyl requires placement of the catheter at a level near the nerve innervation of the surgical site. With morphine, which is much less lipid soluble, the catheter placement is less critical because the drug may cover several interspaces prior to being absorbed. Hydromorphone has intermediate properties.

3. **Drug synergies.** For more than a decade, data have demonstrated an antinociceptive synergy between intrathecal morphine and lidocaine during visceral and somatic nociception at dosages that do not impair motor function. The combination of local anesthetics and opioids offers a synergistic effect that leads to better analgesia than either drug infused alone. Local anesthetic infusion therapy has been shown to be the most effective method of blunting the stress response to tissue trauma. The addition of opioids helps eliminate the problem of tachyphylaxis that may develop with local anesthetics alone.

C. **Neuroaxial infusion therapy: subarachnoid.** The use of spinal blockade in neurosurgical procedures is somewhat limited. Continuous spinal infusion therapy is generally discouraged because of the risk of cerebrospinal fluid leaks and infection as well as the confusion of the neurologic examination.

D. Peripheral nerve blockade. Peripheral nerve infusions of local anesthetic can be beneficial in the intraoperative period as well as for postoperative pain control. Common sites for continuous infusion include the brachial plexus and the femoral nerve. A nerve stimulator or ultrasound is helpful in the proper placement of the catheter. In general, a blunt-tipped needle is preferable to a sharp beveled needle to reduce the risk of nerve injury.

E. PCA. The use of patient-controlled narcotic delivery may be applied to either intravenous opioid delivery or epidural infusion medications such as local anesthetics, opioids, or clonidine. The neurosurgical patient presents a dilemma in the decision-making process. Careful attention must be given equally to the baseline preoperative function in regard to the ability to understand the use of a PCA system and to the expected postoperative cognitive function and the ability to utilize the system. A team approach involving the surgeon, anesthesiologist, and patient is needed when this mode of treatment is considered.

F. Nurse-administered intermittent analgesia. The classic method of postoperative pain relief in the neurosurgical patient is to have a nurse administer intravenous medications. This involves administration either on the patient's demand or at scheduled times at the request of the surgeon or anesthesiologist. This mode of treatment is most appropriate in the patient with altered preoperative or postoperative cognitive function. The disadvantages of this method include delay in treatment, unnecessary suffering, and excessive sedation. It is also labor intensive.

G. TENS. There are no current data to support any change in postoperative outcome with the use of TENS for incisional pain. This method is difficult to use in the neurologic surgery population because of the technical difficulties of application.

H. Psychological counseling. The addition of a psychologist to the postoperative acute pain team is helpful in improving the patient's ability to cope with the emotional stress of pain and disease. Unfortunately, because no good studies on the cost-effectiveness of adding this service exist, reimbursement may be difficult to obtain.

I. Adjuvant drugs. Anticonvulsants are often used after intracranial surgery to prevent seizures. These drugs may also offer some improvement in neuropathic pain syndromes and reduce the opioid requirements. The classic drugs used for neuropathic pain are tegretol and dilantin; however, the most impressive data are with gabapentin. Baclofen has been used to treat spinal-induced spasticity and has been reported in some patients to improve pain of neuropathic origin. Cyclo-oxygenase 2 inhibitors are no longer recommended in the neurosurgical patient. Classic nonsteroidals may reduce opioid needs and improve outcomes. Intramuscular or intravenous ketorolac is generally the drug of choice; however, it should be avoided if the patient is at high risk of hemorrhage. The addition of antiemetics might also be helpful in controlling nausea that can accompany postoperative analgesics. Ondansetron is an attractive choice because it does not tend to potentiate the neurologic cognitive changes of the opioids and other pain medications. Tramadol is a mu- selective agent that has been shown in a few randomized studies to be less effective in the neurosurgical patient than either codeine or morphine. At higher doses up to 75 mg, tramadol had improved efficacy but was not tolerated because of nausea and vomiting.

VI. **Creating a case-specific pain management plan**
   A. **Intracranial procedures.** The patient who has had an intracranial procedure presents one of the most difficult problems in pain management. The use of regional anesthesia is not an option. Oversedating the patient can lead to hypercarbia and hypoxemia. The cognitive function might be impaired because of the surgical area involved. Despite these limitations, controlling pain in this group is crucial because of the increased morbidity and mortality associated with uncontrolled hemodynamic response to pain and surgery. Pain treatment in this patient population must consider multiple factors.
   B. **Procedures of the extremities.** The patient requiring surgery of the extremities gives the anesthesiologist many options. A discussion should occur regarding the patient's postoperative neurologic function and the need for serial functional checks. If the issue of sensory loss is minimal, the use of regional anesthesia is optimal because of the blunting of both pain and the stress response. Other techniques are also acceptable in this population.
   C. **Procedures involving the spine.** When neurologic surgery is performed on the structures of the neuroaxis, regional anesthesia may result in improved outcomes with an effect on both postoperative pain and blood loss. These surgeries have no effect on cognitive response and are appropriate for postoperative PCA.

VII. **Complications of neuroanesthesia pain management**
   A. **Mental status changes.** Serial neurologic checks are often an essential part of the postoperative course. If pain treatment interferes with this assessment, the overall benefit of the pain treatment may be lost. Establishing a team approach with the

surgical team and the nursing team to balance the risks and benefits of pain therapies is crucial.

B. Elevation of arterial carbon dioxide (CO_2). The importance of ICP varies in the neurosurgical population. In patients in whom this is an important factor, it is crucial to have some method of monitoring postsurgical CO_2. Despite the benefits of improved hemodynamics in ensuring the stability of the patient with elevated ICP, the risk of excessive sedation and hypercarbis could be a possible problem, and the patient must be watched closely. Arterial CO_2 and pH are ways to monitor for a possible problem and may be early indicators of impending problems.

C. Reduction of arterial O_2. Hypoxemia may create multiple problems in the patient with neuronal tissue trauma. Anaerobic metabolism occurs when neurons do not have enough oxygen substrate, which can result in a reduction of adenosine triphosphate and subsequent cell death. The use of supplemental oxygen and oxygen saturation as well as serial arterial blood gas monitoring is essential in patients receiving systemic opioids.

D. Hypotension. In the patient with possible spinal cord trauma, the use of regional anesthesia can be helpful in controlling the stress response and subsequent systemic changes. The resultant decrease in mean arterial pressure can decrease perfusion to the neurologic tissue and create ischemia. Careful attention to blood pressure is crucial when using local anesthetics postoperatively.

E. Cerebrospinal fluid leak. The possibility of subarachnoid puncture when placing an epidural catheter must be weighed against the benefit of the catheter. The risks of brain herniation must also be discussed with the surgeon if there is any intracranial disease process.

F. Nerve injury. When using regional techniques in those with coexisting neurologic disease, a risk of nerve injury exists if the patient has abnormal nociception in the area of the proposed procedure. This risk also exists for the patient under general anesthesia or heavy sedation who may be unable to respond to inadvertent intraneural injection.

G. Infection

  1. In the sedated patient, aspiration precautions should be ordered. This should be accompanied by frequent neurologic checks. If aspiration is a risk, sedating medications should be used with caution.

  2. Regional anesthesia should be avoided in the patient with local infection at the site of the proposed regional procedure or in the patient with untreated or uncontrolled systemic infection.

  3. The site of indwelling regional catheters should be checked regularly for infection. If the catheter is tunneled through a gel coat catheter, the risk of infection is more likely to be skin related.

VIII. **Anesthesia methods for neuroaxial pain procedures.** A social emphasis on the importance of treating patients with chronic pain has led to the increase in the number of practitioners performing procedures requiring anesthesia. Neurosurgeons, anesthesiologists, physiatrists, orthopedic surgeons, and neurologists now perform these procedures. Regardless of the practitioner involved, the anesthetic issues are important to achieve a stable course.

A. **Spinal cord stimulation.** This procedure is most commonly performed for pain involving the extremities. Recent expansion of indications includes pelvic pain, occipital neuralgia, angina, and pancreatitis. The procedure is often separated into stages.

1. **The percutaneous trial.** In either the operating room or radiology suite, a temporary stimulation system may be placed under the guidance of a fluoroscope. Anesthesia is difficult because many of these patients have taken oral opioids for long periods and are tolerant to this class of drugs. These patients may require sedation to place the lead in either the lumbar or cervical region but should remain alert and responsive to avoid nerve root injury. The patients also need to be cognitively functional for the computer screening, which involves connecting the epidural lead to the handheld computer and electrically stimulating the nerve tissue to obtain a paresthesia. This requirement for varying levels of sedation makes propofol and remifentanil attractive choices in this group of patients. Regional anesthesia should be avoided. In patients who are stoic, the procedure may be performed under local anesthesia; however, the patient selection for this technique should be very stringent.

2. **The surgical lead.** A surgical lead must be placed in some patients with more anatomically difficult spines or in whom a percutaneous lead has failed. This procedure usually requires a wake-up period so the patient can discuss the perception of stimulation. This may lead to a more difficult task because the procedure itself requires a hemilaminectomy. Some surgeons request a general anesthetic with evoked potential testing for this procedure. NSAIDs should be avoided in this population because of the increased risk of bleeding.

3. **The permanent lead.** In most cases, the permanent implant involves the placement of both the lead and generator. The permanent implant requires the use of a complex anesthetic because the patient needs to be conversing during the lead placement and more sedated for tunneling

and pocket placement. In some cases, the lead placed for the trial procedure is used as a permanent lead. If that is the case, the patient is brought back to the operating room 1 to 4 weeks later for the connection to a permanent generator. This procedure is most often performed under monitored anesthesia care or general anesthesia. This stage requires no period of discussion. Thus, the anesthetic is much less complex. In either method, the placement of the generator pocket determines the patient's positioning. If the generator is placed in a different body area, repositioning and draping may be required, affecting the anesthetic level required.

4. **Intrathecal and epidural drug infusion systems.** The use of neuroaxial infusions to treat pain that is unresponsive to oral or transdermal medications is becoming more common. Catheters may be tunneled and connected to an external infusion source or may be connected to an implantable system that is placed in the subcutaneous tissue.

    a. **Totally implantable infusion systems.** Placing an intrathecal or epidural pump in the subcutaneous tissue involves two steps. First, a catheter must be placed in the epidural or intrathecal space. Once this has been successfully completed, the catheter can be connected to an infusion source. Anesthesia for these procedures might consist of sedation with local infiltration, subarachnoid or epidural block at the time of catheter placement, or general anesthesia. Each method has its risks and benefits. With general anesthesia, the patient is less likely to move, and the risk of nerve injury may be diminished. In the nonresponsive patient, the risk of nerve injury may be increased, however, if the patient cannot respond to development of parasthesia. The spinal or epidural technique avoids the general anesthetic, which may be advantageous for someone at high risk for pulmonary or cardiac complications. Use of sedation with local anesthetic infiltration reduces the risk of undiagnosed nerve injury at the time of catheter insertion. In some patients, the stimulation involved in the tunneling and pocketing component of the procedure might not be successfully blunted with sedation and local infiltration alone, and a conversion to general anesthesia might be required during the course of the procedure.

    b. **Externalized infusion systems.** In patients in whom the need for infusion is short

term or in those with a life expectancy of
<3 months, an externalized system is often
selected. The need for general anesthesia in
this population is rare because of the lack
of pocket creation. Although this procedure
could be completed under neuroaxial blockade or general anesthesia, the more common
scenario is to use monitored anesthesia care
with local infiltration.

B. Radiofrequency nerve ablation. The cost-
effectiveness of radiofrequency ablation has led to
a vast increase in the number of procedures performed annually in the United States and Europe.
Pulsed radiofrequency ablation is a new technique
that has shown promise in treating peripheral nerve
processes without larger procedures. This technique
is also being utilized more commonly in ablating the
sympathetic nervous system and selected peripheral
nerves. The anesthetic in these cases is inherently
difficult. The patient must be sufficiently sedated to
permit the placement of a large radiofrequency cannula and then allowed to awaken rapidly to be able
to answer important stimulation questions involving
sensory, motor, and nociceptive input. The risks of
nerve injury greatly increase in the patient who is
not able to fully discern the computer stimulation
pattern. Because of these issues, the infusion or injection of fast-acting and rapidly- waning drugs is
often utilized. Options include propofol, midazolam,
fentanyl, or local anesthetic as a sole agent.

C. Spinal endoscopy. In 1997, the United States Food
and Drug Administration (FDA) approved the use
of spinal endoscopy. In this method, the physician
uses a fiberoptic scope to visualize and treat disease processes of the spine by an epidural route.
This procedure is stimulating and requires sedation
to be tolerated in most cases. The use of general
anesthesia should be avoided because of the risks of
nerve damage in the patient who is unable to report
paresthesia.

D. Minimally invasive disc procedures. The use
of new percutaneous techniques to treat contained
disc herniations and leaks of the annulus are valuable options in patients who would like to avoid
more invasive techniques such as fusion or artificial
disc replacement. In these cases, there is a need to
converse with the patient at all times. Anesthesia
should be with local anesthesia with or without mild
sedation.

IX. Summary
The neurosurgical patient is a tremendous challenge
to the team providing pain relief. The balance of controlling pain and maintaining safety for the patient in
the postoperative period is a difficult task. It is critical that the anesthesiologist, surgeon, and nursing staff

work together to obtain a good result. As new drugs and techniques become available, it will be important to update our knowledge of the best methods to perform this complex task.

SUGGESTED READINGS

Beilin B, Shavit Y, Trabekin E, et al. The effects of postoperative pain management on immune response to surgery. *Anesth Analg* 2003;97(3):822–827.

Bellieni CV, Burroni A, Perrone S, et al. Intracranial pressure during procedural pain. *Biol Neonat* 2003;84:202–205.

Bruder N, Ravussin P. Cerebral and systemic haemodynamic changes during neurosurgical recovery. *Ann Fr Anesth Reanim* 2004;23: 410–416.

Dunbar PJ, Visco E, Lam AM. Craniotomy procedures are associated with less analgesic requirements than other surgical procedures. *Anesth Analg* 1999;88:335–340.

Kehlet H, Cousins M, Bridenbaugh P. Modification of responses to surgery by neutral blockade. In: Cousins M, Bridenbaugh P, eds. *Neural Blockade in Clinical Anesthesia and Management of Pain*, 5th ed. New York, NY: Lippincott Williams & Wilkins, 1998:129–165.

Leith B. Pharmacological management of pain after intracranial surgery. *J Neurosci Nurs* 1998;30:220–224.

Swenson JD, Davis JJ, Johnson KB. Postoperative care of the chronic opioid-consuming patient. *Anesthesiol Clin North America* 2005;23:37–48.

Verchere E, Grenier B. Pain and postoperative analgesia after craniotomy. *Ann Fr Anesth Reanim* 2004;23:417–421.

Viviand X, Garnier F. Opioid anesthetics (sufentanil and remifentanil) in neuro-anaesthesia. *Ann Fr Anesth Reanim* 2004;23: 383–388.

Yoshimoto H, Nagashima K, Sato S, et al. A prospective evaluation of anesthesia for posterior lumbar spine fusion: the effectiveness of preoperative epidural anesthesia with morphine. *Spine* 2005;30:863–869.

Anesthetic Management

Anesthetic Management of Head Trauma

Takefumi Sakabe and Audrée A. Bendo

Head trauma or traumatic brain injury (TBI) is one of the most serious, life-threatening conditions in trauma victims. Prompt and appropriate therapy is necessary to obtain a favorable outcome. Anesthesiologists manage these patients throughout their perioperative course, taking them from the emergency room to the neuroradiology suite, the operating room, and the neurointensive care unit.

The perioperative management of patients with head injuries focuses aggressively on the stabilization of the patient and the avoidance of the systemic and intracranial insults that cause secondary neuronal injury. These secondary insults, while potentially preventable and treatable, can complicate the course of patients with head injuries and adversely affect outcome.

I. **Head injury practice guidelines.** Evidence-based guidelines for the management of severe TBI were published in 2000 after an extensive review of the literature. Three standards on the basis of Class I evidence and several guidelines on the basis of Class II evidence were recommended. In March 2006, the Brain Trauma Foundation and the Congress of Neurological Surgeons published new guidelines. This review presents literature-based recommendations for the surgical management of TBI.

II. **Classification of head injury.** Head injury is classified into primary injury and secondary injury. This classification is useful when considering therapeutic strategies.

   A. **Primary injury** is the damage produced by a direct mechanical impact and the acceleration–deceleration stress onto the skull and brain tissue, resulting in skull fractures (cranial vault, skull base) and intracranial lesions. The intracranial lesions are further classified into two types: diffuse injury and focal injury.

   1. **Diffuse brain injury** includes two categories.
      a. **Brain concussion** is loss of consciousness lasting <6 hours.
      b. **Diffuse axonal injury** is traumatic coma lasting >6 hours.

   2. **Focal brain injury** includes the following types:
      a. **Brain contusion** is usually located either below or opposite the region of impact.
      b. **Epidural hematoma** is often caused by skull fracture and laceration of the middle meningeal artery.

       c. **Subdural hematoma** is usually caused by the tearing of the bridging veins between the cerebral cortex and draining sinuses. Acute subdural hematoma is often associated with high mortality.

       d. **Intracerebral hematoma** is usually located in the frontal and temporal lobes and visualized as a hyperdense mass on a computed tomographic (CT) scan. **Brain tissue destroyed by the primary impact will not be saved. Therefore, functional outcome is improved by prompt surgical intervention and medical therapy.**

   3. Indications for surgery. Presently, no definitive therapeutic measure exists to treat diffuse axonal injury. Most open and depressed skull fractures and compound skull fractures with dural laceration require early surgical repair. Uncomplicated basal fractures usually do not require operation. The presence of compression of the basal cisterns from a brain contusion indicates operative intervention because of the risk of herniation (usually of the temporal lobe). **Intracranial hematoma is the most common sequela of head trauma requiring surgical treatment.**

B. Secondary injuries develop within minutes, hours, or days of the initial injury and cause further damage to nervous tissue. The common denominators of secondary injury are cerebral hypoxia and ischemia. Secondary injuries are caused by the following disorders:

   1. Respiratory dysfunction (hypoxemia, hypercapnia).

   2. Cardiovascular instability (hypotension, low cardiac output).

   3. Elevation of intracranial pressure (ICP).

   4. Biochemical derangements.

III. Pathophysiology of head trauma. Comprehensive management requires an understanding of the pathophysiologic responses to TBI.

A. Systemic effects of head trauma

   1. Cardiovascular responses to head trauma are commonly observed in the early stage. They include hypertension, tachycardia, and increased cardiac output. Patients with severe head injuries and those suffering from multiple systemic injuries with substantial blood loss, however, may develop hypotension and a decrease in cardiac output. Systemic hypotension (systolic blood pressure of <90 mm Hg) at the time of admission to the hospital is associated with significantly increased morbidity and mortality.

2. **Respiratory responses** to head trauma include apnea and abnormal respiratory patterns. Respiratory insufficiency and spontaneous hyperventilation often occur. Patients may also suffer from aspiration of vomitus and central neurogenic pulmonary edema.
3. **Temperature regulation** may be disturbed, and hyperthermia, if it occurs, can provoke further brain damage.

B. **Changes in cerebral circulation and metabolism.** In **focal brain injury**, cerebral blood flow (CBF) and cerebral metabolic rate for oxygen consumption ($CMRo_2$) decrease in the core area of injury and in the penumbra, an area of hypoperfused tissue that surrounds the damaged tissue. When ICP increases, diffuse and more marked hypoperfusion and hypometabolism ensue.

In **diffuse brain injury**, hyperemia may occur. In most cases, however, CBF decreases within a few hours of head trauma. The combination of hypotension and impaired autoregulation exacerbates cerebral ischemia. The chemical-metabolic regulation of CBF may also be impaired. The combination of these pathophysiologic responses to head injury creates a complicated management scenario.

C. **Acute brain swelling and cerebral edema**
1. **Acute brain swelling** is provoked by a decrease in vasomotor tone and a marked increase in the volume of the cerebral vascular bed. In this situation, increases in blood pressure can easily lead to further brain swelling and an increase in ICP.
2. **Cerebral edema** following head trauma is often a mixture of vasogenic and cytotoxic types caused by blood-brain barrier disruption and ischemia, respectively.

Following head trauma, both acute brain swelling and edema ensue concurrently. When these pathologic conditions occur in association with an intracranial hematoma, the resultant intracranial hypertension causes a further reduction in CBF with cerebral ischemia. Eventually, intracranial hypertension, if untreated, leads to herniation of the brain stem through the foramen magnum.

D. **Excitotoxicity.** Head trauma causes excessive release of glutamate from neurons and glia, increasing the concentration of glutamate in the cerebrospinal fluid (CSF). The biochemical changes associated with the excessive release of glutamate and the activation of glutamate receptors are closely related to an increase in intracellular calcium ion, which triggers a number of events that lead to the damage. These include an activation of phospholipase, protein kinase, proteases, nitric oxide synthase, and

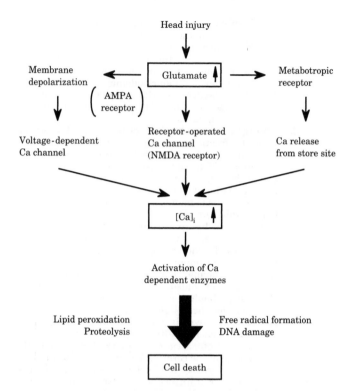

Figure 6-1. Excitotoxicity in head injury. AMPA, alpha-amino-3-hydroxy-5-methyl-4-isoxazoleproprionate; NMDA, N-methyl-D-aspartate; [Ca]ᵢ, intracellular Ca.

other enzymes. Activation of these enzymes also produces lipid peroxidation, proteolysis, free radical formation, deoxyribonucleic acid (DNA) damage, and finally, neuronal death (Figure 6-1).

E. **Inflammatory cytokines and mediators.** The cytokines are major mediators in the initiation of inflammatory and metabolic responses to injury. Cytokines increase in response to cerebral ischemia. Interleukin-6 (IL-6) and tumor necrosis factor alpha are known to be released after TBI. Patients who have Glasgow Coma Scale (GCS) scores of <8 show a higher and more sustained elevation of IL-6. The cytokines released after TBI stimulate the production of free radicals and arachidonic acids and upregulate the activity of the adhesion molecules, which produce disturbances in the microcirculation. All of these changes contribute to secondary brain injury.

IV. Emergency management
  A. Initial assessment of the patient's condition
   1. Neurologic assessment. There is usually little time initially to evaluate the patient's neurologic condition thoroughly. However, a quick neurologic assessment can be performed while stabilizing the patient to achieve adequate ventilation (oxygenation and carbon dioxide [CO_2] elimination) and hemodynamic stability.
      a. GCS (Table 6-1) is a simple and universally accepted method for assessing consciousness and neurologic status in patients with head injuries. The GCS has low interobserver variability and is a good predictor of outcome.
         (1) GCS score of <8 characterizes severe head injury.
         (2) GCS score of 9 to 12 represents moderate injury.
         (3) GCS score of 13 to 15 represents mild injury.
      b. Pupillary responses (size, light reflex) and symmetry of motor function in the extremities should be quickly assessed.
   2. Assessment of injuries to other organs. Trauma patients often suffer from injuries to multiple organ systems. Particular attention should be paid to determine whether there is evidence of intrathoracic or intraperitoneal (intrapelvic) hemorrhage. If bleeding is suspected, the thorax or abdomen should be explored without delay.
  Treatment of hemorrhagic shock takes precedence over neurosurgical procedures. The patient's hemoglobin must be measured immediately, and blood and fresh-frozen plasma should be set up and made available for infusion.
  B. Establishment of airway and ventilation
   1. Tracheal intubation. The first step in emergency therapy is to secure an open airway and ensure adequate ventilation. Because all trauma patients are considered to have a "full stomach" and frequently (approximately 10%) have an associated cervical spine injury as well, cricoid pressure and in-line stabilization of the cervical spine are used during laryngoscopy and intubation.
  If facial fractures and soft tissue edema prevent direct visualization of the larynx, either fiberoptic intubation or intubation with an illuminated stylet may be attempted. In the presence of either severe facial injuries or laryngeal trauma a cricothyrotomy may be required. Nasal intubations are avoided in the presence of a suspected basal skull fracture, severe facial fractures, and bleeding diathesis.

Table 6-1.　Glasgow Coma Scale

Adult Scale		Pediatric Scale		
Parameter	Score	Parameter	Score	
Eye opening		Eye opening		
Spontaneously	4	Spontaneously	4	
To speech	3	To speech	3	
To pain	2	To pain	2	
None	1	None	1	
Best verbal response		Best verbal response[a]		
Oriented	5	Oriented to place	5	>5 y
Confused	4	Words	4	>12 mo
Inappropriate	3	Vocal sounds	3	>6 mo
Incomprehensible	2	Cries	2	<6 mo
None	1	None	1	
Best motor response		Best motor response in upper limbs[a]		
Obeys commands	6	Obeys commands	6	>2 y
Localizes to pain	5	Localizes to pain	5	6 mo–2 y
Withdraws from pain	4	Normal flexion to pain	4	>6 mo
Flexes to pain	3	Spastic flexion to pain	3	<6 mo
Extends to pain	2	Extension to pain	2	
None	1	None	1	

[a]Score highest appropriate for age.

Nasal intubation also adds risk to patients who have basilar skull fractures because of the introduction of contaminated material into the brain. Basilar skull fractures are strongly suspected when hemorrhage of the tympanic cavity, otorrhea, petechiae on the mastoid process (Battle's sign), and petechiae around the eyes (panda sign) are observed.

2. **Drugs to facilitate laryngoscopy and intubation** (see **V.B.1.a.**)

3. **Mechanical ventilation.** As soon as the trachea has been intubated, a nondepolarizing muscle relaxant is administered and mechanical ventilation to a partial arterial pressure of carbon dioxide ($Paco_2$) of approximately 35 mm Hg is instituted. Aggressive hyperventilation ($Paco_2$ of <30 mm Hg) should be avoided unless transtentorial herniation is suspected. Hypoxemia, if present, should be corrected immediately. Hyperoxia may be recommended. If massive aspiration is suspected, bronchial suctioning using a fiberscope is advisable before transferring the patient to either the neuroradiology suite or the operating room.

C. **Cardiovascular stabilization.** Systemic hypotension is one of the major contributors to poor outcome after head trauma. When necessary, fluid resuscitation is initiated immediately and inotropic and vasopressor drugs are administered as required to stabilize the blood pressure.

1. **Fluid resuscitation.** Hypovolemia is often masked by a relatively stable blood pressure secondary to either sympathetic hyperactivity or the reflex response to increased ICP. Therefore, fluid resuscitation should be guided not only by blood pressure but also by urinary output and central venous pressure (CVP).

a. **Crystalloid and colloid solutions.** Isotonic and hypertonic crystalloid solutions and colloid solutions may be given to maintain adequate intravascular volume.

(1) **Lactated Ringer's solution** is slightly hypotonic relative to plasma, which precludes the use of a substantial amount. If administered, serum osmolarity should be measured periodically. When large-volume resuscitation with crystalloid is required, an isotonic crystalloid, such as normal saline, is preferable.

(2) **Hypertonic saline** (3%, 7.5%) can be beneficial in small amounts after TBI. Large volumes may produce a lethal increase in serum sodium concentration.

(3) **Hydroxyethyl starch** (HES) and human plasma products can be administered to maintain intravascular volume for longer periods. No more than 1.5 L of HES should be administered in conjunction with careful monitoring of blood coagulation. The incidence of coagulopathy in patients with head injuries is approximately 20%, and HES in large amounts is known to interfere with blood coagulation. The reported incidence of coagulopathy is less with pentastarch.

b. **Blood and blood products.** Patients who have a low hematocrit may require a transfusion to optimize oxygen delivery; the hematocrit ideally is maintained above 30%. Children require special attention because they can easily become hypovolemic by losing large volumes of blood into an intracranial or subgaleal hematoma or through a scalp laceration, even without blood loss in other organ systems.

c. **Adverse effect of glucose-containing solutions.** Glucose-containing solutions are avoided because hyperglycemia is associated with worsened neurologic outcomes. Glucose should be used only to treat hypoglycemia. The plasma level of 80 to 150 mg/dL is desirable; values above 200 mg/dL should be avoided and treated with insulin.

2. **Inotropics and vasopressors.** If the blood pressure and cardiac output cannot be restored through fluid resuscitation, the administration of intravenous inotropic and vasopressor drugs may be necessary. An infusion of either phenylephrine or dopamine is recommended to maintain cerebral perfusion pressure (CPP), the difference between the mean arterial pressure (MAP) and the ICP, above 60 mm Hg.

D. **Management of elevated ICP.** The reduction of elevated ICP and the maintenance of blood pressure are crucial in the management of intracranial hypertension because CPP is directly related to both MAP and ICP.

1. **Hyperventilation.** When evidence of transtentorial herniation in patients with severe head injuries exists, hyperventilation to a Pa_{CO_2} of 30 mm Hg should be instituted because hyperventilation can rapidly and effectively reduce ICP. Hyperventilation was previously thought to be more effective in children than in adults because of the idea that pediatric patients, unlike adults, responded to TBI with acute brain swelling from hyperemia. The accumulation of

recent data has revealed, however, that hyperemia may not occur as commonly in severe pediatric TBI. The initial response of both adult and pediatric patients to TBI is more often hypoperfusion. Aggressive hyperventilation to a $Paco_2$ of <30 mm Hg can therefore aggravate ischemia through excessive vasoconstriction. To avoid this risk, other measures, including diuretic therapy, barbiturate therapy, and CSF drainage, should be instituted. The $Paco_2$ is allowed to return toward normal as soon as possible.

2. **Diuretic therapy.** Mannitol, 1 g/kg intravenously (i.v.) infused over 10 minutes, is administered to patients in whom transtentorial herniation is suspected. In less acute cases, an infusion of 0.25 to 1 g/kg may be administered over 10 to 20 minutes and repeated every 3 to 6 hours. The serum osmolarity is monitored frequently and should not exceed 320 mOsm/L.

3. **Posture.** A head-up tilt of 10° to 30° facilitates cerebral venous and CSF drainage and lowers ICP. This ICP-reducing effect is negated when systemic blood pressure decreases.

4. **Corticosteroids.** Corticosteroids were previously thought to be of value in reducing brain edema and hence ICP in patients with head trauma. However, recent reports have demonstrated worsened outcomes with the use of corticosteroids. Steroids also increase blood glucose levels, which can adversely affect the injured brain. Corticosteroids, therefore, have no place in the treatment of head injury despite their proven efficacy in spinal cord injury.

5. **Barbiturates.** Barbiturates are known to exert cerebral protective and ICP-lowering effects. High-dose barbiturate therapy may be considered in patients with severe head injuries whose intracranial hypertension is refractory to maximal medical and surgical ICP-lowering therapy. When considering the institution of high-dose barbiturate therapy, hemodynamic stabilization of the patient is a prerequisite. The prophylactic use of barbiturate coma is not indicated.

V. **Anesthetic management**
   A. **Anesthesia.** The major goals of anesthetic management are to (a) optimize cerebral perfusion and oxygenation, (b) avoid secondary damage, and (c) provide adequate surgical conditions for the neurosurgeons. General anesthesia is recommended to facilitate control of respiratory and circulatory function.
      1. **Induction of anesthesia.** Most patients who have severe head injury have already had an endotracheal tube inserted either during triage in the emergency department or for their CT

100 II. Anesthetic Management

examination. The patient who comes to the operating room without endotracheal intubation is treated with immediate oxygenation and securing of the airway. Anesthesiologists must be aware that these patients often have a full stomach, decreased intravascular volume, and a potential cervical spine injury.

Direct arterial pressure monitoring by an indwelling arterial catheter inserted before the induction of anesthesia is recommended. Either the radial artery or the dorsalis pedis artery may be cannulated, depending on other sites of injury.

Several induction techniques are recommended. The patient's presentation and hemodynamic stability determine the choice.

a. **Rapid sequence induction** may be desirable in hemodynamically stable patients, although this procedure can produce an elevation in blood pressure and ICP. During administration of 100% oxygen, an induction dose of thiopental, 3 to 4 mg/kg, or propofol, 1 to 2 mg/kg, and succinylcholine, 1.5 mg/kg, is administered and the trachea is intubated. Etomidate, 0.2 to 0.3 mg/kg, may be administered in patients in whom the circulatory status is concerning. In hemodynamically unstable patients, the dose of induction drugs is substantially decreased or even omitted. However, cardiovascular depression is always a concern, especially in hypovolemic patients.

Succinylcholine has been shown to increase ICP. The prior administration of small doses of a nondepolarizing muscle relaxant may prevent this increase but not predictably. Succinylcholine remains a good choice, however, to facilitate rapid laryngoscopy and to secure the airway. Rocuronium, 0.6 to 1 mg/kg, is an excellent alternative because of its rapid onset of action and lack of effect on intracranial dynamics.

b. **Intravenous induction.** When the patient is stable and does not have a full stomach, anesthesia can be induced by titrating the dose of either thiopental or propofol to minimize circulatory instability. An intubating dose of a nondepolarizing muscle relaxant is given with or without priming to facilitate intubation within a short period of time. For example, rocuronium, 0.6 to 1 mg/kg, allows satisfactory intubating conditions within 60 to 90 seconds. Fentanyl, 1 to 4 mcg/kg i.v., is administered to blunt the hemodynamic response to laryngoscopy and intubation. Lidocaine, 1.5 mg/kg i.v., given 90 seconds before laryngoscopy, can help prevent the increase in ICP.

A large-bore oral gastric tube is inserted after intubation, and gastric contents are initially aspirated and then passively drained during the operation. Nasal gastric tubes are avoided because of the potential presence of a basilar skull fracture.

2. **Maintenance of anesthesia.** The ideal drug for maintenance of anesthesia should reduce ICP, maintain adequate oxygen supply to the brain tissue, and protect the brain against ischemic-metabolic insult. No gold-standard anesthetic drug fulfills these requirements for head injury. The selection of anesthetic drugs is based on a consideration of the intracranial pathology as well as systemic conditions such as cardiopulmonary disturbances and the presence of multisystem trauma.

   a. **Anesthetics**
      (1) **Intravenous anesthetics**
         (a) **Barbiturates.** Thiopental and pentobarbital decrease CBF, cerebral blood volume (CBV), and ICP. The reduction in ICP with these drugs is related to the reduction in CBF and CBV coupled with metabolic depression. These drugs will also have these effects in patients who have impaired CO_2 response.

         Thiopental and pentobarbital have been shown in animal models to protect against focal brain ischemia. In head injury, ischemia is a common sequela. Although barbiturates might be effective in head injury, no prospective, randomized clinical trial has demonstrated that they definitely improve outcome after TBI. In addition, barbiturates can be detrimental in patients with head injuries because of their cardiovascular-depressant effect. Also, when barbiturates are administered for prolonged periods, their duration of action is increased.

         (b) **Etomidate.** As with barbiturates, etomidate reduces CBF, CMR_{O_2}, and ICP. Systemic hypotension occurs less frequently than with barbiturates. Prolonged use of etomidate may suppress the adrenocortical response to stress.

(c) **Propofol.** The cerebral hemodynamic and metabolic effects of propofol are similar to those of barbiturates. Propofol might be useful in patients who have intracranial pathology if hypotension is avoided. Because the context-sensitive half-life is short, emergence from anesthesia is rapid, even after prolonged administration. This may offer an advantage over other intravenous anesthetics in providing the opportunity for early postoperative neurologic evaluation. Because of propofol's potent circulatory depressant effect, however, meticulous care should be exercised to maintain adequate CPP, including the correction of hypovolemia prior to administering propofol. Recent studies have shown a reduction in jugular bulb oxygen saturation during propofol anesthesia. Propofol can also reduce CBF more than $CMRO_2$, producing ischemia under certain conditions. Therefore, care should be taken when hyperventilating patients during propofol anesthesia.

(d) **Benzodiazepines.** Diazepam and midazolam may be useful either for sedating patients or inducting anesthesia because these drugs have minimal hemodynamic effects and are less likely to impair cerebral circulation. Diazepam, 0.1 to 0.2 mg/kg, may be administered for inducting anesthesia and repeated, if necessary, up to a total dose of 0.3 to 0.6 mg/kg. Midazolam, 0.2 mg/kg, can be used for induction and repeated as necessary.

(e) **Narcotics.** In clinical doses, narcotics produce a minimal to moderate decrease in CBF and $CMRO_2$. When ventilation is adequately maintained, narcotics probably have minimal effects on ICP. Despite its small ICP-elevating effect, fentanyl provides satisfactory analgesia and permits the use of lower concentrations of inhalational anesthetics. Some reports have shown that sufentanil increases ICP in patients with severe head injuries. This could result from the autoregulatory response (i.e., cerebral vasodilatation) to the sudden decrease in systemic blood pressure. When these drugs are used, measures to maintain systemic blood pressure need to be implemented.

(2) Inhalational anesthetics

    (a) Isoflurane. A potent metabolic depressant, isoflurane has less effect on CBF and ICP than halothane has. Because isoflurane depresses cerebral metabolism, it may have a cerebral protective effect when the ischemic insult is not severe. Data favor the use of isoflurane over either halothane or enflurane. Isoflurane in concentrations of >1 minimum alveolar concentration should be avoided, however, because it can cause substantial increases in ICP.

    (b) Sevoflurane. In the rabbit cryogenic brain-injury model, the elevation of ICP occurring in association with an elevation in blood pressure was higher in the animals anesthetized with sevoflurane than with halothane. Clinical studies have demonstrated, however, that sevoflurane's effect on cerebral hemodynamics is either similar to or milder than that of isoflurane. The disadvantage of sevoflurane is that its biodegraded metabolite may be toxic in high concentrations. There is no evidence of an adverse effect at clinically used concentrations, however, unless sevoflurane is administered in a low-flow circuit for prolonged periods. Rapid emergence from anesthesia with sevoflurane may be an advantage because it facilitates early postoperative neurologic evaluation.

    (c) Desflurane. Desflurane at high concentrations appears to increase ICP.

(d) **Nitrous oxide (N_2O).** N_2O dilates cerebral vessels, thereby increasing ICP. Patients who have intracranial hypertension or a decrease in intracranial compliance should, therefore, not receive this drug. N_2O should also be avoided in the presence of pneumocephalus or pneumothorax because it diffuses into an airspace more rapidly than the nitrogen diffuses out, thereby increasing the volume within the airspace.

(3) **Local anesthetic.** The infiltration of either lidocaine 1% or bupivacaine 0.25%, with or without epinephrine, in the skin around the scalp incision and the insertion sites for the pin head holder is helpful in preventing systemic and intracranial hypertension in response to these stimuli and avoiding the unnecessary use of deep anesthesia.

(4) **Muscle relaxants.** Adequate muscle relaxation facilitates appropriate mechanical ventilation and reduces ICP. Coughing and straining are avoided because both can produce cerebral venous engorgement.

(a) **Vecuronium** appears to have minimal or no effect on ICP, blood pressure, or heart rate and would be effective in patients with head injuries. This drug is given as an initial dose of 0.08 to 0.1 mg/kg followed by infusion at a rate of 1 to 1.7 mcg/kg/minute.

(b) **Pancuronium** does not produce an increase in ICP but can cause hypertension and tachycardia because of its vagolytic effect, thereby increasing the patient's risk.

(c) **Atracurium** has no effect on ICP. Because of its rapid onset and short duration of action, a bolus dose of 0.5 to 0.6 mg/kg followed by a continuous infusion at a rate of 4 to 10 mcg/kg/minute is administered with monitoring of neuromuscular blockade.

(d) **Rocuronium** is useful for intubation because of its rapid onset of action and lack of effect on intracranial dynamics. For maintenance, drugs with longer durations of action are recommended.

3. **Intraoperative respiratory and circulatory management**
   a. **Mechanical ventilation.** Mechanical ventilation is adjusted to maintain a $Paco_2$ of around 35 mm Hg. The fraction of inspired oxygen (Fio_2) is adjusted to maintain a Pao_2 of >100 mm Hg.

   Patients, especially those who have pulmonary contusion, aspiration, or central neurogenic pulmonary edema, may require positive end-expiratory pressure (PEEP) to maintain adequate oxygenation. Excessive PEEP should be avoided, however, because the elevation in intrathoracic pressure can compromise cerebral venous drainage and increase ICP.

   b. **Circulatory management.** CPP should be maintained between 60 and 110 mm Hg. The transducer for direct monitoring of arterial blood pressure is zeroed at the level of mastoids to reflect the cerebral circulation.

   When hypotension persists despite adequate oxygenation, ventilation, and fluid replacement, careful elevation of the blood pressure with a continuous infusion of an inotrope or vasopressor may be necessary. Phenylephrine, 0.1 to 0.5 mcg/kg/minute, and dopamine, 1 to 10 mcg/kg/minute, are appropriate drugs in this setting. A bolus dose of vasopressor must be used cautiously because abrupt increases in blood pressure can elevate ICP to dangerous levels, especially in patients who have disordered autoregulation.

   Hypertension is treated cautiously because the elevation in blood pressure may reflect compensatory hyperactivity of the sympathetic nervous system in response to elevated ICP and compression of the brain stem (Cushing's reflex). Adequate oxygenation, ventilation, volume replacement, and analgesia should be first assessed and corrected. When necessary, an antihypertensive drug, such as either labetalol or esmolol, which has minimal cerebral vasodilating effects, should be administered. When treating hypertension, maintenance of CPP is a major concern.

4. **Intraoperative management of elevated ICP**
   a. **Patient's posture.** A slight head-up tilt of 10° to 30° is desirable. CPP might not be improved, however, if systemic blood pressure decreases substantially. When the surgeon requests either rotation or flexion of the head and the neck, the anesthesiologist must ensure the adequacy of venous return.

   b. **Ventilation.** The Pa_{CO_2} is maintained at around 35 mm Hg. Hyperventilation is best avoided unless monitoring ensures adequate brain oxygenation.
   c. **Circulation.** Both hypotension (systolic blood pressure of <90 mm Hg) and hypertension (systolic blood pressure of >160 mm Hg) should be corrected when indicated.
   d. **Diuretics**
       (1) **Mannitol** decreases cerebral volume and reduces ICP.
       (2) **Furosemide** may be coadministered in severe cases as well as in the patient who has compromised cardiac function and the potential for heart failure. Furosemide, 0.1 to 0.2 mg/kg, is given 15 minutes before mannitol administration. When furosemide and mannitol are administered, careful monitoring of intravascular volume either by CVP or pulmonary artery pressure is necessary.

       Ventilation, oxygenation, depth of anesthesia, and last dose of diuretics should be assessed in the patient if protrusion of the brain is observed after craniotomy. If all are adequate, additional thiopental (or pentobarbital) may be indicated. More vigorous hyperventilation is also an option with careful monitoring of brain oxygenation. If these measures fail, decompressive craniectomy maybe necessary.
   e. **CSF drainage.** If an intraventricular catheter is in place, CSF drainage is an effective and reliable technique for reducing ICP.

B. Monitoring
   1. **Standard monitoring** includes heart rate and rhythm (electrocardiogram), noninvasive and direct arterial blood pressure measurement, pulse oximetry, end-tidal CO_2, body temperature, urinary output, CVP, and neuromuscular blockade. Arterial blood gases, hematocrit, electrolytes, glucose, and serum osmolarity should be measured periodically.
   2. **Monitoring for air embolism.** Detection of venous air embolism by Doppler ultrasound should be considered for surgical procedures in which veins in the operative site are above the level of the heart.
   3. **Brain monitoring** as with an electroencephalogram, evoked potentials, jugular venous bulb oxygen saturation (Sj_{O_2}), flow velocity measured by transcranial Doppler (TCD), brain tissue P_{O_2} (btP_{O_2}), and ICP may be used.

a. **Sjo$_2$.** The Sjo$_2$ provides continuous information about the balance between global cerebral oxygen supply and demand. An Sjo$_2$ of <50% for >15 minutes is a poor prognostic sign and is often associated with a poor neurologic outcome. The decrease in Sjo$_2$ could be caused by excessive hyperventilation, decreased CPP, cerebral vasospasm, or a combination. The major causes of a decrease in Sjo$_2$ and their treatment are listed in Table 6-2.

b. **Flow velocity** of basal cerebral arteries as measured by the TCD technique is helpful in assessing the cerebral circulatory state at the bedside. However, it does not provide an absolute value for the CBF. High-normal values may indicate hyperemia or vasospasm. The TCD waveform can differentiate between these two conditions. A disadvantage of this monitor is that the application of the Doppler probe is not always possible during the surgical procedure.

c. **Near-infrared spectroscopy,** currently available in clinical practice, provides relative information about changes of oxy- and deoxyhemoglobin and the cytochrome oxidase redox status in the brain tissue of interest in a noninvasive and continuous fashion.

d. **ICP.** The association between severity of ICP elevation and poor outcome is well known. Monitoring ICP is useful, therefore, not only as a guide to therapy, but also for assessing

Table 6-2.   Major causes of decreased Sjo$_2$[a] and treatment

Cause	Clinical condition	Treatment
Cao$_2$ ↓	Hypoxemia	Correction of hypoxemia
	Anemia	Blood transfusion
CBF ↓	Hypotension	Fluid replacement; inotropics and vasopressors
	Hyperventilation	Correction of Paco$_2$
	Intracranial hypertension	Mannitol, furosemide, barbiturate, propofol
CMRo$_2$ ↑	Hyperthermia	Cooling
	Seizures	Barbiturate, propofol

Cao$_2$, oxygen content in arterial blood; CBF, cerebral blood flow; CMRO$_2$, cerebral metabolic rate for oxygen consumption.
[a]Sjo$_2$ $\propto$ [Cao$_2$—CMRo$_2$/CBF].

the response to the therapy and determining the prognosis.

e. **btPo₂.** A probe for the determination of $btPo_2$ is available. A $btPo_2$ of <10 mm Hg is assumed to convey the risk of hypoxic injury. The disadvantages of $btPo_2$ monitoring include the facts that it (a) only provides focal monitoring, (b) cannot be used in the surgical field during operation, and (c) has a critical threshold that is not well determined.

VI. **Cerebral protection**

A. **Hypothermia.** A reduction of body temperature to 33°C to 35°C may confer cerebral protection. Protective mechanisms include a reduction in metabolic demand, excitotoxicity, free radical formation, and edema formation. In an animal ischemia model, mild hypothermia of approximately 34°C to 36°C markedly attenuated ischemic injury. In clinical practice, controversy concerning the effectiveness of hypothermia in head injury still continues. The multi-institutional study of postoperative mild hypothermia in patients with head injury was terminated by its Safety Monitoring Board after enrolling 392 patients (see Clifton G et al.). The results showed no difference in mortality between patients with hypothermia and normothermia, and patients with hypothermia experienced more medical complications. Subgroup analysis revealed that younger patients (45 years of age or younger) who were hypothermic on admission and assigned to the hypothermic group tended to have better outcomes than those assigned to the normothermic group. A new study of this group with an earlier induction of hypothermia and more consistent critical care has been initiated.

When induction of hypothermia is elected, meticulous care is necessary to avoid adverse side effects such as hypotension, cardiac arrhythmias, coagulopathies, and infections. Rewarming should be carried out slowly. Temperature monitoring at two or more sites is recommended and may include the tympanic membrane, nasopharyngeal area, esophagus, and blood.

VII. **Postoperative management**

A. **Emergence and extubation.** Anesthesiologists often receive requests to awaken patients promptly to allow early postoperative neurologic assessment. Patients who had a normal level of consciousness before the operation and who have undergone an uneventful procedure can be awakened and their tracheas extubated in the operating room, assuming that emergence criteria have been satisfactorily met. Smooth emergence with control of systemic blood pressure and avoidance of coughing is necessary to prevent postoperative cerebral edema and hematoma formation.

B. Contraindications to extubation. Extubation in the operating room is discouraged for patients whose level of consciousness was depressed preoperatively and in whom brain swelling is either marked during operation or expected to occur postoperatively. Patients who have sustained multiple traumatic injuries are also candidates for postoperative ventilation. Patients who are hypothermic during emergence should be mechanically ventilated postoperatively and their tracheas extubated after careful rewarming.

VIII. Summary. The major goal of perioperative management of patients with head injuries is to prevent secondary damage. Therapeutic measures based on established guidelines and recommendations must be instituted promptly and continued throughout the perioperative course. Appropriate selection of anesthetics and meticulous general management of respiration, circulation, metabolism, fluid replacement, and temperature are all essential to improve outcome.

SUGGESTED READINGS

The Brain Trauma Foundation and the Congress of Neurological Surgeons. Guidelines for the surgical management of traumatic brain injury. *Neurosurgery* 2006;58(3) Suppl S2-1–S2-62.

Bullock RM, Chesnut RM, Clifton GL, et al. Guidelines for the management of severe traumatic brain injury. *J Neurotrauma* 2000; 17:451–553.

Carney NA, Chesnut R, Kochanek PM. Guideline for the acute medical management of severe traumatic brain injury in infants, children, and adolescents. *J Neurotrauma* 2003;54:S235–S310.

Clifton GL, Miller ER, Choi SC, et al. Lack of effect of induction of hypothermia after acute brain injury. *N Engl J Med* 2001;344: 556–563.

Clifton GL, Miller ER, Choi SC, et al. Hypothermia on admission in patients with severe brain injury. *J Neurotrauma* 2002;19: 293–301.

Doppenberg EMR, Choi SC, Bullock R. Clinical trials in traumatic brain injury: lessons for the future. *J Neurosurg Anesthesiol* 2004; 16:87–94.

Fritz HG, Bauer R. Secondary injuries in brain trauma: effect of hypothermia. *J Neurosurg Anesthesiol* 2004;16:43–52.

Gabriel EJ, Ghajar J, Jagoda J, et al. Guidelines for prehospital management of traumatic brain injury. *J Neurotrauma* 2002;19: 111–174.

Mackenzie CF. Threats and opportunities in pre-hospital management of traumatic brain injury. *J Neurosurg Anesthesiol* 2004;16: 70–74.

Polderman KH, Joe RTT, Peerdeman SM, et al. Effects of therapeutic hypothermia on intracranial pressure and outcome in patients with severe head injury. *Intensive Care Med* 2002;28:1563–1573.

Robertson CS. Management of cerebral perfusion pressure after traumatic brain injury. *Anesthesiology* 2001;95:1513–1517.

Thiagarajan A, Goverdhan PD, Chari P, et al. The effect of hyperventilation and hyperoxia on cerebral venous oxygen saturation in patients with traumatic brain injury. *Anesth Analg* 1998;87:850–853.

Anesthesia for Supratentorial Tumors

Nicolas J. Bruder and Patrick A. Ravussin

I. **Anesthesia for supratentorial tumors**
   A. **Background.** Approximately 35,000 new brain tumors are diagnosed per year in the United States. In adults, 85% are primary (9% of all primary tumors); 60% are primary and supratentorial (gliomas approximately 35%; meningiomas approximately 15%; pituitary adenomas approximately 8%). Approximately 12% of intracranial tumors are metastases. Their incidence increases with age, and approximately one-sixth of patients with cancer develop a brain metastasis which is symptomatic in most cases and often the controlling variable for survival.
   B. **General considerations**
      1. **Concerns and problems**
         a. **Patient symptoms** result from local mass effect and generalized increased intracranial pressure (ICP) effects.
         b. **Main surgical concern** is brain exposure without retraction or mobilization damage.
         c. **Main anesthetic concern** is the avoidance of secondary brain damage (Table 7-1). Therefore, understanding the following is vital: pathophysiology of ICP and cerebral perfusion; effects of anesthesia on ICP, cerebral perfusion, and metabolism; and therapeutic options for decreasing ICP, brain bulk, and tension perioperatively.
         d. **Specific problems** are massive intraoperative hemorrhage, seizures, air embolism (head-elevated/sitting position or if venous sinuses are traversed), monitoring brain function and environment, and rapid versus prolonged anesthetic emergence. A concurrence of intra- and extracranial pathologies might also occur (e.g., cardiovascular or pulmonary disease; paraneoplastic phenomena with metastases; chemotherapy/radiotherapy effects).
      2. **Pathophysiology of rising ICP.** The usual intracranial space-occupying components—brain tissue, intravascular blood, cerebrospinal fluid (CSF)—are contained in an unyielding skull. Any volume increase (tumor in this chapter) must be compensated by parallel volume reduction of one or more of these components, mainly CSF or blood (the brain is largely incompressible). The ability

Table 7-1.   Secondary insults to the already injured brain

Intracranial	Systemic
• Increased intracranial pressure	• Hypercapnia/hypoxemia
• Epilepsy	• Hypo-/hypertension
• Vasospasm	• Hypo-/hyperglycemia
• Herniation: falx, tentorium, foramen magnum, craniotomy	• Low cardiac output
	• Hypo-osmolality
• Midline shift: tearing of cerebral vessels	• Shivering/pyrexia

to compensate for the presence of a mass and maintain homeostasis depends on the volume of the mass and its rate of growth (the ICP volume curve shifts to the left for rapidly expanding masses). Homeostatic mechanisms: *early* (limited capacity)—intracranial to extracranial blood shift; *late* (larger capacity)—CSF displacement (ineffective if CSF flow is obstructed); *exhaustion*—rapid ICP rise → impaired cerebral circulation → brain herniation (end stage of compensation).

3. **Intracerebral perfusion and cerebral blood flow (CBF)**
   a. **Regulation of CBF** is through gradients in wall pressure of cerebral arterioles (result of cerebral perfusion pressure [CPP]) and partial pressure of arterial carbon dioxide ($Paco_2$) concentration (result of ventilation) (Figure 7-1).
   b. **Autoregulation of CBF** keeps the CBF constant despite changing CPP via alterations in cerebral vasomotor tone (i.e., cerebrovascular resistance [CVR]). Characteristics are: dominant to ICP homeostasis; normally functional for CPP of 50 to 150 mm Hg; impaired/affected by intracranial (e.g., blood in CSF, trauma, tumors) and extracranial (e.g., chronic systemic hypertension) pathologies and anesthetic drugs. Autoregulation is not immediate in that a sudden increase in blood pressure gives rise to a temporary increase in CBF.
   c. **Formulas.** CBF = CPP/CVR, CPP = MAP − ICP. Note that normally, ICP ≈ CVP (central venous pressure).
   d. **Inadequate perfusion.** Depends on both the reduction of CBF and its duration when CBF falls under 20 mL/100 g/minute. Inadequate perfusion is also linked to CPP <50 mm Hg with intact autoregulation. Action is to restore CPP and CBF (↑ MAP [mean arterial pressure], ↓ ICP, ↑ cardiac output); reduce cerebral metabolic demand (deepen anesthesia and hypothermia and treat epilepsy).

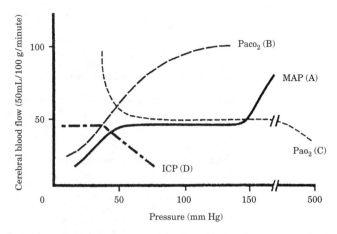

Figure 7-1.   Pressure-cerebral blood flow relationships. (A) Cerebral blood flow (CBF) autoregulation. CBF is maintained at 50 mL/100 g/minute for mean arterial pressure (MAP)/cerebral perfusion pressure = 50 to 150 mm Hg. (B) Linear relationship between partial pressure of arterial carbon dioxide ($Paco_2$) and CBF for $Paco_2$ = 20 to 80 mm Hg. (C) Pao_2 and CBF. (D) Intracranial pressure (ICP) and CBF.

      e. **Vasodilatory and vasoconstrictive cascades.** If autoregulation is intact:
          ↓ MAP → cerebral arteriolar vessel dilatation →↑ CBV (cerebral blood volume) →↑ ICP →↓ CPP (vicious circle!). Conversely, ↑ MAP →↑ CPP →↓ ICP via cerebral vasoconstriction (positive circle).
      f. **$Paco_2$.** Hypocarbia results in vasoconstriction, reducing CBF, CBV, and therefore ICP, making hyperventilation a favorite tool for the acute control of intracerebral hyperemia and elevated ICP. However, the relative reduction of CBF is larger than the reduction of cerebral metabolic rate for oxygen consumption ($CMRo_2$), inducing a risk of cerebral ischemia.
  4. **Anesthesia and intracranial pressure, perfusion, and metabolism.** Anesthesia affects the intracranial environment *through* drug and nondrug effects, all sensitive to the intra- and extracranial state (e.g., cerebral compliance, intracranial pathology, volemic state).
      a. **Intravenous anesthetics** (barbiturates, propofol, etomidate) reduce $CMRo_2$ dose dependently by depressing electrical and neurotransmitter synthesis (not basal metabolic) activity of the neurons with a ceiling effect at electroencephalographic (EEG) burst

suppression. They are cerebral vasoconstrictors → ↓ CBF, CBV, and ICP. Cerebral flow-metabolism coupling, autoregulation, and $Paco_2$ vessel reactivity remain intact. In contrast to volatile anesthetics, propofol suppresses the cerebrostimulatory effects of nitrous oxide.

b. **Volatile anesthetics** (e.g., isoflurane, sevoflurane, desflurane) decrease $CMRo_2$. They are all cerebral vasodilators (desflurane > isoflurane > sevoflurane). For <1 to 1.5 minimum alveolar concentration (MAC) and in the normal brain (flow/metabolism coupling intact), CBF decreases compared to the awake state and autoregulation is maintained. Above 1 to 1.5 MAC, there is a dose-related increase in CBF with impaired autoregulation (Figures 7-2 and 7-3). Maintained $Paco_2$ reactivity allows hypocapnic control of this type of vasodilatation. A situation to avoid is brain pathology + high volatile MAC → impaired/abolished carbon dioxide (CO_2) reactivity.

c. **Nitrous oxide** (N_2O) is cerebrostimulatory → ↑ $CMRo_2$, CBF, and sometimes ICP, particularly with volatile anesthesia. For the

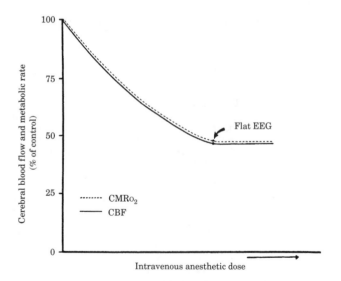

Figure 7-2. Cerebral blood flow (CBF)—cerebral metabolic rate for oxygen consumption ($CMRo_2$) coupling during increasing dose of an intravenous anesthetic. A normal $CMRo_2$ of 4 mL/100 g/minute is coupled to a CBF of 50 mL/100 g/minute. EEG, electroencephalogram.

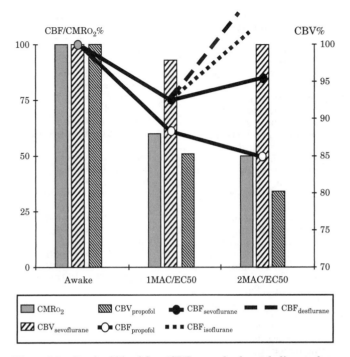

Figure 7-3. Cerebral blood flow (CBF)—cerebral metabolic rate for oxygen consumption ($CMRo_2$)—cerebral blood volume (CBV) during increasing doses of an intravenous (propofol) and volatile anesthetics. Changes are noted as a percentage value from the awake state. Despite similar changes in $CMRo_2$, changes in CBF and CBV are markedly different among intravenous and volatile agents and among sevoflurane, isoflurane, and desflurane above 1.5 minimum alveolar concentration (MAC). EC50, median effective concentration.

normal brain, this cerebral vasodilatation can be controlled by hypocapnia or intravenous anesthetics (volatiles—*no* attenuating effect). $CMRo_2$ and CBF are higher for 1 MAC anesthesia with nitrous oxide-volatile versus volatile only.

d. **Opioids** have been associated with short-term ↑ ICP (large doses). However, opioids are only modest direct cerebral vasodilators; therefore, reflex cerebral vasodilatation after ↓ MAP/CPP probably causes the transient ↑ ICP. Opioids modestly ↓ $CMRo_2$ without affecting flow-metabolism coupling, autoregulation, or vessel CO_2 sensitivity. Remifentanil is particularly suitable for rapid emergence.

Table 7-2.   Intracranial hypertension and brain bulging: prevention and treatment

Prevention	Treatment
• Preoperative: adequate anxiolysis and analgesia • Preinduction: hyperventilate on demand, head-up position, head straight, no jugular vein compression • Avoid overhydration • Osmotic diuretics (mannitol, hypertonic saline); steroids for tumor • Loop diuretics (furosemide) • Optimize hemodynamics: MAP, central venous pressure, pulmonary capillary wedge pressure, heart rate; use beta-blockers, clonidine, or lidocaine if necessary • Ventilation: PaO_2 >100; $PaCO_2 \sim 35$ mm Hg, low intrathoracic pressure • Use of intravenous anesthetics for induction and maintenance	• Cerebrospinal fluid drainage (lumbar catheter or ventricle) • Osmotic diuretics • Hyperventilation • Augment depth of anesthesia using intravenous anesthetics (propofol, thiopental, etomidate) • Muscle relaxation • Improve cerebral venous drainage: head up, no positive end-expiratory pressure, reduce inspiratory time • Mild controlled hypertension if cerebral autoregulation intact (MAP ~ 100 mm Hg)

MAP, mean arterial pressure.

  e. **Neuromuscular blocking agents (NMB).** The effect of succinylcholine on ICP is controversial, but fasciculations may increase ICP. Succinylcholine may be used for difficult intubation or rapid sequence induction in patients with brain injuries. Other NMB have no effect on ICP.
  f. **Other drugs.** Avoid vasodilating antihypertensive agents (nitroglycerin, nitroprusside, hydralazine) → cerebral vasodilatation. Take into account pharmacologic interactions, particularly with antiepileptic agents.
5. **Reducing ICP, brain bulk, and tension** (Table 7-2). The effectiveness of these techniques depends on intact intracerebral homeostatic mechanisms and/or structures.
  a. **Intravenous anesthetics** →↓ $CMRO_2$, CBF →↓ CBV, ICP →↓ brain bulk. Cerebral vasoconstriction depends on intact $CMRO_2$-CBF coupling (Figure 7-2) and is dose related up to neuronal electrical silence (EEG burst suppression). Like autoregulation,

CMR_{O_2}-CBF coupling is impaired by brain contusion and other intracerebral pathologies.

b. **Hyperventilation** $\rightarrow$ hypocarbia $\rightarrow$ cerebral vasoconstriction (acute effect lasting for a maximum of 24 hours). For intact autoregulation, CBF is linearly related to Pa_{CO_2} from 20 to 70 mm Hg (3% to 4% change/mm Hg Pa_{CO_2}). Factors impairing CO_2 reactivity are head injury, other intracerebral pathology, high-inspired volatile anesthetic concentrations, N_2O (especially with already dilated vessels). Typical target: Pa_{CO_2} of 30 to 35 mm Hg; based on arterial blood gas analysis rather than end-tidal CO_2 (ET_{CO_2}: possibility of large arterio-alveolar CO_2 gradients in neurosurgical patients). Side effects of hyperventilation include linear reduction in coronary artery flow and cardiac venous return as well as hypokalemia.

c. **Diuretics.** Osmotic diuretics (e.g., mannitol, hypertonic saline) $\rightarrow$ acutely $\uparrow$ blood osmolality $\rightarrow \downarrow$ brain water content (mainly healthy brain tissue with intact blood-brain barrier) $\rightarrow \downarrow$ brain bulk, ICP, $\uparrow$ compliance. Also: better blood rheology ($\downarrow$ endothelial edema; $\downarrow$ erythrocyte edema $\rightarrow \uparrow$ erythrocyte deformability). Typical regimen: mannitol, 0.5 to 1 g/kg intravenously (i.v.), (split between rapid precraniotomy dose and slower infusion until brain dissection is complete). ICP effect: prompt, lasts for 2 to 3 hours, removes approximately 90 mL brain water at peak effect. Problems: hypernatremia, acute hypervolemia. Compensate urinary losses due to mannitol with isotonic saline.

d. **CSF drainage.** Can be accomplished either by direct puncture of the lateral ventricle by the surgeon or lumbar spinal catheter by the anesthesiologist preoperatively; this is effective only without caudal block to CSF outflow. Acute brain herniation might occur; therefore, lumbar CSF drainage should be used cautiously and only when the dura is open and the patient is at least mildly hyperventilated. Draining 10 to 20 mL CSF effectively reduces brain tension; up to 50 mL can be drained if necessary.

e. **Use the vasoconstrictive cascade.** Mild $\uparrow$ MAP $\rightarrow \uparrow$ CPP $\rightarrow \downarrow$ CBV.

f. **Avoid other factors** causing cerebral vasodilatation: hypovolemia, hypoxia, patient positioning (head-down, extreme turning of the neck $\rightarrow \downarrow$ cerebral venous drainage, rotation of the head on one side and jugular venous

Table 7-3.   Preoperative neurologic evaluation

History
- Seizures, level of consciousness
- ↑ICP: headache, nausea, vomiting, blurred vision
- Focal neurology: hemiparesis, sensory deficits, etc.
- Hydration: duration of bed rest, fluid intake, diuretics, syndrome of inappropriate secretion of antidiuretic hormone
- Medication: steroids, antiepileptic drugs
- Associated illnesses, trauma

Physical Examination
- Mental status, level of consciousness
- Papilledema (↑ICP), Cushing response (hypertension, bradycardia)
- Pupil size, speech deficit, Glasgow Coma Scale score, focal signs

Investigations (Computed Tomographic/Magnetic Resonance Imaging Scans)
- Size and location of the tumor: e.g., silent or eloquent area?, near major vessel?
- Intracranial mass effects: midline shift, ↓ ventricle size, temporal lobe herniation, cerebrospinal fluid space surrounding the brain stem, edema, hydrocephalus

ICP, intracranial pressure.

thrombosis on the other side → major brain swelling), volatile anesthetics >1 to 1.5 MAC.

C. General anesthetic management

  1. **Preoperative assessment.** Anesthetic strategy is based on the patient's neurologic and general state and the planned surgery; both should be discussed with the neurosurgeon.

   a. Neurologic state of patient. Assess (Table 7-3): ICP increases and intracranial compliance (computed tomographic [CT] scan or magnetic resonance imaging [MRI]); size of ICP/CBF homeostatic reserve (margin before brain ischemia/neurologic impairment); autoregulation impairment (diffuse brain pathology, coma); presence of neurologic damage (permanent/reversible); present drug therapy (especially antiepileptic drugs and their side effects); neurodiagnostic studies.

   b. General state of patient. Cardiovascular system: brain perfusion/oxygenation depends on it; acute intracranial pathologies affect cardiac and lung function (worst situation: neurogenic pulmonary edema); supratentorial surgery (meningioma, metastasis) may result in significant bleeding (hypovolemia, hypotension → ↓ CPP/CBF and ↑ ICP). Respiratory system: hyperventilation to

↓ ICP, CBF, CBV, and brain tension depend on it; 40% of brain metastases are from lung (primary tumor, its chemotherapy/radiotherapy). The head-up/sitting position affects the cardiac and respiratory systems. Other systems: paraneoplastic or chemotherapy-/radiotherapy-associated syndromes (hematology, coagulation); renal system, diuretics, and decreased fluid intake; altered endocrine system (intracranial processes; pituitary adenoma or its therapy; steroids); gastrointestinal tract (steroids and mucosa; motility effects of ↑ ICP). Coagulation profile must be normal: stop aspirin at least 7 days and clopidogrel 10 days before surgery.

- c. **Biology.** Coagulation, hemoglobin, platelet count, potassium, sodium.
- d. **Planned operative intervention.** Clarify surgical approach (tumor size/position, proximal structures and likelihood of vascular involvement, radical excision), resultant patient positioning (supine, prone, sitting, lateral), and tumor type.
  - (1) **Meningiomas.** The combination of large size, difficult location, and radical excision (total resection is virtually curative) makes for long, technically demanding operations, often with significant bleeding (surrounding structures, meningioma vascularity). Anesthetic priority: maximal brain tension reduction to facilitate surgical access; compensate blood losses with isotonic saline or colloids (hematocrit >28%).
  - (2) **Gliomas.** Often simple debulking with easy surgical access and little risk of bleeding. Risk of postoperative intracranial hypertension due to edema.
  - (3) **Others.** Third ventricle colloid cysts, which may result in obstructive hydrocephalus and therefore ↑ ICP at induction. Colloid cysts, basal cistern epidermoids, and transcranially resected pituitary tumors need maximal brain relaxation for exposure at skull base.
  - (4) **Pituitary adenoma by transsphenoidal resection.** Essentially an extracranial operation in a head-up position.
- e. **Determination of anesthetic strategy.** Points to be addressed:
  - (1) **Vascular access.** Consider the risk of bleeding or venous air embolism, hemodynamic and metabolic monitoring, and

infusion needs for vasoactive and other substances.

(2) **Fluid therapy.** Target normovolemia/normotension; avoid hyposmolar (Ringer's lactate) and glucose-containing solutions (hyperglycemia → ↑ ischemic brain injury).

(3) **Anesthetic regimen.** "Simple" procedures (low risk of ICP problems or ischemia, little need for brain relaxation): volatile-based technique okay (<1.5 MAC). "High-risk" procedures (anticipated ICP problems, significant risk of intraoperative cerebral ischemia, need for deep brain relaxation): use total intravenous anesthesia with propofol.

(4) **Extracranial monitoring** such as cardiovascular or renal, venous air embolism.

(5) **Intracranial monitoring.** General or local environment versus specific functions: metabolic (jugular venous bulb oxygen saturation [Sjo_2], brain tissue oxygen partial pressure [$btPo_2$]), neurophysiologic (EEG/evoked potential), functional (transcranial Doppler).

2. **Preoperative preparation**
   a. **Premedication.** Risk assessment: *sedation* → hypercapnia, hypoxemia, upper airway obstruction → ↑ ICP; *stress* → ↑ CPP/CBF/$CMRo_2$, ↑ ICP and the development of vasogenic edema with impaired autoregulation. Best: titrated intravenous analgesia/sedation (e.g., midazolam, 0.5 to 2 mg, ± fentanyl, 25 to 100 mcg, or sufentanil, 5 to 20 mcg) under direct anesthesiologic supervision for vascular access placement, and so on. Patients without signs of ↑ ICP can benefit from oral premedication with a small benzodiazepine dose (e.g., 5 mg midazolam). Continue steroids (supplement with pituitary axis suppression) and other regular medication (anticonvulsants, antihypertensives, other cardiac drugs). Consider starting anticonvulsant therapy if not already initiated (e.g., loading dose of phenytoin, 15 mg/kg, or fosphenytoin, 20 mg/kg, over 30 minutes) and H_2 blockers (for ↓ gastric emptying, ↑ acid secretion with steroids, ↑ ICP).
   b. **Vascular access.** Two large-bore peripheral intravenous catheters are typical for full craniotomy.
      (1) **Central venous access.** Recommended for significant risk of venous air embolism (radiographically control catheter tip

position at transition of vena cava/right atrium) or bleeding, long-lasting procedures (>6 hours), major cardiovascular compromise (if severe, consider pulmonary artery catheter or transesophageal echocardiography), and continuous infusion of vasoactive drugs. Jugular cannulation technique (conventional or retrograde) must be meticulous, impairment of cerebral venous drainage must be avoided (hematoma, head-down position → ↑ ICP!).

(2) **Arterial cannulation.** Obligatory for full craniotomy due to the need for close monitoring and control of CPP (obtain by transducing arterial pressure at mid-ear/circle of Willis level, CPP = MAP - ICP); frequent determination of arterial $Paco_2$ (hyperventilation) and plasma glucose, potassium, and so on, values. Note that $ETco_2$ monitoring is no substitute for $Paco_2$ measurement (correlates poorly, especially with ventilation–perfusion mismatch).

(3) **Jugular venous bulb monitoring (JVBM).** Permits monitoring (intermittent or continuous with fiberoptic oximetry) of cerebral oxygen extraction (Sao_2–$Sjvo_2$), allowing conclusions about the adequacy of global cerebral perfusion (assuming $CMRo_2$ is constant). But frequently difficult to interpret during surgery due to the rotation of the head. Technique: retrograde cannulation of jugular vein; catheter tip should be radiographically verified to be in the jugular venous bulb.

c. **Monitoring**

(1) **Cardiovascular.** Electrocardiographic (myocardial ischemia, arrhythmias); arterial and CVP (see preceding text); pulse oximetry. Others: $ETco_2$ (trend monitor for $Paco_2$, detection of venous air embolism); temperature via esophageal thermistor (modest, passive hypothermia, [approximately $35°C$] might confer significant neuronal protection during focal ischemia at small systemic cardiorespiratory risk); urinary catheter.

(2) **Air embolism.** Sensitively detected by precordial Doppler, end-tidal nitrogen or CO_2 (alternative: transesophageal echocardiography).

(3) **Neuromuscular block.** Do not monitor on hemiplegic extremities (↑ acetylcholine receptor density of lower motor neuron units innervated by dysfunctional or nonfunctional upper motor neurons → resistance to nondepolarizing myorelaxants → effective overdose for normal neuromuscular units). Contralateral hemiparesis to a supratentorial tumor is not associated with hyperkalemia as in paraplegic or patients with burns; succinylcholine is therefore not contraindicated.

(4) **Blood chemistry.** Monitor glucose regularly; hyperglycemia →↑ neuronal damage during ischemia. During general anesthesia, steroids →↑ blood glucose levels; brain retraction → focal cerebral ischemia. Others: K, hematocrit, coagulation.

(5) **Intracranial environment, cerebral function.** JVBM (see preceding text); EEG monitoring (information on $CMRo_2$, cerebral ischemia, "depth of anesthesia"). Others: evoked potentials (intactness of specific central nervous system [CNS] pathways); $btPo_2$ (information on adequate oxygen supply to brain areas at risk of ischemia).

(6) **ICP monitoring.** Currently rare for elective neurosurgery due to improvements in perioperative ICP control but still has an important role in neurotraumatology.

3. **Induction of anesthesia**

a. **Goals.** Ventilatory control (early mild hyperventilation; avoid hypercapnia, hypoxemia); sympathetic/blood pressure control (avoid CNS arousal: adequate antinociception, anesthesia); optimal position on ICP–volume curve (avoid venous outflow obstruction).

b. **Typical induction scheme.** Detailed in Table 7-4.

c. **Myorelaxants.** Modern nondepolarizing drugs have minimal effects on intracerebral hemodynamics. Interaction (↑ doses by 50% to 60%) between pancuronium/vecuronium/rocuronium/cisatracurium and chronic (>7 days) phenytoin/carbamazepine treatment can occur due to increased metabolism and resistance to myorelaxants; no neuromuscular transmission monitoring on hemiplegic extremities (see preceding text). Note that because neurosurgical patients are susceptible to myorelaxant hangover (difficult to detect by

Table 7-4. Suggested anesthesia induction and maintenance scheme

Induction
- Adequate preoperative anxiolysis in the anesthetic room
- Electrocardiogram, capnometer, pulse oximeter, noninvasive blood pressure
- Venous, arterial lines: insert under LA
- Furosemide 1 mg/kg
- Preoxygenation, then fentanyl, 1–2 mcg/kg, (or alfentanil, sufentanil, remifentanil)
- Propofol, 1.25–2.5 mg/kg, or thiopental, 3–6 mg/kg, then nondepolarizing myorelaxant
- Control ventilation (Paco$_2$ ∼ 35 mm Hg)
- Intubation

Maintenance
- Propofol, 50–150 mcg/kg/min, or sevoflurane, 0.5%–1.5%, or desflurane, 3%–6%
- Maintain analgesia: fentanyl, 1–2 mcg/kg/h, (or alfentanil, sufentanil, remifentanil)
- LA, fentanyl 2 mcg/kg (skull-pin head holder placement, skin incision)
- Position: head-up, jugular veins free
- Mannitol, 0.5–0.75 g/kg, insert lumbar drain
- Ensure adequate volemia (NaCl 0.9% or hydroxyethyl starch 6%—not regular Ringer's lactate!)

LA, local anesthesia.

manual relaxometry), avoid long-acting myorelaxants (e.g., pancuronium); use middle-to short-acting drugs (e.g., vecuronium, cisatracurium, mivacurium, rocuronium).

d. **Patient positioning.** Pin holder application is a maximal nociceptive stimulus. Block by deeper analgesia (fentanyl bolus, 1 to 3 mcg/kg, sufentanil bolus, 0.2 to 0.3 mcg/kg, alfentanil, 10 to 20 mcg/kg, remifentanil, 0.25 to 1 mcg/kg) or anesthesia (e.g., propofol bolus, 0.5 mg/kg) and/or local anesthetic infiltration of the pin site. Alternative: antihypertensives (esmolol, 0.5 mg/kg, labetalol, 0.075 to 0.15 mg/kg). Remember that pin insertion can introduce venous air embolism! Avoid extreme positions; pad and/or fix regions susceptible to pressure, abrasion, or movement injury. Fix the endotracheal tube securely to avoid accidental extubation and abrasions with movement, and tape the eyes occlusively to avoid corneal damage. A mild head-up position helps venous drainage; mild knee flexion decreases back strain. Avoid severe lateral extension/flexion of head on neck (maintain more than two fingers' space between chin and nearest bone). Extreme flexion of the head may induce quadriparesis or massive swelling of the face and tongue making rapid extubation impossible. If the head is turned laterally, elevate contralateral shoulder (with a wedge or roll) to prevent brachial plexus stretch injury. Lateral/sitting/prone position: specific precautions. Verify cautiously all potential pressure points (eyes + + +), peripheral arterial pulses, nerve compression, and ventilation.

4. **Maintenance of anesthesia (Table 7-4)**
   a. **Goals**
      (1) **Controlling brain tension *through* control of CMRo$_2$ and CBF.** Preventing CNS arousal (depth of anesthesia, antinociception); treating consequences of CNS arousal (sympatholysis, antihypertensives); the "chemical brain retractor concept" (Table 7-5).
      (2) **Neuroprotection.** Maintenance of an optimal intracranial environment (adequate CPP, Paco$_2$, Sao$_2$: matching cerebral substrate demand and supply); specific neuroprotection is controversial and should not induce adverse effects or delayed recovery.
   b. **Choice of technique.** Controversy: intravenous or volatile anesthesia for neurosurgery? No study to date has shown significant outcome differences for intravenous versus volatile-based neuroanesthesia. But operative conditions are worse with volatile anesthetic inspired concentration (Fi) >1.5 MAC.
      (1) **Volatiles.** *Con*: CBF-CMRo$_2$ uncoupling; ↑ CBF/ICP/brain bulk. Pro: easy, extensive, successful use; control; predictability (early awakening). *Recommendation*: use for "simple" cases (no ischemia, ICP, or brain bulk problems);

Table 7-5. The chemical brain retractor concept

- Mild hyperosmolality[a]
- Mild hyperventilation

combined with:

- Adequate head-up positioning
- Lumbar cerebrospinal fluid drainage
- Intravenous anesthetic agent (propofol)
- Mild controlled hypertension[b]
- Avoidance of brain retractors
- Venous drainage: jugular veins free

[a]Before bone flap removal, give mannitol, 0.5–0.75 g/kg, or 7.5% NaCl, 3–5 mL/kg (NaCl 0.9% = 304 mOsm/kg).
[b]Mean arterial pressure ∼ 100 mm Hg.

early moderate hyperventilation; Fi < 1.5 MAC; avoid combination with N_2O ($\uparrow$ cerebrostimulation).

(2) **Intravenous techniques.** *Con*: more onerous use; prolonged/unpredictable awakening (mitigated by target-controlled infusion [TCI]; short-acting, infusion duration—insensitive drugs [e.g., propofol, remifentanil]). *Pro*: intact CBF—CMR_{O_2} coupling; $\downarrow$ CBF/ICP/ brain bulk; propofol blunts N_2O cerebrostimulation. *Recommendation*: use for cases with high risk of ICP/brain bulk problems or intraoperative cerebral ischemia; use TCI and short-acting drugs.

c. **Management of increases in ICP and brain bulk** (Table 7-2)

d. **Other measures.** When CNS and hemodynamic arousal are evident despite adequate anesthesia/analgesia, consider sympatholysis (esmolol, 0.5 to 1 mg/kg; labetalol, 0.075 to 0.15 mg/kg; clonidine, 1 to 1.5 mcg/kg).

e. **Antibioprophylaxis.** Oxacillin or second-generation cephalosporin before skin incision.

f. **Fluid therapy.** Goals: normovolemia, normotension, normoglycemia, hematocrit approximately 30%, mild hyperosmolality (<320 mOsm/L at end of procedure). *Recommendations*: avoid glucose-containing solutions, Ringer's lactate (hypo-osmolar); use 0.9% sodium chloride (NaCl) or 6% hydroxyethyl starch.

5. **Emergence from anesthesia** causes respiratory, cardiovascular, metabolic/endocrine, and neurologic changes. Emergence is associated with hemodynamic arousal lasting 10 to 25 minutes, weakly correlating with rises in oxygen consumption and mediated by elevated catecholamine levels and nociceptive stimuli. Treatment: antinociception, sympatholysis. Oxygen consumption is increased (up to 5 times) by rewarming (shivering/nonshivering thermogenesis) and pain. As a result of all of these factors, 20% of elective craniotomy patients develop raised ICP in the early postoperative period. Systemic hypertension is frequent and has been associated with an increased risk of postoperative intracranial hemorrhage.

a. **Aims of emergence.** Maintain intra- or extracranial homeostasis (MAP-CPP-CBF-ICP, CMR_{O_2}, Pa_{CO_2}, Pa_{O_2}, temperature). Avoid factors leading to intracranial bleeding (e.g., coughing, intratracheal suctioning, ventilator fight, $\uparrow$ blood pressure). The patient should be calm, cooperative, and responsive to verbal commands soon after emergence.

Table 7-6. Early vs. delayed awakening: pros and cons

Early Awakening	Delayed Awakening
Pros	*Pros*
• Earlier neurologic examination and reintervention	• Less risk of hypoxemia and/or hypercarbia
• Baseline neurology for subsequent examinations	• Better respiratory, hemodynamic control
• Less hypertension, catecholamine burst	• Easier to transfer to the ICU
• Performed by anesthesiologist who knows patient	• Stabilization in same state as during surgery
• Surgery/recovery period separated, ↓ costs	• → Better late hemostasis
Cons	*Cons*
• Increased risk of hypoxemia, hypercarbia	• Less neurologic monitoring
• Respiratory monitoring during transfer to ICU	• More hypertension, catecholamine release → ↑ bleeding

ICU, intensive care unit.

   b. **Early versus late emergence.** Ideal: rapid
      emergence to permit early assessment of
      surgical results and postoperative neurologic
      follow-up. However, early emergence is still
      not appropriate for some categories of patients
      (see in the subsequent text and Tables 7-6 and
      7-7).
   c. **Indications for late emergence.** Obtunded
      consciousness or inadequate airway con-
      trol preoperatively; intraoperative catastro-
      phe; significant risk of brain edema, ↑ ICP, or
      deranged intracerebral hemo- or homeostasis
      postoperatively. Risk factors for latter: long
      (>6 hours) and extensive surgery (particu-
      larly with bleeding), repeat surgery, surgery
      involving or close to vital brain areas, and

Table 7-7. Check-list before trying an early landing

- Adequate preoperative state of consciousness
- Cardiovascular stability, normal body temperature, and
  adequate oxygenation
- Limited brain surgery, no major brain laceration
- No extensive posterior fossa surgery involving cranial nerves
  IX–XII
- No major arteriovenous malformation removal (avoiding
  malignant postoperative edema)

surgery associated with significant brain ischemia (e.g., long vascular clipping times, extensive retractor pressure). If delayed emergence is chosen, adequate sedation and analgesia should be ensured, preferably with short-acting drugs.

d. **Preconditions for early emergence.** Anesthesiologic: should be planned (Table 7-7); use pharmacologically adequate anesthetic technique for early awakening; pay meticulous attention to intraoperative homeostasis (oxygenation, temperature, intravascular volume, cardiovascular function, CNS metabolism); avoid trauma of mechanical brain retraction (pharmacologic ICP/brain bulk control; see Table 7-5). Neurosurgical: minimization of blood loss (obsessive hemostasis); minimal surgical invasiveness (microsurgery, small operative fields). Craniotomy may be painful after the operation. Postoperative analgesia should be anticipated before awakening, especially if remifentanil is used for maintenance. Under these conditions, early emergence can be associated with less hemodynamic, metabolic, and endocrine activation than for delayed emergence.

e. **Differential diagnosis of unplanned delayed emergence.** Within 10 to 20 minutes of cessation of pharmacologically adequate anesthesia with short-acting agents, the patient should be awake enough to obey simple verbal commands. If not, consider and treat or rule out nonanesthetic causes (seizure, cerebral edema, intracranial hematoma, pneumocephalus, vessel occlusion/ischemia, metabolic or electrolyte disturbances). Suspected opioid overhang (fentanyl or sufentanil): try carefully titrated antagonization with small doses of naloxone or naltrexone.

f. **Neurologic evaluation.** Perform a baseline simple examination to assess motor responses of arms and legs, size of pupils and reactivity to light, adequate understanding of simple words and verbal response, and orientation to time and space.

D. **Specific anesthetic management**
1. **Predicted difficult airway.** Avoiding hypoxia is more important than preventing ICP increases. Method of choice: fiberoptic intubation. Technique: well-prepared, informed, cooperative patient; good local anesthesia (nasopharynx, airways); supplemental judicious light sedation (bolus midazolam, 0.5 to 1 mg ± fentanyl, 25 to 50 mcg; alternatively: low-dose propofol infusion at 1 to 2 mg/kg/hour) but avoid deep sedation and hypercapnia; treat

hypertension promptly (esmolol, labetalol, clonidine).

2. **Infectious tumors (abscesses)** are part of the differential diagnosis of supratentorial mass lesions. They are often accompanied by low-grade fever. Risk factors: contiguous infections (sinus, ear); right-to-left cardiac shunt; immunosuppression (extrinsic/intrinsic); intravenous drug abuse. Initial treatment: antibiotics (infection); corticosteroids (brain swelling). Definitive diagnosis/treatment: craniotomy, abscess aspiration. Surgical and anesthetic management: as for supratentorial neoplasms; aseptic precautions and sterile technique are vital for immunocompromised patients with acquired immunodeficiency syndrome. Note the association between human immunodeficiency virus infection and cerebral non-Hodgkin's lymphomas.

3. **Craniofacial/skull base surgery.** Increasingly used for orbital, posterior nasal sinus wall tumors. *Particularities*: complex, multidisciplinary surgery; tracheostomy/oral intubation frequent. Extensive bony involvement →↑ bleeding, hemorrhagic diathesis, venous air embolism (head-up position). Sensory ± motor neurophysiologic cranial nerve monitoring is common (motor monitoring: avoid neuromuscular blockade). Repeat procedures may be necessary and a difficult intubation (skull base exposure requires extensive temporalis muscle mobilization, which can lead to mandibular pseudoankylosis and limited mouth opening) can result.

II. **Anesthesia for intracranial hematomas**
   A. **General considerations.** The effects of intracranial hematomas on neurostatus and ICP depend particularly on the speed with which they arise. *Slow*: chronic subdural hematomas—subtle neurologic signs, small ↑ ICP; anesthetic technique: similar to supratentorial tumors. Most often seen in elderly patients (>70 years). *Fast*: acute epidural (e.g., traumatic), subdural, or intracerebral hematoma—massive neurologic impairment, potentially acutely life-threatening ↑ ICP; anesthetic technique: aggressive ↓ ICP and measures to preserve brain oxygenation and perfusion, followed by urgent surgical decompression. Situation frequently seen in head trauma or due to anticoagulation or antiplatelet agents. Coagulation should be corrected before surgery (factors II, VII, IX, and X, and vitamin K for patients treated with vitamin K antagonists; platelet transfusion for patients taking clopidogrel).
   B. **Anesthetic management of acute intracranial hematoma**
      1. **Induction.**
         a. **Basics.** Ensure oxygenation and then secure airway and hyperventilate with 100% oxygen.

Swift, atraumatic intubation (always dangerous if a fractured cervical spine is suspected or confirmed by x-ray); aim for a minimal ICP rise by avoiding coughing and arterial hypertension due to light anesthesia. In polytraumatized, hypotensive, and hypovolemic patients, one should decrease hypnotic, analgesic doses and restore circulating volume. If the patient has a full stomach, use aspiration prophylaxis and cricoid pressure (cautiously if suspected fractured cervical spine).

   b. **Pharmacologic range of options.** Intubation without further use of drugs in the deeply unconscious patient; judicious sedative use (e.g., etomidate, 0.2 to 0.5 mg/kg; propofol, 0.5 to 1.5 mg/kg; or thiopental, 2 to 4 mg/kg) with myorelaxation for a semiconscious, struggling patient; "classical" rapid sequence induction for the (still) conscious and stable patient. *Controversy*: what myorelaxant scheme to use? Succinylcholine, perhaps preceded by a small dose of nondepolarizing myorelaxant, remains the classical and time-tested scheme.

   c. **Control of ICP and brain swelling.** Next priority after securing ventilation and airway; should be started as early as possible and continued through to intensive care treatment. Start with large doses of mannitol, 0.7 to 1.4 g/kg (Table 7-2).

2. **Anesthesia maintenance.** Aims: control of ICP and brain swelling; maintenance of cerebral perfusion and oxygenation by matching CMR_{O_2} and CBF.

   a. **Monitoring**

      (1) **Cardiovascular monitoring** for these frequently hemodynamically unstable patients should include invasive arterial pressure monitoring, preferably commenced before induction (close hemodynamic control, repeated laboratory determinations). Electrocardiographic monitoring: interactions between brain damage and myocardial injury, risk of arrhythmias.

      (2) **ICP monitoring.** Generally installed once hematoma is evacuated, mainly for use in intensive care unit.

      (3) **Laboratory analyses.** Blood gas analysis (acid–base balance, ventilation, etc.); glucose (hyperglycemia and brain ischemia); coagulation profile (brain tissue damage → ↑ circulating thromboplastin); blood osmolality as guidance for use of osmotic diuretics (e.g., with mannitol, maximum should be 320 mOsm/kg).

b. **Anesthetic technique.** Intravenous anesthetics ($\rightarrow \downarrow$ CMRo$_2$, $\downarrow$ CBF, $\uparrow$ CVR) are the mainstay of anesthesia for acute intracranial hematoma. Volatile anesthetics are *not* recommended because of risk of $\uparrow\uparrow$ ICP/brain tension (to the point of acute transtentorial/craniotomy herniation, even with preexisting hypocapnia) and much smaller CMRo$_2$ reduction and neuroprotection against focal ischemia than with intravenous anesthetics (propofol, barbiturates). The following different situations must be evaluated and treated:

   (1) Deep coma and signs of brain herniation: myorelaxation and repeated small doses of thiopental titrated to blood pressure

   (2) Coma but no sign of herniation, increased ICP: propofol TCI or small doses of thiopental and opioids titrated to blood pressure; myorelaxation

   (3) Conscious patient but mass effect on CT-scan: rapid sequence induction, followed by propofol TCI, opioids, and myorelaxation

c. **Cardiovascular control.** Avoid arterial hypotension (by using doses of intravenous anesthetics that are too large) to prevent $\downarrow$ CPP ($\rightarrow$ cerebral ischemia and/or reflex cerebral vasodilatation $\rightarrow \uparrow$ ICP not controlled by hypocapnia [vasodilatory cascade]). *Controversy:* control of arterial hypertension and acute intracranial hematoma (Table 7-2): carefully balance maintenance of CPP to areas of brain rendered ischemic due to compression by hematoma against risk of more vasogenic brain edema or bleeding. Jugular venous bulb oxygen saturation monitoring may help assess adequacy of global CPP. btPo$_2$ can help assess adequacy of local O$_2$ delivery. Globally adequate CPP does not rule out regional CPP inadequacies $\rightarrow$ regional ischemia. If arterial pressure requires reduction, first improve analgesia (i.e., opioids) and/or depth of anesthesia (propofol, barbiturates, etomidate) before instituting specific antihypertensive treatment (usually antisympathetic drugs [e.g., esmolol, labetalol, clonidine]). Avoid cerebral vasodilators. Decrease blood pressure no >15% to 20%. Anticipate severe hypotension after brain decompression due to disappearance of the Cushing response: rapid fluid loading, neosynephrine, noradrenaline, or epinephrine ready to use.

d. **Emergence.** Patients with acute cerebral hematoma have significant brain injury with significant actual and potential brain swelling. They should therefore undergo slow weaning and delayed extubation in the neurointensive care unit. Chronic subdural hematoma patients frequently have minimal neurologic impairment preoperatively and can therefore often be awakened and their tracheas extubated immediately after surgery.

III. **Conclusions.** The main objectives of anesthesia for excision of a cerebral tumor include the following:
  • Preserving uninjured cerebral territories by global maintenance of cerebral homeostasis and cardiovascular stability as well as neuroprotection.
  • Balancing CBF autoregulation and MAP and preserving cerebral vasoreactivity to Pa_{CO_2}.
  • Achieving and maintaining brain relaxation by means of:
    — ↓ CMR_{O_2}, CBF, and CBV
    — moderate hyperventilation ($Pa_{CO_2} \sim 35$ mm Hg)
    — strict maintenance of CPP
    — osmotherapy
    — CSF drainage
  • Timely awakening to facilitate early and continuing neurologic assessment and permit prompt diagnosis and treatment of complications.

SUGGESTED READINGS

Basali A, Mascha E, Kalfas I, et al. Relation between perioperative hypertension and intracranial hemorrhage after craniotomy. *Anesthesiology* 2000;93:48–54.

Bruder N, Ravussin P. Recovery from anesthesia and postoperative extubation of neurosurgical patients: a review. *J Neurosurg Anesthesiol* 1999;11:282–293.

Cheng MA, Todorov A, Tempelhoff R, et al. The effect of prone positioning on intraocular pressure in anesthetized patients. *Anesthesiology* 2001;95:1351–1355.

de Nadal M, Munar F, Poca MA, et al. Cerebral hemodynamic effects of morphine and fentanyl in patients with severe head injury: absence of correlation to cerebral autoregulation. *Anesthesiology* 2000;92:11–19.

Kaisti KK, Langsjo JW, Aalto S, et al. Effects of sevoflurane, propofol, and adjunct nitrous oxide on regional cerebral blood flow, oxygen consumption, and blood volume in humans. *Anesthesiology* 2003;99:603–613.

Kaisti KK, Metsahonkala L, Teras M, et al. Effects of surgical levels of propofol and sevoflurane anesthesia on cerebral blood flow in healthy subjects studied with positron emission tomography. *Anesthesiology* 2002;96:1358–1370.

Petersen KD, Landsfeldt U, Cold GE, et al. Intracranial pressure and cerebral hemodynamics in patients with cerebral tumors: a randomized prospective study of patients subjected to craniotomy in propofol-fentanyl, isoflurane-fentanyl, or sevoflurane-fentanyl anesthesia. *Anesthesiology* 2003;98:329–336.

Richard A, Girard F, Girard DC, et al. Cisatracurium-induced neuromuscular blockade is affected by chronic phenytoin or carbamazepine treatment in neurosurgical patients. *Anesth Analg* 2005;100:538–544.

Rosner MJ, Daughton S. Cerebral perfusion pressure management in head injury. *J Trauma* 1990;30:933–940.

Todd MM, Hindman BJ, Clarke WR, et al. Mild intraoperative hypothermia during surgery for intracranial aneurysm. *N Engl J Med* 2005;352:135–145.

Todd MM, Warner DS, Sokoll MD, et al. A prospective, comparative trial of three anesthetics for elective supratentorial craniotomy. Propofol/fentanyl, isoflurane/nitrous oxide, and fentanyl/nitrous oxide. *Anesthesiology* 1993;78:1005–1020.

Verchere E, Grenier B, Mesli A, et al. Postoperative pain management after supratentorial craniotomy. *J Neurosurg Anesthesiol* 2002;14:96–101.

Warner DS. Experience with remifentanil in neurosurgical patients. *Anesth Analg* 1999;89:S33–S39.

Werner C, Kochs E, Bause H, et al. Effects of sufentanil on cerebral hemodynamics and intracranial pressure in patients with brain injury. *Anesthesiology* 1995;83:721–726.

Anesthesia for Posterior Fossa Surgery

Deborah J. Culley and Gregory Crosby

Operations in the posterior fossa are often demanding, delicate, and long. Anesthesia for these cases can also be challenging. In addition to the anesthetic management issues that apply to supratentorial surgery, posterior fossa surgery presents special problems related to positioning, cranial nerve dysfunction, and prevention of and monitoring for venous air embolism (VAE).

I. Preoperative considerations

A. The reticular activating system, cranial nerves, and structures vital for control of the airway and cardiovascular and respiratory systems are contained within a very small space in the posterior fossa. Accordingly, patients may present with dysphagia, laryngeal dysfunction, respiratory irregularities, or altered states of consciousness. In some cases, chronic aspiration owing to loss of airway reflexes can further compromise respiratory function.

B. Hydrocephalus caused by obstruction of ventricular outflow is a common cause of increased intracranial pressure (ICP) with posterior fossa lesions. This is evident on the preoperative computed tomographic scan or magnetic resonance imaging scan and can be treated by ventricular drainage, endoscopic third ventriculostomy, or hypertonic osmotherapy with mannitol and furosemide administered either pre- or intraoperatively.

II. Positioning

A. General issues

1. Posterior fossa surgery often requires unusual patient positioning. The prone, lateral, park bench, and sitting positions are commonly used. Regardless of the position chosen, care in positioning is of utmost importance because most problems are presumably avoidable with careful positioning and padding of vulnerable areas.

2. In the prone position, facial skin ulcerations can occur from uneven pressure distribution when the horseshoe headrest is used, and blindness can result from pressure on the globe of the eye.

3. In the lateral and park bench positions, there is a risk of brachial plexus injury if the up arm is pulled caudally to gain access to the retromastoid area.

4. Excessive neck rotation can also stretch and damage the brachial plexus, and extreme neck flexion is associated with the risk of quadriplegia.

5. Injury to the ulnar nerve at the elbow and peroneal nerve at the knee is also possible.

B. The sitting position

1. Advantages of the sitting position include good surgical exposure, improved ventilation, better access to the airway, greater comfort for the surgeon, and possibly reduced blood loss.

2. Disadvantages include the risk of VAE and pneumocephalus and the potential for hemodynamic instability. Additional complications include sciatic nerve injury from extreme flexion of the hip, massive swelling of the face and tongue from extreme neck flexion and/or rotation, and midcervical quadriplegia (ostensibly caused by a combination of stretch or compression of the cord by extreme neck flexion and hypotension).

3. The main contraindication to the use of the sitting position, however, is the presence of a documented right-to-left intracardiac or pulmonary shunt, which would facilitate systemic embolization of air.

C. VAE

1. VAE can occur whenever pressure within an open vessel is subatmospheric. Clinically significant VAE is unusual unless the surgical site is >20 cm above the level of the heart. Hence, VAE is a particular problem during surgery in the seated position, but it also occurs, albeit less frequently, in patients operated on in the lateral or prone position.

2. When open vessels cannot collapse, which is the case with major venous sinuses as well as bridging and epidural veins, the risk of VAE increases substantially. Most studies indicate that the incidence of VAE during posterior fossa procedures in the sitting position is 40% to 45%. For seated cervical laminectomy or surgery in the prone or lateral positions, VAE occurs in approximately 10% to 15% of cases.

3. Massive air embolism produces abrupt and catastrophic hemodynamic changes. Fortunately, this type of VAE is rare.

4. More commonly, air entrainment occurs slowly over a longer period of time and may produce little or no respiratory or hemodynamic compromise.

    a. As air is cleared to the pulmonary circulation, pulmonary vascular resistance and pulmonary artery (PA) and right atrial pressures increase.

    b. This vascular obstruction increases deadspace ventilation, resulting in the decrease in end-tidal carbon dioxide (ET_{CO_2}) and increase in partial pressure of arterial carbon dioxide (Pa_{CO_2}) that are characteristic of VAE. In addition, nitrogen appears in the exhaled gas.

        c. Hypoxemia develops owing to the partially occluded pulmonary vasculature and the local release of vasoactive substances.

        d. If unchecked, cardiac output decreases as a result of right heart failure and/or reduced left ventricular filling.

    5. Despite firmly held opinions and anecdotes, there is little evidence that the sitting position—at least when used in large centers doing large numbers of sitting cases—is less safe than alternative surgical positions. It is therefore difficult to argue that the sitting position should be abandoned purely because of the risk of VAE.

D. Paradoxic air embolism (PAE)

    1. When air enters the venous circulation, there is a risk that the air could pass via the pulmonary vascular bed or a patent foramen ovale (PFO) to the arterial side and embolize to coronary or cerebral vessels. The incidence of clinically significant PAE is unknown, and only a handful of cases have been reported (most without complications).

    2. Approximately 25% of the population have a probe-PFO, and the incidence of VAE is approximately 45%. Therefore, approximately 10% to 15% of patients operated in the sitting position are at potential risk for PAE.

    3. Precordial echocardiography has been used preoperatively to identify patients at risk because of a PFO. While detection of a PFO indicates that a patient is at risk for PAE, failure to identify a PFO is not reassuring because precordial echo has a high false-negative rate. Hence, echocardiography is not presently recommended as a routine part of the preoperative evaluation of such patients.

III. Anesthetic management

A. Premedication

    1. There is no contraindication to premedication of patients who have small cranial nerve or cerebellar lesions. If the patient has either elevated ICP or symptomatic hydrocephalus, heavy premedication should be avoided.

B. General monitoring issues

    1. For most posterior fossa cases, routine operative monitoring, usually with the addition of an intraarterial catheter for blood pressure monitoring, suffices.

    2. For sitting cases, two additional issues arise. First, blood pressure should be measured at the level of the head because blood pressure measured at the level of the heart will underestimate that perfusing the brain. Second, monitoring for and prevention of VAE are major considerations.

C. Monitoring for VAE

    1. Hemodynamic changes. Monitoring of hemodynamics may not provide sufficient advanced warning in the case of massive air embolism because the hemodynamic changes are abrupt and catastrophic.

2. **Doppler and ETco₂ monitoring.** Clinically, several monitoring options are available. In general, Doppler and ET_{CO_2} monitoring are considered the acceptable minimum.

3. **Precordial Doppler**

   a. This device can detect 1 mL of air or less, which makes it more sensitive than any other monitor except transesophageal echocardiography (TEE). The Doppler is not quantitative, however, and it requires experience to recognize which of the various sounds it emits is indicative of air.

   b. The Doppler probe should be placed after the patient is in the operative position. The probe is usually positioned at the middle third of the sternum on the right side but, because the position of the right atrium varies with the patient's position, proper placement must be confirmed. Hearing heart tones is not enough.

   c. To test for proper placement of the probe, agitated saline is injected through a right atrial catheter or peripheral intravenous line; alternatively, the injection of 0.5 to 1 mL of air, carbon dioxide (CO_2), or circuit gas is acceptable. The probe is properly placed if this maneuver produces characteristic Doppler sounds signaling air embolism.

   d. Because of its sensitivity, a properly positioned Doppler, combined with end-tidal gas monitoring, is essential for all posterior fossa procedures in the seated position.

4. **End-tidal gas monitoring**

   a. For reasons already stated, VAE is associated with a decreasing ET_{CO_2} and the presence of end-tidal nitrogen (ET_{N_2}).

   b. While theoretically quantitative, ET_{N_2} monitoring is less useful in practice because the ET_{N_2} concentration produced by even a large air embolus is small and just reaches the threshold of the sensitivity of clinically available end-tidal gas monitors.

   c. ET_{CO_2} monitoring is of intermediate sensitivity but provides a qualitative estimate of the size of a VAE. In general, the larger the embolus, the greater the decrease in ET_{CO_2}. A decrease in ET_{CO_2} is not specific for VAE, however, because a decrease in cardiac output from any cause has the same effect.

   d. The ET_{CO_2} monitoring is particularly useful for corroborating evidence of VAE from the Doppler and judging the clinical and physiologic significance of the embolus.

5. **Central venous catheter (CVP)**
   a. As a monitor for VAE, the CVP is insensitive and easily superseded by other devices. It has another utility, however.
   b. The CVP can help in positioning the Doppler. Also, the aspiration of air both confirms the diagnosis of VAE and serves as a treatment.
   c. To facilitate rapid aspiration of air, a multiorificed catheter is recommended. Because air tends to localize at the junction between the superior vena cava and the right atrium, greatest air retrieval occurs when the catheter orifices traverse this region.
   d. Catheter position can be confirmed in a number of ways. The catheter can be advanced until a right ventricular pressure trace is obtained and then withdrawn several centimeters. Alternatively, a chest x-ray can be obtained to confirm position. One simple method involves using the electrocardiogram, but its use has a risk of microshock. The right arm lead is connected to the catheter by a fluid column of sodium bicarbonate or via the J wire used to place the catheter. The tip is advanced until a biphasic P wave appears, at which point the catheter is withdrawn a few centimeters.
   e. One should always attempt to insert a CVP catheter in posterior fossa cases requiring the sitting position, but whether the inability to do so should result in cancellation of the case is controversial.

6. **PA pressure**
   a. Because PA pressures rise with significant VAE, the PA catheter can be useful for both diagnosis and therapy.
   b. However, it is difficult to aspirate air from the distal port of a PA catheter, and the middle port may not be an optimal location. Aspiration is more effective with a CVP catheter.
   c. In addition, as a diagnostic tool, the PA catheter offers no advantage over ET_{CO_2} monitoring.

7. **Transesophageal echocardiography (TEE)**
   a. TEE is more sensitive than Doppler ultrasound and is specific because the air bubbles are visualized directly. It is the only monitor that can detect PAE.
   b. TEE is expensive, requires special expertise, and demands near constant attention. For these reasons, in most centers, it is not a routine monitor for VAE.

D. **Prevention of VAE**
1. Positive end-expiratory pressure (PEEP)
   a. The use of PEEP to prevent VAE in the sitting position is controversial. High levels of PEEP (>10 cm H_2O) are needed to increase

venous pressure at the head, and studies are inconsistent as to whether PEEP decreases the incidence of VAE. PEEP can, however, reduce venous return, cardiac output, and mean arterial blood pressure, which may be detrimental.

   b. Experimental data also indicate that the discontinuation of PEEP is associated with the entrainment of venous air and promotes right-to-left shunting of air. Overall, PEEP is not recommended.

2. Volume loading

   a. Although hypovolemia has been proposed as a predisposing factor for VAE, evidence for a prophylactic effect of volume loading on the incidence of VAE and PAE is not strong enough to warrant its routine use. Adequate hydration is the goal.

3. Deliberate hypoventilation

   a. While some studies suggest that moderate hypoventilation may reduce the risk of VAE, hypoventilation also increases cerebral blood flow and cerebral blood volume, which may impair surgical exposure.

   b. Until the benefits of hypoventilation are confirmed, mild hyperventilation is the more common practice.

E. Anesthetic technique

1. There is no evidence that any one anesthetic drug or technique is superior to another for posterior fossa surgery. Moreover, hemodynamic changes associated with the assumption of the sitting position are minor regardless of the anesthetic technique.

2. The use of nitrous oxide (N_2O) is controversial. Because of the risk of VAE and the ability of N_2O to expand air bubbles, some practitioners argue that N_2O should be avoided in sitting position cases. This is a debatable position, however, because (a) N_2O has not been shown to increase the risk of VAE in sitting cases and (b) morbidity has not been shown to increase if N_2O is used provided it is discontinued the moment VAE is suspected. We subscribe to the latter reasoning; N_2O is used but discontinued if VAE occurs. Sensitivity of the embolism-detection device does not change.

3. The airway requires special attention. Often with posterior fossa cases, substantial neck flexion is required for optimal surgical exposure. Such flexion can advance the tip of the endotracheal tube into a mainstem bronchus or cause kinking of the endotracheal tube in the posterior pharynx.

   a. Some clinicians use a wire-reinforced tube while others prefer nasotracheal intubation. We use neither routinely but emphasize that careful assessment of tube patency and position is of utmost importance because access to the airway is quite limited.

  b. This assessment should be conducted after positioning the patient but before making the skin incision. Palpation of the cuff above the sternal notch is useful in confirming the position of the tube.

  c. If evidence of partial obstruction of the tube (e.g., high airway pressures, slow upstroke of the $ETCO_2$ tracing) exists, demonstrate that a suction catheter passes freely through the endotracheal tube, and insist on repositioning of the head and neck if it does not.

4. In most cases, controlled mild hyperventilation is desirable to improve surgical exposure and reduce retraction pressure on the brain. However, changes in respiration may be more sensitive to brain stem manipulation than hemodynamic changes. As such, the use of spontaneous ventilation may be appropriate in rare circumstances, when manipulation or ischemia of respiratory centers is likely. This should only be undertaken after discussion with the surgeon since hypoventilation that occurs with spontaneous ventilation during general anesthesia may cause brain engorgement and make surgical exposure more difficult.

F. Intraoperative considerations

  1. Cardiovascular reflexes

  a. Operations on or near the brain stem (e.g., during acoustic neuroma surgery) can produce abrupt, often profound, cardiovascular responses that may signal potential damage to the brain stem.

  b. Stimulation of the floor of the fourth ventricle, medullary reticular formation, or trigeminal nerve results in hypertension, usually in association with bradycardia. Bradycardia also results from stimulation of the vagus nerve.

  c. If such changes occur, the surgeon should be alerted immediately so that he or she can avoid the manipulation that provokes the response.

  d. Masking such changes with pharmacologic treatment is undesirable unless the changes are recurrent and severe. Hypertensive responses are typically so abrupt and transient that by the time a drug is administered, the stimulus is gone and treatment becomes unnecessary.

  e. Bradycardia can be both treated and prevented with glycopyrrolate or atropine, but the tachycardia produced by the former is less marked.

  2. Brain stem monitoring

  a. Cranial nerve injury is a significant risk of operations in the area of the cerebellopontine angle and lower brain stem. Therefore, intraoperative stimulation and recording from cranial nerves V, VII, VIII, XI, and XII are often utilized.

b. Monitoring techniques include somatosensory evoked potentials (SSEPs), brain stem auditory evoked potentials (BAEPs), and the spontaneous and evoked electromyogram (EMG).

c. This monitoring can be a challenge for the anesthesiologist because muscle relaxants complicate interpretation of the EMG, and N_2O and high-dose inhalation anesthesia may interfere with SSEPs. The BAEPs are robust and minimally influenced by anesthetics.

d. Although direct intracranial stimulation of the facial nerve produces facial movement even in well-paralyzed patients, "spontaneous" (i.e., surgical manipulation-induced) EMG discharges are subtle. Hence, some electrophysiologists request that, with the exception of succinylcholine for intubation, no muscle relaxants be given. The clinical necessity for this "pure" state has not been documented, however, and some centers are satisfied with a continuous infusion of relaxant to maintain a constant level of modest twitch suppression.

3. **Treatment of VAE**

a. Except in rare cases of severe hemodynamic instability, changing the patient's position is seldom required and often inconvenient. (The surgeon cannot identify a source of air entrainment if the wound faces the floor!) Other measures should be used first.

b. Alert the surgeons; they should irrigate the field with saline.

c. If N_2O is being used, discontinue it immediately.

d. Aspirate the right atrial catheter.

e. Provide cardiovascular support as needed.

f. Modify the anesthetic technique as needed.

g. Ask an assistant to compress both jugular veins lightly to minimize air entrainment.

h. Change patient position if the preceding measures fail to prevent ongoing VAE.

G. **Emergence from anesthesia**

1. **General objectives**

a. As with other types of intracranial neurosurgery, prompt, smooth emergence and avoidance of coughing, straining, and abrupt increases in blood pressure are desirable.

b. The feasibility of extubation depends on the usual factors plus preexisting neurologic impairments, the nature and extent of the surgery, and the likelihood of brain stem edema or injury. Even if extubation is not planned, one should attempt to awaken the patient for postoperative neurologic evaluation.

2. **Ventilation/airway abnormalities**

   a. Because of disease- or surgery-induced dysfunction of cranial sensory or motor nerves, patients may have difficulty swallowing, vocalizing, or protecting the airway. In addition, damage to or edema of the respiratory centers from intraoperative manipulation can result in hypoventilation or erratic respiratory patterns. Therefore, longer-term ventilation and airway protection might be required in some patients.

   b. Severe tongue and facial edema can occur owing to position-induced venous or lymphatic obstruction. The endotracheal tube should be left in place until the edema resolves.

   c. Pulmonary edema may result from large VAE. Although pulmonary edema is usually responsive to conservative measures such as supplemental oxygen (O_2) and diuretics, continued postoperative ventilation may be appropriate until evaluation is completed.

3. **Cardiovascular issues**

   a. Hypertension is common after posterior fossa surgery and may contribute to edema formation and intracranial hemorrhage. Hence, one should be prepared to control postoperative hypertension.

4. **Neurologic complications**

   a. A variety of untoward neurologic complications can occur after posterior fossa operations. These include altered levels of consciousness, varying degrees of paresis, and specific cranial nerve deficits (e.g., visual disturbances, facial nerve paresis, impaired swallowing or phonation).

   b. Treatment is supportive, but evaluation of delayed emergence should proceed lest a treatable nonanesthetic cause go unrecognized. If cerebral paradoxical air embolism is suspected, hyperbaric oxygen therapy may be warranted.

5. **Pneumocephalus**

   a. Air is retained in the cranial cavity after all craniotomies regardless of position. When the patient is in the sitting position, cerebrospinal fluid drains easily, and a larger amount of air may be trapped when the wound is closed. In most cases, the air is reabsorbed uneventfully over several days and no treatment is necessary. There is little evidence that anesthetic technique influences either the incidence or the volume of pneumocephalus.

  b. Tension pneumocephalus can occur when the brain re-expands and compresses the air. This situation is difficult to diagnose but should be suspected if emergence is delayed after an otherwise uneventful operation or if either cardiovascular collapse or neurologic deterioration occurs postoperatively.

  c. In such rare circumstances, surgical evacuation may be indicated.

SUGGESTED READINGS

Black S, Ockert DB, Oliver WC, et al. Outcome following posterior fossa craniectomy in patients in the sitting or horizontal positions. *Anesthesiology* 1988;69:49.

Blanc P, Boussuges A, Henriette K, et al. Iatrogenic cerebral air embolism: importance of an early hyperbaric oxygenation. *Intensive Care Med* 2002;28:559.

Drummond JC, Patel PM. Neurosurgical anesthesia. In: Miller RD, ed. *Anesthesia*. 6th ed. Philadelphia, PA: Elsevier Churchill Livingstone, 2005:2127–2173.

Patel SJ, Wen DY, Haines SJ. Posterior fossa: surgical considerations. In: Cottrell JE, Smith DS, eds. *Anesthesia and Neurosurgery*. 4th ed. St. Louis, MO: Mosby, 2001:319–334.

Porter JM, Pidgeon C, Cunningham AJ. The sitting position in neurosurgery: a critical appraisal. *Br J Anaesth* 1999;82:117–128.

Schmitt HJ, Hemmerling TM. Venous air emboli occur during release of positive end-expiratory pressure and repositioning after sitting position surgery. *Anesth Analg* 2002;94:400.

Smith DS, Osborn I. Posterior fossa: anesthetic considerations. In: Cottrell JE, Smith DS, eds. *Anesthesia and Neurosurgery*. 4th ed. St. Louis, MO: Mosby, 2001:335–352.

Stendel R, Gramm HJ, Schroder K, et al. Transcranial Doppler ultrasonography as a screening technique for detection of a patent foramen ovale before surgery in the sitting position. *Anesthesiology* 2000;93:971–975.

Anesthetic Management of Intracranial Aneurysms

Philippa Newfield and Audrée A. Bendo

The anesthetic and perioperative management of the surgical and endovascular treatment of intracranial aneurysms is designed to facilitate the conduct of the procedure and the patient's recovery and minimize the risk of aneurysmal rupture, cerebral ischemia, neurologic deficit, and associated systemic morbidity to improve functional survival.

I. **Aneurysms**
   A. **Types**
      1. **Saccular aneurysms** (<2.5 cm in diameter) are formed by the disintegration of the artery's elastic layer at the flow separator region from the pounding of the arterial pulse wave.
      2. **Giant aneurysms** measure up to 10 cm in diameter and represent 5% of all aneurysms.
      3. **Other types of aneurysms** include fusiform (associated with severe atherosclerosis or degenerative processes in childhood), dissecting (from a tear in the luminal endothelium that permits a blood column to dissect between the endothelium and the media), traumatic (developing in the 2 to 3 weeks after severe head injury), and mycotic (infectious).
   B. **Location.** Ninety percent of aneurysms occur on the anterior circulation, most commonly the internal carotid-posterior communicating artery (more common in women), anterior communicating artery (more common in men), and middle cerebral artery (MCA) bifurcation. Ten percent occur on the posterior circulation, most commonly at the basilar apex. The internal carotid artery bifurcation is affected in children.
   C. **Epidemiology.** The annual incidence of aneurysmal subarachnoid hemorrhage (SAH) is approximately 6 to 8/100,000 in most western populations. The rate of rupture of an intracranial aneurysm is 0.05% to 6% per year, depending on the size and location of the aneurysm. Aneurysms are 11 times more likely to rupture in patients who have had a previous SAH than in those who have an asymptomatic aneurysm. Smoking and hypertension are risk factors. The incidence in men outnumbers women until age 50; women predominate thereafter; and aneurysms commonly present in the sixth decade of life. Approximately 20% of patients have more than one aneurysm.

Table 9-1.   Predictors of mortality after subarachnoid hemorrhage

Poor neurologic condition at hospital admission, a function of rate and volume of bleed
Depressed level of consciousness after initial bleed
Older age
Preexisting illness
Elevated blood pressure
Thick clot in the brain substance or ventricles on initial computed tomographic scan
Repeat hemorrhage
Basilar aneurysmal location

Aneurysmal SAH accounts for 10% of all cerebrovascular accidents.

D.   Natural history. One patient in six will die within minutes of an SAH. Of the patients who survive to be admitted to the hospital, 25% will die thereafter, and just over 50% will recover completely. Without treatment, at least 50% of ruptured aneurysms will rerupture within 6 months and then at a rate of 3% per year.

E.   Prognostic factors. The rate and volume of bleeding affect the patient's neurologic condition at hospital admission and determine outcome. Patients who remain conscious and complain only of severe headache after SAH do better than patients who are comatose upon arrival at the hospital. Older age, poor general health, evidence of clots in either the brain substance or the ventricles, and repeat hemorrhage all affect outcome adversely (Table 9-1).

F.   Genetics and associated diseases. Of patients who have SAH, 5% to 10% will have one or more first-order relatives who have also had a ruptured aneurysm. The inheritance is probably dominant with variable penetrance. Conditions associated with intracranial aneurysms include polycystic kidney disease (5% of aneurysms series, 33% of polycystic kidney series), coarctation of the aorta (1% of aneurysm patients, 5% of coarctation patients, all of whom are hypertensive), sickle cell disease, drug abuse (cocaine: generalized vasoconstriction and hypertension; intravenous use: mycotic aneurysms), and hypertension (30% to 40% of patients with SAH). Rarer associations are with fibromuscular dysplasia, Marfan's syndrome, tuberous sclerosis, Ehlers-Danlos syndrome, hereditary hemorrhagic telangiectasia, moyamoya disease, and pseudoxanthoma elasticum. Choriocarcinoma and cardiac myxomas are associated with multiple cerebral aneurysms.

II.   SAH. Rupture of an intracranial aneurysm causes the sudden onset of an excruciating headache. Patients may also complain of malaise and be irritable, combative, and uncooperative.

A. **Diagnosis**

   1. **History** includes the patient's report that this is the "worst headache of my life" as well as malaise, nausea, and vomiting.

   2. **Physical examination** identifies change in level of consciousness, focal neurologic deficits, fever, meningismus, nuchal rigidity (may be absent early after SAH), photophobia, ophthalmic hemorrhages (poor prognostic sign), fluid (hypovolemia), and electrolyte (hyponatremia) imbalance.

   3. **Imaging** should be performed: computed tomographic (CT) scan for amount of subarachnoid, intracerebral, and intraventricular blood; cerebral angiography for exact location and configuration of aneurysm and neck.

   4. **Lumbar puncture** is recommended for analysis of cerebrospinal fluid (CSF) if the CT scan is negative.

   5. **Common misdiagnoses** include flu, meningitis, cervical disc disease, migraine, myocardial infarction, malingering, and intoxication.

B. **Grading**

   1. **Botterell** in 1956 introduced a system for grading patients after SAH to facilitate assessment of surgical risk, prediction of outcome, and prompt evaluation of the patient's condition. The Grades I to V describe the patient's level of consciousness and degree of neurologic impairment, with each higher grade representing greater severity.

   2. **Hunt and Hess** modified Botterell's system in 1968 to include a provision for the effect of serious systemic illness (Table 9-2a).

   3. The **World Federation of Neurological Surgeons** (WFNS) 1988 grading scale, based on the Glasgow Coma Scale, demonstrated that the preoperative level of consciousness correlated most directly with outcome (Table 9-2b).

III. **Complications of SAH** (Table 9-3)

A. **Rebleeding,** the occurrence of further hemorrhage after the initial SAH, is one of the major causes of neurologic deterioration after SAH. The cardinal signs are deterioration in the level of consciousness, development of focal neurologic deficits (aphasia, hemiplegia), abnormal vital signs (hypertension, bradycardia, arrhythmias, irregular respirations), and the presence of hemorrhage on ophthalmic examination.

   1. These subsequent episodes of aneurysmal rupture are usually more severe than the first hemorrhage. The mortality associated with a second hemorrhage rises precipitously with significant morbidity in the surviving patients. Late rebleeding is fatal in 67% of cases. All

Table 9-2a.   Clinical grading after subarachnoid hemorrhage: Hunt and Hess modification

Grade	Description	Mortality (%)
Grade 0	Unruptured aneurysm	—
Grade I	Asymptomatic or minimal headache with normal neurologic examination	2
Grade II	Moderate to severe headache, nuchal rigidity, no neurologic deficit other than cranial nerve palsy	5
Grade III	Lethargy, confusion, or mild focal deficit	15–20
Grade IV	Stupor, moderate to severe hemiparesis, possible early decerebrate rigidity, vegetative disturbances	30–40
Grade V	Deep coma, decerebrate rigidity, moribund appearance	50–80

Serious systemic diseases (hypertension, coronary artery disease, chronic pulmonary disease, diabetes) and severe vasospasm on angiography cause assignment of the patient to the next less favorable category.
Hunt WE, Hess EM. *J Neurosurg* 1968;28:14, with permission.

Table 9-2b.   World Federation of Neurological Surgeons Clinical Grading Scale

WFNS Grade	GCS Score	Motor Deficit
I	15	Absent
II	14−13	Absent
III	14−13	Present
IV	12−7	Present or absent
V	6−3	Present or absent

WFNS, World Federation of Neurological Surgeons; GCS, Glasgow Coma Scale.
Drake CG, Hunt WE, Kassell N, et al. *J Neurosurg* 1988;68:985, with permission.

rebleeding accounts for 22% of the mortality from SAH.

2. The incidence of rebleeding is highest (4%) during the first 24 hours after SAH and then declines to 1% to 2% per day for the next 13 days. Approximately 20% to 30% of ruptured aneurysms rebleed within the first 30 days after SAH. The cumulative risk of rebleeding is 19% at 2 weeks, 50% at 6 months, and then decreases to 3% per year for up to 15 years. During the ensuing 5 months after the initial SAH, 10% to 15% of patients will rebleed. **The overall incidence of rebleeding is 11%.**

3. The incidence of **aneurysmal rupture during induction of anesthesia** is 0.5% to 2% and carries a mortality of 75%. The incidence of

Table 9-3.   Complications of aneurysmal subarachnoid hemorrhage

Central nervous system
Rebleeding
Vasospasm
Disordered autoregulation
Intracranial hypertension
Hydrocephalus
Seizures
Systemic disorders
Hypovolemia
Hyponatremia, hypokalemia, hypocalcemia
Electrocardiographic abnormalities
Respiratory abnormalities: pulmonary edema, pneumonia, pulmonary embolus
Hepatic dysfunction
Renal dysfunction
Thrombocytopenia
Gastrointestinal bleeding

intraoperative aneurysmal rupture varies from 6% to 18%, depending on the institution and the size and location of the aneurysm. In order of decreasing incidence, the causes of rupture during operation include aneurysm dissection, brain retraction, hematoma evacuation, and dural and arachnoid opening.

4. **Pathophysiologic sequelae** of rebleeding include intracranial hypertension and compromised cerebral perfusion; acute hydrocephalus from the sudden deposition of subarachnoid clot that obstructs the flow of CSF through the basal cisterns; cerebral infarction from either direct, hematoma-induced destruction of tissue or shifts in the intracranial contents with vascular compromise; impaired autoregulation (the ability of the normal brain to maintain cerebral blood flow [CBF] at a fairly constant level between a mean arterial pressure [MAP] of 50 and 150 mm Hg); and a reduction in the cerebral metabolic rate for oxygen consumption (CMR_{O_2}).

5. **Predisposing factors for rebleeding:**
   a. Large volume of blood in the subarachnoid space from the initial SAH
   b. Poor neurologic status owing to the devastation caused by the initial SAH
   c. Short interval from the initial hemorrhage
   d. Female gender: women rebleed twice as frequently as men
   e. Older age and poor general medical condition
   f. Systemic hypertension: the risk of rebleeding is directly related to the patient's systolic blood pressure
   g. Multiple previous episodes of rebleeding that increase the likelihood of subsequent rupture and death
   h. Presence of either an intracerebral or intraventricular hematoma
   i. Abnormal clotting parameters
   j. Posterior circulation aneurysms

6. **The size of the hematoma from the episode of rebleeding** is the most critical factor in determining outcome. Patients who have a large subdural hematoma and a marked midline shift on CT scan have a poorer prognosis, as do those who have associated intracerebral and intraventricular hemorrhage.

7. **Early surgical or endovascular obliteration of the aneurysm** is the only definitive means to prevent rebleeding. Either operation or endovascular obliteration within 24 to 48 hours of SAH is therefore favored because of the association with improved outcome. At 1-year

follow-up, the results of the International Subarachnoid Aneurysm Trial comparing operative aneurysmal clip ligation with endovascular
metal coiling demonstrated that the risk of rebleeding was low in both groups: 1% for the
surgical group and 2.4% for the endovascular
group. The effects of rebleeding were taken
into account in determining that the relative
risk of either death or significant disability for
endovascular patients is 22.6% lower than for
surgical patients. This represented an absolute
risk reduction of 6.9%. Most of the 2,143 patients randomized into the trial were in good
condition (WFNS Grades I and II) after SAH
and had small anterior-circulation aneurysms
(92% <11 mm in size) for which endovascular
coiling and neurosurgical clipping were both
considered therapeutic options.

8. **Prevention of rebleeding.** The following are
preferred methods:

   a. Control systolic hypertension and increases
   in transmural pressure (MAP minus intracranial pressure [ICP]).

   b. Administer short-acting antihypertensive
   drugs (esmolol, labetalol) to control either
   labile hypertension or transient spikes in
   blood pressure from therapeutic interventions.

   c. Maintain the patient's "normal" blood pressure as the lower acceptable limit to avoid
   either initiation or exacerbation of vasospasm from a decrease in cerebral perfusion pressure (CPP), the difference between
   MAP and ICP.

   d. Administer narcotic analgesics and sedatives in titrated doses to reduce pain and
   anxiety while avoiding oversedation and
   hypoventilation.

   e. Avoid the rapid drainage of CSF from lumbar or ventricular puncture, which may
   lead to a fall in ICP, a relative rise in
   transmural pressure, and the potential for
   aneurysmal rerupture. CSF drainage may
   be instituted to lower ICP, however, if cerebral perfusion is seriously compromised
   because of intracranial hypertension.

   f. Maintain euvolemia.

   g. Avoid seizures that may themselves lead to
   hypertension.

   h. Maintain transmural pressure across the
   wall of the aneurysm during the induction
   of anesthesia for aneurysmal clip ligation by
   the prevention of sudden increases in systemic blood pressure and decreases in ICP.
   Adjust ventilation to maintain normocapnia

(Paco$_2$ of 35 to 40 mm Hg) until the dura is opened. The presence of a large hematoma may mandate hyperventilation to improve intracranial compliance during induction. Give mannitol and begin spinal drainage after the bone flap has been turned.

    i. Decrease the turgor of the aneurysmal sac during manipulation of the aneurysm by the neurosurgeon's temporary proximal occlusion of the parent vessel. The patient's blood pressure is maintained in the high-normal range to enhance distal and collateral perfusion. The blood pressure is quickly returned to the patient's low-normal range if the temporary clip is removed before the aneurysm has been secured to prevent aneurysmal rupture. Hypotension induced with either isoflurane or sodium nitroprusside (SNP) is not favored, however, because the CBF-lowering effect of the hypotension may adversely affect patients who have developed or are in the process of developing cerebral vasospasm.

    j. Control blood pressure during emergence from anesthesia to prevent bleeding from other unsecured aneurysms, muslin-wrapped aneurysms, and sites of surgical hemostasis.

9. Management of rebleeding after SAH is designed to maintain CPP, limit intracranial hypertension, decrease intracranial volume, control systemic blood pressure, reduce transmural pressure across the wall of the aneurysm, and optimize cerebral oxygen delivery through the maintenance of normal arterial oxygen saturation and normal hemoglobin concentration.

    a. If the aneurysm bleeds before, during, or after the **induction of anesthesia**, the patient is hyperventilated with 100% oxygen. Thiopental lowers the blood pressure and affords some cerebral protection, but excessive lowering of the systemic pressure at this juncture can be detrimental if it interferes with cerebral perfusion. Immediate craniotomy to accomplish "rescue clipping" after rupture during induction of anesthesia has been successful.

    b. **Intraoperative rupture** of the aneurysm mandates rapid surgical control. The MAP may be reduced to 50 mm Hg briefly to facilitate temporary proximal and distal control of the parent vessel in preparation for clip ligation of the neck of the aneurysm. Once the parent vessel is controlled, the blood pressure is increased to normal to enhance collateral circulation during the period of temporary occlusion. Alternatively, the ipsilateral carotid artery may be manually compressed for up to 3 minutes to produce a bloodless field. Blood loss is replaced immediately because it is essential to maintain normovolemia if the blood pressure needs to be reduced.

10. **Emergency reoperation** may be necessary for evacuation of a hematoma or to control postsurgical bleeding or ventricular drainage. In an emergency, an external ventricular drain may be inserted at the patient's bedside to decompress the ventricules.

11. Although the use of epsilon-aminocaproic acid and other **antifibrinolytic drugs** halved the rebleeding rate in the initial 2 weeks after SAH, the incidence of vasospasm and hydrocephalus increased, resulting in no improvement in overall outcome. Instead of using antifibrinolytic drugs, neurosurgeons use either early endovascular obliteration or early operation with definitive clipping of the aneurysm. This mandates the rapid and efficient accomplishment of diagnosis, evaluation, and initial treatment.

B. **Vasospasm or delayed ischemic deficit**

1. **Vasospasm** is the reactive narrowing of the larger conducting arteries in the subarachnoid space that are surrounded by clots after SAH and affected by spasmogenic breakdown products of the red blood cells within the clot. The subsequent delayed ischemic deficit and infarction caused by vasospasm are major causes of disability and death after SAH, accounting for 30% of SAH-induced morbidity and mortality. Vasospasm has been considered the causative factor in 28% of all deaths and 39% of all disability after SAH and is therefore responsible for the great human cost and extensive utilization of limited health care resources.

   a. Patients of all neurologic grades have a 50:50 chance of developing significant angiographic vasospasm. Symptoms of delayed ischemia occur in 20% to 25% of patients, and 30% to 50% of patients have evidence of infarction from vasospasm on CT scan. Death from vasospastic infarction occurs in 5% to 17% of patients.

   b. The incidence of vasospasm peaks between the 4th and 9th day after SAH and decreases over the next 2 to 3 weeks.

   c. Vasospasm is directly related to the severity of the hemorrhage from the aneurysmal rupture which correlates well with the location and volume of blood noted on the post-SAH CT scan. The **risk of vasospasm** is increased by SAH-induced cerebral dysautoregulation and abnormal carbon dioxide (CO_2) responsiveness, a Glasgow Coma Scale score of <14 on hospital admission, an early increase in mean MCA flow velocity on transcranial Doppler (TCD) ultrasonography, and anterior cerebral and internal carotid artery aneurysms. The timing of surgery and the method of occlusion—surgical versus endovascular—have no effect on the subsequent development of vasospasm. The intraoperative transfusion of packed red blood cells is a risk factor for poor outcome, and postoperative transfusion is correlated with the development of angiographically confirmed vasospasm. The mechanism may involve either the depletion or the inactivation of nitric oxide, an endogenous vasodilator, which transfused red cells lack.

2. **Diagnosis of vasospasm**
   a. **Clinical signs** include either progressive impairment in the level of consciousness or the appearance of new focal neurologic deficits >4 days after the initial SAH that are not associated with any other structural or metabolic cause. The onset may be either sudden or insidious and accompanied by increased headache, meningismus, and fever. It is important to rule out other causes of clinical deterioration after SAH including rebleeding, hydrocephalus, subdural hematoma, cerebral infarction and edema, meningitis, seizures, electrolyte and acid–base disturbances, and adverse reactions to medications.
   b. **TCD ultrasonography** may be used to determine the efficacy and duration of treatment. Both a large increase in blood flow velocity (MCA velocity >120 cm/second) and a rapid rise in blood flow velocity (>50 cm/second in 24 hours) reflect a reduction in vessel caliber. A peak flow velocity of 140 to 200 cm/second indicates moderate vasospasm; a peak flow velocity >200 cm/second is associated with severe vasospasm. Critically high blood flow velocities (>120 cm/second) correlate strongly with vasospasm on angiography. Because TCD is operator dependent and reflects technical factors, ICP, cardiac output, and the artery being assessed, it is important to correlate TCD results with sequential neurologic examination and ICP, blood pressure, and cardiac output.
   c. **Cerebral angiography** is the most reliable modality for diagnosing and evaluating

vasospasm. Although some angiographic evidence of vasospasm occurs in 70% to 80% of cases, only one-third of patients develop the clinical picture. Signs and symptoms of decreased CBF usually occur when the reduction in the diameter of the arterial lumen exceeds 50%, the definition of angiographically severe vasospasm.

d. **Xenon-enhanced CT,** a relatively inexpensive technique, demonstrates the decrease in regional cerebral blood flow (rCBF) in patients who have clinical vasospasm. This technique can quantify rCBF accurately, be repeated within 20 minutes, fuse rCBF data with conventional CT scan anatomy, and distinguish ischemia from other causes of neurologic deterioration after SAH.

e. **Jugular bulb oximetry** detects changes in cerebral oxygen extraction (AVDo$_2$). Patients who develop clinical vasospasm have a significant rise in AVDo$_2$ approximately 1 day before the onset of signs of neurologic deficit. Increases in AVDo$_2$ may therefore predict impending clinical vasospasm while an improvement in AVDo$_2$ reflects the patient's response to treatment.

f. **CBF-measuring modalities** include positron emission tomography, which demonstrates a fall in CMRo$_2$ after SAH and single-photon emission computed tomography (SPECT). Angiographic vasospasm, delayed ischemic deficit, and increased TCD velocities are associated with regions of hypoperfusion on SPECT.

3. **Treatment of vasospasm** involves pharmacologic and mechanical modalities.

a. **Early operation** for clip ligation of the aneurysmal neck permits the removal of a fresh clot by irrigation and suction. The surgeon may instill recombinant tissue plasminogen activator (rTPA) directly into the subarachnoid space to dissolve the remaining clot. This fibrinolytic drug can reduce vasospasm, but it also may cause bleeding by dissolving normal clots. Therefore, only patients at great risk of developing clinically significant vasospasm are candidates for this treatment.

b. **Early operative clip ligation and endovascular occlusion** of the aneurysm both facilitate the subsequent treatment of vasospasm. While patients who had better clinical grades (WFNS Grades I to III) on hospital admission and whose aneurysms were occluded with endovascular coils were less likely to develop symptomatic vasospasm as compared with those undergoing surgical clip ligation, there was no significant difference in overall outcome between those two groups at the longest follow-up period.

c. The prophylactic use of the **calcium antagonist** nimodipine within 96 hours of SAH is now a standard aspect of care after SAH. Although nimodipine reduces the incidence of vasospasm, the improvement in mortality has not been statistically significant when compared with control groups. Because nimodipine tends to decrease blood pressure, patients may require hydration and the administration of pressor drugs during the induction of anesthesia and careful attention to fluid balance intra- and postoperatively.

d. **Enoxaparin,** a low-molecular-weight heparin given as one subcutaneous injection of 20 mg/day, has been shown to improve overall outcome at 1 year after SAH by reducing delayed ischemic deficit and cerebral infarction. Patients receiving enoxaparin also had fewer intracranial bleeding events and a lower incidence of severe shunt-dependent hydrocephalus.

e. **Other drugs** used to treat vasospasm include tirilazad, an antioxidant and free radical scavenger whose clinical trials have demonstrated mixed results; nicaraven, a free radical scavenger associated with a trend toward improved mortality, good outcome, and smaller infarct size at 3 months; ebselen, an antioxidant and anti-inflammatory drug whose neuroprotective properties have caused it to be effective in the treatment of acute stroke; and fasudil, a kinase inhibitor used intra-arterially to treat vasospasm. The use of endothelin antagonists has been associated with an increase in the incidence of pneumonia and hypotensive episodes.

f. **"Triple-H therapy,"** hypertensive hypervolemic hemodilution, augments cerebral perfusion in vasospastic areas of the brain in which autoregulation is impaired through increases in blood pressure, cardiac output, and intravascular volume. Relative hemodilution to a hematocrit of 30% to 35% promotes blood flow through the cerebral microvasculature. The early institution of triple-H therapy is crucial to prevent the progression from vasospasm-induced mild ischemia to infarction. The expansion of intravascular volume is important after SAH because the total circulating blood volume and total circulating red cell volume are reduced secondary to supine diuresis, peripheral pooling, negative nitrogen balance, decreased erythropoiesis, iatrogenic blood loss, and increased natriuresis from the elaboration of natriuretic hormone.

(1) The guidelines for optimal volume expansion include a central venous pressure (CVP) of 10 mm Hg and a pulmonary capillary wedge pressure (PCWP) of 12 to 16 mm Hg. The vagal and diuretic response to intravascular volume augmentation may necessitate the administration of atropine, 1 mg intramuscularly (i.m.) every 3 to 4 hours, and aqueous vasopressin (Pitressin), 5 units i.m., to reduce urine output to <200 mL/hour. Hydrocortisone has also been used to attenuate the excessive natriuresis and consequent hyponatremia seen in patients after SAH and to prevent the decrease in total blood volume. The use of albumin to augment intravascular volume after the administration of normal saline has failed to increase the CVP above 8 mm Hg may improve clinical outcome at 3 months and reduce hospital costs.

(2) Vasopressor drugs, including dopamine, dobutamine, and phenylephrine, may be necessary to increase blood pressure. If the aneurysm has not been secured, systolic pressure is maintained at 120 to 150 mm Hg. After the aneurysm has been secured, systolic blood pressure may be increased to 160 to 200 mm Hg. Invasive hemodynamic monitoring including the direct measurement of systemic arterial blood pressure, CVP, pulmonary artery pressure, PCWP, and cardiac output improves the safety and efficacy of treatment with induced hypertension.

(3) The complications of triple-H therapy include rebleeding, transformation to hemorrhagic infarction, cerebral edema, intracranial hypertension, hypertensive encephalopathy, myocardial infarction, pulmonary edema, congestive heart failure, coagulopathy, dilutional hyponatremia, and the complications of central catheterization.

g. **Transluminal balloon angioplasty,** the mechanical dilatation of a cerebral vessel at a segment of spastic narrowing by the use of an inflatable intravascular balloon, may effect improvement in the patient's level of consciousness and focal ischemic deficits. Early intervention is crucial to success. The superselective intra-arterial infusion of papaverine has also been successful in dilating distal vessels, but because papaverine can be neurotoxic, verapamil, nimodipine, and nicardipine have been used instead. The complications of angioplasty include rupture of the aneurysm, rupture of intracranial vessels, intimal dissection, and cerebral ischemia and infarction.

4. **Prevention of vasospasm** requires attentive critical care, maintenance of normovolemia and electrolyte balance, monitoring of the level of consciousness and neurologic function in a critical care area until the peak time for the development of vasospasm has passed, and prevention of secondary cerebral insults and medical complications. After SAH, patients require 3 to 4 L of fluid per day to maintain normovolemia. Hypotonic solutions (e.g., lactated Ringer's solution) are avoided and hyponatremia is treated with either normal or hypertonic saline as necessary. The blood pressure is controlled before the aneurysm has been secured but not treated thereafter unless the elevation reaches critically high levels. Mannitol, ventricular drainage (with avoidance of a sudden drop in ICP and consequent rise in transmural pressure), and mild hyperventilation are used to maintain ICP in the normal range. The goal is to keep the CPP above 60 to 70 mm Hg.

IV. **Central nervous system (CNS) complications.** The CNS is directly affected by SAH and the resultant hematoma, vascular disruption, and edema, all of which decrease CBF and CMR_{O_2}. The patient's clinical grade correlates with the extent of neurologic impairment caused by the intracranial pathophysiology.

A. The cerebral vasculature's responsiveness to changes in CO_2 tension (Pa_{CO_2}) is preserved after SAH. A decline in CO_2 reactivity usually does not occur without extensive disruption of cerebral homeostasis.

B. SAH interferes with **cerebral autoregulation.** The upper and lower limits of autoregulation are higher in hypertensive patients.

C. Intracranial aneurysms themselves, particularly giant ones, and the SAH-induced hematoma and edema all have the potential for causing **intracranial hypertension** with a resultant decrease in the patient's level of consciousness and the potential for brain stem herniation and death. After SAH, the patient's Hunt and Hess clinical grade reflects the ICP. Grade I and II patients have normal ICP (but not necessarily normal elastance), whereas Grades IV and V patients have intracranial hypertension.

D. **Hydrocephalus** occurs in 10% of patients after SAH from obstruction of the CSF drainage pathways by either intraventricular or intraparenchymal blood and the subsequent development of arachnoidal adhesions that prevent reabsorption of CSF. Whether the aneurysm has been occluded by either surgical or endovascular means does not affect the patient's subsequent risk for the development of hydrocephalus.

1. **Acute hydrocephalus** occurs in 15% to 20% of patients. It is characterized by the onset of lethargy and coma within 24 hours of SAH and is associated with poor clinical grade on admission, either thick subarachnoid blood or intraventricular hemorrhage on initial CT scan, alcoholism, female gender, older age, increased aneurysm size, pneumonia, meningitis, and a preexisting history of hypertension. The development of acute ventricular dilatation immediately after SAH, a cause of the assignment of a spuriously poor neurologic grade, may require external ventricular drainage (EVD) to normalize ICP, especially if the patient's level of consciousness is depressed. Good results have been achieved when EVD is performed in conjunction with early occlusion of the aneurysm. While half of the patients who develop acute hydrocephalus go on to require a ventriculoperitoneal shunt, EVD can reduce the need for permanent shunting. Other predictors of the need for permanent shunting are poor grade on admission, rebleeding, and intraventricular hemorrhage.

2. **Chronic hydrocephalus,** which develops weeks later in 25% of patients who survive SAH, is an important cause of failure to improve in patients who are initially comatose and of secondary slow decline in those who were originally in good condition. Symptoms include impaired consciousness, dementia, gait disturbance, and incontinence. A CT scan is indicated a month after SAH to ascertain ventricular size.

E. The post-SAH incidence of **seizures** ranges from 3% to 26%. Early seizures occur in 1.5% to 5% of patients; late seizures occur in 3%. Seizures are detrimental to patients after SAH because they increase CBF and $CMRo_2$ and may precipitate rebleeding from the attendant rise in blood pressure. Patients at highest risk for the development of seizures have either thick cisternal blood or lobar intracerebral hemorrhage on CT scan. Other risk factors include rebleeding, vasospasm and delayed ischemic deficit, MCA aneurysms, subdural hematoma, and chronic neurologic impairment. The value of prophylactic anticonvulsant therapy is controversial, however, because most seizures occur in the first 24 hours after SAH and frequently before hospitalization. Neurosurgeons usually institute seizure prophylaxis with phenytoin, fosphenytoin, or levetiracetam for 1 to 2 weeks after SAH. Patients who have either an intracranial hemorrhage or more than one early seizure receive anticonvulsants for at least 6 months.

V. **Systemic sequelae of SAH**
  A. **Fluid and electrolyte balance**
    1. Most patients (30% to 100%) develop a decrease in intravascular volume after SAH that correlates with clinical grade and the presence of intracranial hypertension.
    2. Hyponatremia occurs from the release of atrial natriuretic factor from the hypothalamus. Treatment includes hydration with either normal or hypertonic (3%) saline to improve cerebral perfusion.
    3. Many patients (50% to 75%) develop hypokalemia and hypocalcemia and require replacement.
  B. **Cardiac sequelae**
    1. **Electrocardiographic (ECG) abnormalities** occur in 50% to 100% of patients after SAH. The most common are T-wave inversion and ST segment depression. Other changes include U waves, QT interval prolongation, and Q waves. These abnormalities are similar to those seen with cardiac ischemia and infarction and may predispose the patients to life-threatening arrhythmias. Prolongation of the corrected QT interval (QTc) makes patients particularly vulnerable to ventricular arrhythmias. The routine measurement of QTc may identify patients at risk for potentially lethal arrhythmias, a risk exacerbated by hypokalemia.
    2. **Rhythm disturbances,** seen in 30% to 80% of patients, include premature ventricular complexes (most commonly), sinus bradycardia and tachycardia, atrioventricular dissociation, atrial extrasystole, atrial fibrillation, brady- and tachyarrhythmias, and ventricular tachycardia and fibrillation. Arrhythmias occur most frequently within the first 7 days of SAH. The peak occurrence is between the 2nd and 3rd day.
    3. The **etiology** has been attributed to injury to the posterior hypothalamus with release of norepinephrine and resultant subendocardial ischemic changes and electrolyte disturbances. This increase in sympathetic tone can persist for the first week after SAH.
    4. The extent of myocardial dysfunction correlates with the severity of the neurologic injury after SAH.
    5. **Prophylactic adrenergic blockade** has improved cardiac outcome in some patients.

6. In determining whether to proceed with surgery on an emergent basis after SAH, the measurement of serial cardiac isoenzymes and the assessment of ventricular function by echocardiography help elucidate the degree of ischemia.

7. The use of a **pulmonary artery catheter** to monitor PCWP and cardiac output may facilitate management of both the patient's cardiac dysfunction and the response to triple-H therapy for the treatment of vasospasm.

8. The presence of either a severe arrhythmia, as occurs in 5% of the patients who have arrhythmias, or significant cardiogenic pulmonary edema may necessitate the **postponement of surgery** until treatment has been instituted although delay could put patients at risk for rebleeding and compromise the treatment of vasospasm.

C. **Respiratory system**
1. Pulmonary conditions including cardiogenic and neurogenic pulmonary edema, pneumonia, adult respiratory distress syndrome, and pulmonary emboli account for 50% of deaths from medical complications at 3 months after SAH. Medical complications themselves cause 23% of all deaths.

2. The majority (60%) of patients become symptomatic from pulmonary edema between days 0 and 7 after SAH; the largest number of cases presents on day 3. The incidence of pulmonary edema is greater in patients older than 30 years. Poor clinical grade at the time of admission also correlates with more respiratory dysfunction, suggesting neurogenic influences.

3. Treatment includes antibiotics, supportive care, and correction of intracranial (intracranial hypertension, cerebral edema, hydrocephalus) and fluid and electrolyte abnormalities.

D. **Other medical complications**
1. **Hepatic dysfunction** (hepatic failure and hepatitis) occurs in 25% of patients after SAH, correlates positively with poor clinical grade, and is frequently observed in patients who develop pulmonary edema.

2. **Renal dysfunction** is noted in 8% of patients after SAH and occurs more frequently in septic patients who are receiving antibiotics.

3. **Thrombocytopenia** occurs in 4% of patients after SAH and is associated with sepsis, severe neurologic deficits, and antibiotic use. Disseminated intravascular coagulation and leukocytosis have also been reported.

4. **Gastrointestinal bleeding** occurs in almost 5% of patients and should be part of the differential diagnosis of any unexpected episode of hypotension and tachycardia.

VI.   Surgical intervention

A.   Early aneurysmal clip ligation in the first 24 to 48 hours after SAH has advantages: prevention of rebleeding, reduction in vasospasm from removal of blood from the subarachnoid space ("intracranial toilet"), and ability to treat vasospasm through volume expansion and deliberate hypertension with relative safety. Other advantages include reductions in medical complications, patient anxiety, and the cost of hospitalization.

B.   The International Study on the Timing of Aneurysm Surgery, published in 1990, documented that early (0 to 3 days after SAH) and late (11 to 14 days) surgery yielded similar overall morbidity and mortality. The fact that results were better in the subset of North American patients who were alert and underwent early operation has made early surgical intervention a common practice.

VII.   Anesthesia for surgical intervention

A.   Preoperative evaluation includes the following:

1.   Review of neurodiagnostic studies (magnetic resonance imaging, CT scan, and cerebral angiogram)
2.   History and focused physical and neurologic examination
3.   Notation of ward blood pressures and association between blood pressure decrease and neurologic deterioration
4.   Assessment of fluid and electrolyte balance
5.   Cardiac history and ECG with determination of need for echocardiogram, cardiac isoenzymes, cardiac nuclear scanning, perioperative cardiovascular monitoring
6.   Notation of current drug regimen

B.   Premedication includes the following:

1.   Calcium channel-blocking drugs, anticonvulsants, and steroids are continued.
2.   Drugs to reduce gastric acidity (cimetidine, ranitidine) and speed gastric emptying (metoclopramide) are given before the induction of anesthesia.
3.   Sedatives, hypnotics, anxiolytics, and narcotics are used sparingly to avoid respiratory depression and the masking of neurologic deterioration. The anesthesiologist can administer small doses of intravenous narcotic (morphine, 1 to 4 mg; fentanyl, 25 to 50 mcg) and benzodiazepine (midazolam, 1 to 2 mg) to good-grade patients under direct supervision. Poor-grade patients do not receive premedication unless an endotracheal tube is in place, in which case they could require muscle relaxation, sedation, and blood pressure control.

C.   Monitoring during anesthesia includes:

1.   Cardiac rate, rhythm, and ischemia via ECG with V_5 lead

2. Direct intra-arterial blood pressure with pressure transducer at brain level to reflect cerebral perfusion
3. CVP through the antecubital, jugular, or subclavian route
4. PCWP and cardiac output in patients who have cardiac compromise or severe vasospasm
5. Intermittent arterial blood gases, glucose, electrolytes, osmolality, hematocrit
6. Brain temperature by tympanic or nasopharyngeal thermistor
7. CBF velocity by TCD ultrasonography
8. Electrophysiologic monitors: electroencephalogram (EEG); brain stem, auditory, somatosensory, and motor-evoked potentials
9. Jugular bulb venous oxygen saturation
10. Neuromuscular blockade, oxygen saturation, urine output, end-tidal CO_2

D. **Intravenous access.** The need for adequate intravenous access mandates the insertion of two large-bore intravenous catheters in addition to the CVP or pulmonary artery catheter before (a) positioning for operation, which may limit access to arteries and veins, and (b) interventions that will affect blood pressure, ICP, and transmural pressure.

E. **Induction of Anesthesia**
1. The induction period is critical because the rupture of the aneurysm at this juncture can be fatal. A smooth induction requires limitation of the hypertensive response to laryngoscopy and intubation, obliteration of coughing and straining on the endotracheal tube, and maintenance of adequate CPP while minimizing the change in transmural pressure across the wall of the aneurysm.
2. The ICP of good-grade patients (Grades 0, I, II) is usually normal; a decrease in blood pressure of 20% to 30% below the patient's normal value is not detrimental in the absence of evidence of cerebral ischemia. Poor-grade patients (Grades IV and V) already have the potential for ischemia secondary to intracranial hypertension and impaired perfusion. Decreasing the blood pressure of these patients may exacerbate the cerebral ischemia. Measures are still necessary, however, to blunt the sympathetic response to laryngoscopy and intubation.
3. Good-grade patients do not require hyperventilation during induction (Pa_{CO_2} 35 to 40 mm Hg) because they have normal intracranial elastance. Poor-grade patients who have intracranial hypertension benefit from moderate hyperventilation to a Pa_{CO_2} of 30 mm Hg during induction.

4. The intravenous induction of anesthesia confers loss of consciousness while maintaining cardiovascular and intracerebral homeostasis during catechol-releasing maneuvers by the administration of thiopental, 3 to 5 mg/kg, etomidate, 0.1 to 0.3 mg/kg, or propofol, 1 to 2 mg/kg; fentanyl, 3 to 5 mcg/kg, or remifentanil, 0.5 mcg/kg; lidocaine, 1.5 mg/kg; and midazolam, 0.1 to 0.2 mg/kg. The patient is ventilated by mask with 100% oxygen (Table 9-4).

5. If the patient does not have an increase in intracranial elastance, the introduction of isoflurane or sevoflurane before laryngoscopy deepens the anesthesia.

6. Additional fentanyl, 1 to 2 mcg/kg; propofol, 0.5 mg/kg; or lidocaine, 1.5 mg/kg, is given before brief gentle laryngoscopy and intubation to preserve hemodynamic and intracranial stability.

F. **Muscle relaxants**

1. **Vecuronium,** 0.1 mg/kg, a nondepolarizing muscle relaxant of intermediate duration, does not increase the heart rate (and blood pressure) or the ICP in the presence of a reduction in intracranial compliance.

2. **Succinylcholine** has increased ICP and caused ventricular fibrillation in patients after SAH. Susceptible patients include those who are comatose

Table 9-4. Induction of anesthesia for endovascular and operative treatment of intracranial aneurysms

Optimal head position	
Deep plane of anesthesia	
Fentanyl	0.5–1 mcg/kg
Remifentanil	0.5 mcg/kg
Thiopental	3–5 mg/kg
Propofol	1–2 mg/kg
Vecuronium	0.1 mg/kg
Low-dose inhaled anesthetic	0.5 minimum alveolar concentration
Controlled ventilation	100% oxygen
$Paco_2$ 35–40 mm Hg (normal ICP)	
$Paco_2$ 30–35 mm Hg (elevated ICP)	
Before laryngoscopy	
Lidocaine	1.5 mg/kg
Thiopental	2–3 mg/kg
Propofol	0.5 mg/kg
Brief, gentle laryngoscopy	
Intubation	

ICP, intracranial pressure.

but nonparetic; have flaccid paralysis, spasticity, or clonus after head injury; or move their extremities in response to pain but not command. For these patients, rocuronium, 0.6 mg/kg, which does not adversely affect CBF or ICP, is useful for rapid-sequence induction.

G. **Cardioactive drugs**
1. **Cardioactive drugs** counteract the hypertensive response to laryngoscopy and intubation. Esmolol, 0.5 mg/kg, and labetalol, 2.5 to 5 mg, block the chronotropic and inotropic effects of sympathetic stimulation without affecting CBF or ICP. Intravenous lidocaine is also useful for this purpose.
2. **SNP,** a direct-acting cerebral vasodilator, increases cerebral blood volume (CBV) and ICP. Although SNP, 100 mcg intravenously (i.v.), can prevent the hypertensive response to laryngoscopy and intubation, it may be detrimental in patients who have a reduction in intracranial compliance.
3. **Nitroglycerin** also increases CBV from the dilatation of capacitance vessels and therefore may increase ICP.
4. **The calcium channel-blocking drugs** nicardipine, 0.01 to 0.02 mg/kg, and diltiazem, 0.2 mg/kg or 10 mg, facilitate rapid control of hypertension intraoperatively. Neither drug decreases local CBF or blood flow velocity.

H. **Maintenance**
1. **Intravenous drugs** including propofol, narcotics, and nondepolarizing muscle relaxants are used together or in combination with 0.5 minimum alveolar concentration (MAC) of a volatile anesthetic for maintenance of anesthesia. It is important to be able to manipulate blood pressure, minimize brain retractor pressure through cerebral relaxation, and facilitate rapid emergence and timely neurologic assessment.
2. All inhalational anesthetics are cerebral vasodilators and have the potential for increasing ICP; all of them, with the exception of **nitrous oxide** (N_2O), depress cerebral metabolism. N_2O should be avoided, especially during the induction of anesthesia, in patients who have decreased intracranial compliance. It is introduced only after giving cerebral vasoconstricting drugs and establishing hypocapnia. Alternatively, the use of N_2O may be dispensed with altogether, especially if there is concern about the possibility of venous air embolism.
3. **Isoflurane** increases CBF minimally but has increased ICP despite hypocapnia in patients who have space-occupying lesions. Isoflurane is therefore used in low concentrations or avoided altogether in patients known to have a decrease

in intracranial compliance. The cerebral vascular effects of desflurane (4% to 6%) are similar to those of isoflurane. Sevoflurane is also a cerebral vasodilator but might not increase ICP when administered after the establishment of hypocapnia. The low blood-gas solubility coefficient of desflurane and sevoflurane permits rapid emergence and prompt postoperative neurologic evaluation.

4. **Fentanyl** and **remifentanil** improve cerebral relaxation during craniotomy in hyperventilated patients receiving isoflurane. Either fentanyl, bolus: 25 to 50 mcg i.v.; infusion: 1 to 2 mcg/kg/hour, or remifentanil, bolus: 0.25 mcg/kg; infusion: 0.05 to 2 mcg/kg/hour (depending on whether remifentanil is combined with 60% N_2O, 0.4 to 1.5 MAC of isoflurane, or propofol, 100 to 200 mcg/kg/minute) may be combined with isoflurane or sevoflurane or administered with an infusion of either thiopental, 1.0 to 1.5 mg/kg/hour, or propofol, 40 to 60 mcg/kg/minute, for the maintenance of anesthesia.

5. **Thiopental** may be useful as the primary anesthetic in a dose of up to 3 mg/kg/hour when the brain is "tight." The disadvantages of this approach are the potential for a slow recovery from anesthesia and the potential for systemic hypotension, which may be counteracted by volume expansion and enhancement of cardiac performance by monitoring pulmonary artery pressure and cardiac output.

I. **Emergence**

1. Good-grade patients may be awakened in the operating room and their tracheas extubated at the end of the operation. The avoidance of coughing, straining, hypercarbia, and hypertension is essential. Hypertension in the immediate postoperative period, secondary to preexisting hypertension, pain, urinary retention from a malfunctioning catheter, and CO_2 retention from residual anesthesia usually returns to normal within 12 hours. Antihypertensive drugs are administered as necessary.

2. If patients have received remifentanil intraoperatively, longer-acting narcotics are administered before the conclusion of the operation to confer analgesia in the immediate postoperative period.

3. The blood pressure of patients whose aneurysms have been wrapped rather than clipped or who have other untreated aneurysms is maintained within 20% of their normal range (120 to 160 mm Hg systolic) to avoid rupture during emergence.

4. Hypervolemia and relative hemodilution are maintained in the postoperative period.

5. Both poor preoperative status (Grade III to V) and a catastrophic intraoperative event (e.g., brain swelling, aneurysmal rupture, ligation of a feeding vessel) mandate continued intubation, sedation, and postoperative ventilatory support.

6. When the patient either fails to awaken or has a new neurologic deficit at the conclusion of the operation, the residual effects of sedatives, narcotics, muscle relaxants, and inhalational drugs should be reversed or dissipated, the $Paco_2$ normalized, and other causes of depressed consciousness (e.g., hypoxia, hyponatremia) ruled out or treated. Both the persistence of diminished responsiveness and a new neurologic deficit for 2 hours after surgery require a CT scan to diagnose the presence of hematoma, hydrocephalus, pneumocephalus, infarction, or edema. An angiogram is helpful in demonstrating vascular occlusion.

VIII. **Intraoperative management**
A. **Fluid administration**
   1. Patients have an SAH-induced decrease in circulating blood volume and therefore require hydration with isotonic crystalloid solution before the induction of anesthesia to preserve cerebral perfusion.
   2. Full restoration of the intravascular volume to a state of modest hypervolemia occurs after the aneurysm has been clipped. Glucose-free crystalloid solutions are administered because both focal and global ischemic deficits can be exacerbated by hyperglycemia. Normal saline and other isotonic solutions are preferable to lactated Ringer's solution, which is hypo-osmolar to plasma and can lead to cerebral edema if the blood-brain barrier is disrupted.
   3. Blood and blood products are indicated to maintain the hematocrit at 30% to 35%. Blood is available in the operating room when the dissection of the aneurysm commences. The use of 5% albumin can confer some rheologic advantage. The administration of >500 mL of hetastarch can, however, interfere with hemostasis and cause intracranial bleeding.
B. **Cerebral volume reduction**
   1. The volume of the intracranial contents is reduced and brain relaxation improved to facilitate the surgical approach to the aneurysm after the opening of the dura.
   2. Moderate hyperventilation to a $Paco_2$ of 30 to 35 mm Hg is maintained until the dura is incised at which time the $Paco_2$ is reduced to 25 to 30 mm Hg to decrease CBF, CBV, and brain bulk. With a preoperative increase in intracranial

elastance, the Pa_{CO_2} is reduced to 25 to 30 mm Hg during induction. Higher Pa_{CO_2} values are necessary in patients who have vasospasm and during the period of induced hypotension.

3. Mannitol starts working within 10 to 15 minutes of the administration of 0.25 to 1 gm/kg, which should occur after turning the bone flap to avoid any decrease in CBV and ICP. Furosemide, 0.25 to 1.0 mg/kg, potentiates the action of mannitol and diminishes the dose.

4. CSF may be drained through a lumbar sub-arachnoid catheter inserted after the induction of anesthesia, a ventricular catheter, or intraoperative cannulation of the basal cisterns. Leakage of CSF is avoided while the cranium is closed to prevent a decrease in ICP and the concomitant rise in transmural pressure. If the ICP is elevated preoperatively, the escape of CSF from the subarachnoid puncture before craniotomy may also cause tonsillar herniation.

C. **Temporary proximal occlusion**

1. **Controlled hypotension** during microscopic dissection of the aneurysm with SNP, esmolol, or isoflurane has been advocated in the past to reduce the risk of rupture by decreasing aneurysmal wall tension and augmenting the malleability of the aneurysmal neck. Such artificial lowering of the blood pressure also decreases bleeding. Controlled hypotension can, however, compromise rCBF in patients who have SAH-induced dysautoregulation. Because patients with SAH have a higher incidence of cerebral ischemia, infarction, and postoperative neurologic deficit, neurosurgeons prefer to avoid the use of induced hypotension. An exception may be made to gain control of the parent vessel if the aneurysmal sac ruptures during surgical manipulation. Relative contraindications to induced hypotension include the presence of intracerebral hematoma, occlusive cerebrovascular disease, coronary artery disease, renal dysfunction, anemia, and fever.

2. Neurosurgeons now favor **temporary proximal occlusion** of the aneurysm's parent vessel to reduce the risk of rupture during aneurysmal manipulation. The application of temporary clips decreases the turgor of the aneurysmal sac through "local hypotension" and a reduction in blood flow.

3. The **risks** of distal ischemia and infarction, cerebral edema, and damage to the parent vessel are directly related to the duration of temporary occlusion and the integrity of the collateral

circulation. The chance of developing a new neurologic deficit after temporary proximal occlusion is exacerbated by older age, poor preoperative neurologic status, and aneurysms involving the distributions of the basilar and middle cerebral arteries.

4. Drugs suggested for **cerebral protection** during temporary occlusion include mannitol, vitamin E, and dexamethasone. Thiopental, 3 to 5 mg/kg, may be administered as a bolus immediately before temporary occlusion.

5. **Mild hypothermia** to 32°C to 34°C has been investigated as a cerebral protective adjunct during aneurysm surgery. The preliminary results from the International Hypothermia in Aneurysm Surgery Trial, completed in 2003, failed to demonstrate any alteration in outcome for patients who were cooled before aneurysmal clip ligation.

6. The **duration of temporary occlusion** is 20 minutes or less because studies have shown a higher incidence of neurologic deficit and infarction postoperatively when the duration exceeds that limit. Some neurosurgeons even recommend removal of the temporary clip at 10 minutes of occlusion to reestablish perfusion and then reapplication after an additional dose of thiopental.

7. To **enhance collateral circulation** during temporary proximal occlusion, the patient's blood pressure is maintained in the high-normal range. This may require dopamine or phenylephrine, although patients who have coronary artery disease may be at risk for the development of cardiac ischemia.

D. **Intraoperative aneurysmal rupture**

1. **Rupture** of the aneurysm during induction of anesthesia and operation (7% before dissection, 48% during dissection, 45% during clip ligation) markedly increases mortality and morbidity because of the ischemia attendant upon the hypotension and surgical maneuvers to secure the aneurysmal neck including temporary proximal and distal occlusion. Normotension is maintained during this time to maximize collateral perfusion.

2. **Diagnosis** of rupture during or after induction is based on an abrupt increase in blood pressure with or without bradycardia. The ICP might increase as well. The TCD may demonstrate the rupture and the efficacy of management.

3. **Therapy** is designed to maintain cerebral perfusion, control ICP, and reduce bleeding by lowering the systemic pressure with thiopental or SNP

after restoring the intravascular volume with crystalloid, colloid, blood, and blood products.

4. Intraoperative rupture of the aneurysm requires **rapid surgical control.** After restoration of intravascular volume, the MAP may be reduced briefly to 40 to 50 mm Hg to facilitate clip ligation of the aneurysmal neck or temporary proximal and distal occlusion of the parent vessel. Once the parent vessel is occluded, the blood pressure is increased to enhance collateral circulation.

IX. **Endovascular treatment.** See Chapter 16A.

A. Interventional neuroradiologists are now able to treat aneurysms with **endovascular technology** as an alternative to operation, depending on the age of the patient and the size and location of the aneurysm. Most commonly, the Guglielmi detachable metal coil is threaded into the aneurysmal sac through a catheter inserted into the cerebral vascular tree through the femoral artery, cannulation of which can be extremely stimulating.

B. For good-grade patients who have small, anterior-circulation aneurysms, endovascular coil treatment is significantly more likely than neurosurgical treatment to result in survival free of disability 1 year after the SAH. Institutions that offer endovascular services also have lower rates of in-hospital mortality for both endovascular and surgical cases. Long-term follow-up data are necessary to determine whether endovascular or operative treatment is safer and more effective in this subgroup of patients.

C. The **challenges** of anesthesia for interventional neuroradiology include work in a location remote from the operating room, the need for communication with a team perhaps unfamiliar with the requirements of patients undergoing anesthesia for neurosurgical procedures, and the need for the anesthesiologist to have a thorough understanding of the technicalities, pace, and interventions planned by the interventional neuroradiologists. The anesthesiologist must also be familiar with the plan for anticoagulation (degree, duration, timing of reversal) and the potential intraprocedural requirement for induced hypotension, hypertension, and hypercapnia. Above all, the attention to the patient's comfort and safety, the precautions (two large-bore intravenous catheters, comfortable pillow, padding of all pressure points), and the monitoring (standard monitors plus direct intra-arterial blood pressure measurement when manipulation of blood pressure is required) for both conscious sedation and general anesthesia in the interventional suite must be identical to those indicated when patients are anesthetized in the operating room.

D. Anesthesia for endovascular procedures includes conscious sedation and general anesthesia. **Conscious sedation** offers the advantage of conferring the ability to perform intermittent neurologic examination. Some interventional neuroradiologists prefer **general anesthesia** because the quality of the images improves when patients are rendered motionless. Because access to the airway is limited, it is important to secure the airway before the procedure begins. Endotracheal intubation offers the combination of absolute control of ventilation, adequate conditions for intracranial manipulation, and excellent images. The **choice of anesthetic drugs** includes either total intravenous anesthesia or a combination of intravenous and inhalational anesthetics with or without muscle relaxation. The rapid return to consciousness at the conclusion of the procedure is important to facilitate neurologic evaluation.

E. Complications include both hemorrhagic and occlusive catastrophes. Differentiation between the two is important. If the problem is **hemorrhagic**, immediate administration of protamine to reverse the anticoagulation and maintenance of the blood pressure in the low-normal range are indicated. **Occlusive** problems require deliberate hypertension titrated to the neurologic examination either with or without direct thrombolysis. Other emergent interventions include volume expansion, head-up tilt, hyperventilation, diuretics, anticonvulsant drugs, hypothermia to 33°C to 34°C, and the infusion of thiopental to achieve encephalographic (EEG) burst suppression.

X. Hypothermic circulatory arrest for giant and vertebrobasilar aneurysms

A. Giant cerebral aneurysms are larger than 2.5 cm in diameter, lack an anatomic neck, and have perforating vessels traversing the aneurysmal wall. They represent 5% of all aneurysms and cause headache, visual disturbance, cranial nerve palsies, and signs and symptoms of an intracranial mass lesion.

B. Surgical treatment of giant aneurysms, associated with significant perioperative morbidity and mortality, uses proximal and distal temporary occlusion to collapse the aneurysm and empty the aneurysmal sac during circulatory arrest with adenosine under profound hypothermia. Circulatory arrest affords good visualization, a bloodless field, and easy aneurysmal manipulation and clip placement. Endovascular techniques may be an option only if the aneurysm is not wide necked and there is no need to debulk it.

C. Decreasing the cerebral metabolic rate for oxygen consumption affords **cerebral protection** during circulatory arrest. **Barbiturates** reduce the active component (maintenance of neuronal activity) of the cerebral metabolic rate and may be administered before cooling and arrest as either a single dose of 30 to 40 mg/kg over 30 minutes or as a continuous infusion. **Hypothermia** reduces the active and basal (maintenance of cellular integrity) components of cerebral oxygen consumption and confers protection during anoxic conditions. The tolerable period of circulatory arrest doubles for every 8°C temperature reduction. At 15°C to 18°C, clinical circulatory arrest has been used safely for up to 60 minutes.

1. Brain temperature may be measured directly and correlates closely with esophageal, tympanic membrane, and nasopharyngeal thermistors but not rectal or bladder temperatures.

2. Hypothermia increases blood viscosity with the sludging of red blood cells. The deliberate lowering of the hematocrit through phlebotomy and simultaneous volume repletion with crystalloid avoids this complication while preserving platelet-rich autologous blood for transfusion during rewarming.

D. **Monitors** include direct arterial and CVP measurement, EEG to indicate burst suppression, somatosensory evoked potentials to measure sensory conduction to the cortex, brain stem auditory evoked potentials, and transesophageal echocardiography to assess ventricular function.

E. The major **postoperative complications** associated with hypothermic circulatory arrest are coagulopathy and intracranial hemorrhage. Risks may be reduced by the following:

1. The surgeon dissects the aneurysm and achieves hemostasis before the initiation of hypothermic circulatory arrest.

2. The activated clotting time (ACT) is maintained between 400 and 450 seconds after heparinization. After rewarming, protamine is used to reverse heparinization to achieve an ACT of 100 to 150 seconds.

3. Previously phlebotomized blood is transfused, and additional blood products (fresh frozen plasma, cryoprecipitate, platelets) are given as needed.

4. Hemostasis is achieved before dural closure.

SUGGESTED READINGS

Bendo AA, Kass IS, Hartung J, et al. Anesthesia for neurosurgery. In: Barash PG, Cullen B, Stoelting R, eds. *Clinical Anesthesia*, 2nd ed, Philadelphia, PA: Lippincott Williams & Wilkins, 2006:746–789.

Bernadini GL, DeShaies EM. Critical care of intracerebral and subarachnoid hemorrhage. *Curr Neurol Neurosci Res* 2001;1:568–576.

Classen J, Vu A, Kreiter KT, et al. Effect of acute physiologic derangements on outcome after subarachnoid hemorrhage. *Crit Care Med* 2004;32:832.

deGans K, Nieuwkamp DJ, Rinkel GJE, et al. Timing of aneurysm surgery in subarachnoid hemorrhage. *Neurosurgery* 2002;50:336–342.

Dorsch NW. Therapeutic approaches to vasospasm in subarachnoid hemorrhage. *Curr Opin Crit Care* 2002;8:128–133.

Ferch R, Pasqualin A, Pinna G, et al. Temporary arterial occlusion in the repair of ruptured intracranial aneurysms: an analysis of risk factors for stroke. *J Neurosurg* 2002;97:836–842.

Hashimoto T, Gupta DK, Young WL. Interventional neuroradiology—anesthetic considerations. *Anesthesiol Clin N Am* 2002;20:347.

International Subarachnoid Aneurysm Trial (ISAT) Collaborative Group. International Subarachnoid Aneurysm Trial (ISAT) of neurosurgical clipping versus endovascular coiling in 2143 patients with ruptured intracranial aneurysms: a randomized trial. *The Lancet* 2002;360:1267–1273.

Janjua N, Mayer SA. Cerebral vasospasm after subarachnoid hemorrhage. *Curr Opin Crit Care* 2003;9:113–119.

Kimme P, Fridrikssen S, Engdahl O, et al. Moderate hypothermia for 359 operations to clip cerebral aneurysms. *Br J Anaesth* 2004;93:343–347.

Liu AY, Lopez JR, Do HM, et al. Neurophysiological monitoring in the endovascular therapy of aneurysms. *Am J Neuroradiol* 2003;24:1520–1527.

McKhann GM, Mayer S, Le Roux P. Perioperative and intensive care of patients with aneurysmal subarachnoid hemorrhage. In: Le Roux P, Winn HR, Newell DW, eds. *Management of Cerebral Aneurysms.* Philadelphia, PA: Elsevier Science, 2004:303–333.

Newfield P, Hamid RKA, Lam AM. Anesthetic management—intracranial aneurysms and A-V malformations. In: Albin M, ed. *Textbook of Neuroanesthesia with Neurosurgical and Neuroscience Perspectives.* New York, NY: McGraw-Hill, 1997:859–900.

Niskanen M, Koivisto T, Rinne J, et al. Complications and postoperative care in patients undergoing treatment for unruptured intracranial aneurysms. *J Neurosurg Anesthesiol* 2005;17:100–105.

Osborn IP. Anesthetic considerations for interventional neuroradiology. *Int Anesthesiol Clin* 2003;41:69–77.

Rabinstein AA, Pichelmann MA, Friedman JA, et al. Symptomatic vasospasm and outcomes following aneurysmal subarachnoid hemorrhage: a comparison between surgical repair and endovascular coil occlusion. *J Neurosurg* 2003;98:319–325.

Sen J, Belli A, Alban H, et al. Triple-H therapy in the management of aneurysmal subarachnoid hemorrhage. *Lancet Neurol* 2003;2:614–621.

Solenski NJ, Haley EC Jr, Kassell NF, et al. Medical complications of aneurysmal subarachnoid hemorrhage: a report of the multicenter cooperative aneurysm study. *Crit Care Med* 1995;23:1007–1117.

Sommargren CE. Electrocardiographic abnormalities in patients with subarachnoid hemorrhage. *Am J Crit Care* 2002;11:48–56.

Tregiarri MM, Walder B, Suter PM, et al. Systematic review of the prevention of delayed ischemic neurological deficits with hypertension, hypervolemia, and hemodilution therapy following subarachnoid hemorrhage. *J Neurosurg* 2003;98:978.

Yamada M, Nishikawa K, Kawahara F, et al. Anesthetic management for clipping a giant basilar aneurysm with moderate hypothermia, extracorporeal circulation assistance, and propofol infusion. *J Neurosurg Anesthesiol* 2003;15:274–277.

Ischemic Cerebrovascular Disease

Ian A. Herrick, Miguel F. Arango, and
Adrian W. Gelb

Patients presenting for carotid endarterectomy (CEA) are often elderly, have advanced cerebrovascular disease, and frequently have significant coexisting diseases involving other organ systems. Anesthetic management of these patients requires both an understanding of the physiologic stress imposed by the surgical procedure (disruption of the major cerebral hemispheric blood supply) and an appreciation of the physiologic constraints imposed by the coexisting diseases.

I. Guidelines for performing CEA

A. Several prospective, randomized studies have reported superior outcome for medically stable patients who have symptomatic, high-grade carotid stenoses (70% to 99%) after CEA combined with best medical therapy compared to medical treatment alone.

B. On the basis of these studies, both the American Heart Association and the Canadian Neurosurgical Society have formulated guidelines for performing CEA (Table 10-1).

C. Subgroup analyses of the results of these multicenter trials have expanded the selection criteria for patients likely to benefit from CEA to include older patients and those who have complex carotid disease (e.g., tandem extracranial–intracranial stenoses). As a result, anesthesiologists can expect to care more frequently for older patients and those at increased risk for complications.

D. Endovascular treatment for carotid stenosis—carotid angioplasty and stenting (CAS)—has been developed over the past several years. Although CAS are increasingly used in clinical practice, the utility and durability are still undergoing clinical trials which will better define indications.

E. CEA remains the preferred surgical intervention for the prevention of stroke among patients who have extracranial cerebrovascular disease.

II. Physiologic considerations

A. **Cerebral blood flow (CBF) and metabolism**

1. The brain is highly active metabolically but is essentially devoid of oxygen and glucose reserves, making it dependent on the continuous delivery of oxygen and glucose by cerebral circulation.

Table 10-1.   Surgery guidelines for carotid endarterectomy

- Appropriate candidate for CEA
    Symptomatic 70%–99% stenosis with
        TIA(s) or nondisabling stroke
        Surgically accessible stenosis
        Stable medical and neurologic condition
- Uncertain candidate for CEA[a]
    Symptomatic <70% stenosis with[b]
        TIA(s) or nondisabling stroke
        Surgically accessible stenosis
        Stable medical and neurologic condition
    Asymptomatic >60% stenosis with
        Surgically accessible stenosis
        Stable medical condition
- Inappropriate candidate for CEA
    Asymptomatic ≤60% stenosis
    Symptomatic or asymptomatic with
        Intracranial stenoses more severe than the extracranial
            stenosis
        Uncontrolled diabetes mellitus, hypertension, congestive
            heart failure, or unstable angina pectoris
        A major neurologic deficit or decreased level of
            consciousness

The percentage stenosis should be defined by cerebral angiography and the NASCET method. The surgeon's rate of surgical complications (stroke or death) should be <6% for CEA in cases of symptomatic stenoses (appropriate or uncertain candidates), and <3% in cases of asymptomatic stenoses (uncertain candidates).
[a]Guidelines uncertain = insufficient evidence to support a definitive recommendation.
[b]Guideline for symptomatic <70% stenosis expected to be clarified this year with publication of NASCET results for this group of patients.
TIA, transient ischemic attack; CEA, carotid endarterectomy; NASCET, North American Symptomatic Carotid Endarterectomy Trial.
Adapted from Findlay JM, et al. Guidelines for the use of carotid endarterectomy: current recommendations from the Canadian Neurosurgical Society. *Can Med Assoc J* 1997;157:653.

2. CBF is provided by the internal carotid arteries (approximately 80%) and the vertebral arteries (approximately 20%), which anastomose at the base of the brain to form the circle of Willis.
3. Patients who have advanced occlusive cerebrovascular disease may be dependent on other collateral channels to maintain adequate CBF.
4. Normally, CBF is autoregulated to match the brain's metabolic requirements and maintain normal neuronal function.
B. **Cerebral perfusion**
1. CBF is related to cerebral perfusion pressure (CPP) and cerebrovascular resistance (CVR) according to the equation CBF = CPP/CVR.
2. The following factors affect CBF:

        a. CPP equals mean arterial blood pressure (MAP) minus intracranial pressure or central venous pressure, whichever is higher.

        b. CVR is a function of blood viscosity and the diameter of the cerebral resistance vessels.

    3. Optimization of CBF during CEA is hampered by the fact that the only factors readily amenable to intraoperative manipulation are arterial blood pressure and arterial carbon dioxide tension (Pa_{CO_2}), which impact on CPP and CVR, respectively.

C. Carbon dioxide tension Pa_{CO_2}

    1. Within the range of Pa_{CO_2} from 20 to 80 mm Hg, CBF changes by 1 to 2 mL/100 g/minute for every 1 mm Hg change in Pa_{CO_2}.

    2. The most common approach to ventilatory management during CEA is to maintain normocapnia. This is achieved by ventilation to a Pa_{CO_2} that produces a normal pH in the absence of coexisting metabolic acidosis.

D. Blood pressure

    1. CBF remains remarkably constant within the range of MAP from 50 to 150 mm Hg. Beyond this range, the limit of vasomotor activity is exceeded and CBF directly depends on changes in CPP.

    2. In patients who have preexisting chronic hypertension, both the upper and lower limits of autoregulation are shifted to higher pressures.

    3. In patients who have cerebrovascular disease, the CBF response to changes in Pa_{CO_2} during carotid cross-clamping is impaired. Under these conditions, improvement in CBF is likely to depend largely on increases in CPP, emphasizing the relatively greater importance of blood pressure control during CEA surgery.

    4. During CEA, blood pressure should be maintained within the normal preoperative range. Mild increases in systolic blood pressure of up to 20% above normal at the time of cross-clamping are acceptable, but hypotension and severe hypertension should be avoided.

III. Preanesthetic assessment

  A. The patient's state of health is determined from the medical history, pertinent physical examination, and chart review.

  B. Coexisting diseases are assessed and optimized. Common coexisting diseases include coronary artery disease, arterial hypertension, peripheral vascular disease, chronic obstructive pulmonary disease, diabetes mellitus, and renal insufficiency.

  C. For patients who have diabetes, perioperative blood glucose should be carefully managed to avoid both hypo- and hyperglycemia. Current evidence suggests that hyperglycemia adversely affects outcome after temporary focal or global cerebral ischemia.

D. Cardiac complications are a major source of mortality after CEA. Preoperative factors reported to correlate with increased perioperative cardiac morbidity include poorly controlled hypertension, congestive heart failure, and recent myocardial infarction.

E. Cerebral angiograms should also be reviewed to identify patients at increased risk from the presence of significant contralateral carotid artery disease or poor collateral circulation.

F. A risk stratification scheme for perioperative complications has been proposed for patients undergoing CEA (Table 10-2).

IV. Anesthetic management. CEA can be safely performed under general anesthesia, regional anesthesia, or local anesthetic infiltration. Experienced centers report similar morbidity and mortality, and available evidence is insufficient to establish the definitive superiority of any one technique.

A. Regional anesthesia

1. Superficial and deep cervical plexus blocks are the most commonly used regional anesthetic techniques for CEA.

   a. A superficial cervical plexus block is performed by injecting a local anesthetic subcutaneously along the posterior border of the sternocleidomastoid muscle where the cutaneous branches of the plexus fan out to innervate the skin of the lateral neck.

   b. A deep cervical plexus block is a paravertebral block of the C2-4 nerve roots. This technique involves injecting local anesthetic at the vertebral foramina (transverse processes) of the C2-4 vertebrae to block the neck muscles, fascia, and greater occipital nerve.

   c. Many regional anesthesia textbooks describe the techniques in detail and should be reviewed before performing the blocks.

2. Intraoperative monitors include the following:

   a. Intra-arterial cannula for blood pressure measurement

   b. Continuous electrocardiogram (ECG)

   c. Pulse oximetry

   d. Capnography sampled via nasal prongs for monitoring respiratory rate

3. Supplemental oxygen should be provided through a mask or nasal prongs positioned to avoid the site of surgery.

4. Carefully titrated sedation using small, repeated, intravenous doses of fentanyl, 10 to 25 mcg, and/or midazolam, 0.5 to 2 mg, should render the patient comfortable and cooperative during the operation. Propofol is a reasonable alternative

Table 10-2.   Preoperative risk stratification for patients undergoing carotid endarterectomy

Risk Group	Characteristics	Total Morbidity and Mortality (%)
1	Neurologically stable, no major medical or angiographic risk	1
2	Neurologically stable, significant angiographic risk, no major medical risk	2
3	Neurologically stable, major medical risk, ± major angiographic risk	7
4	Neurologically unstable, ± major medical or angiographic risk	10

Type of Risk	Risk Factors
Medical risk	Angina
	Myocardial infarction (<6 mo)
	Congestive heart failure
	Severe hypertension (>180/110 mm Hg)
	Chronic obstructive pulmonary disease
	Age >70 y
	Severe obesity
Neurologic risk	Progressing deficit
	New deficit (<24 hr)
	Frequent daily TIA(s)
	Multiple cerebral infarcts
Angiographic risk	Contralateral ICA occlusion
	ICA siphon stenosis
	Proximal or distal plaque extension
	High carotid bifurcation
	Presence of soft thrombus

TIA, transient ischemic attack; ICA, internal carotid artery.
Adapted from Sundt TM Jr, Sandok BA, Whisnant JP. Carotid endarterectomy. Complications and preoperative assessment of risk. *Mayo Clinic Proc* 1975;50:301–306. Reproduced with permission from Herrick IA, Gelb AW. Occlusive cerebrovascular disease: anesthetic considerations. In: Cottrell JE, Smith DS, eds. *Anesthesia and Neurosurgery*, 3rd ed. St Louis, MO: Mosby, 1994:484.

administered as intermittent intravenous bolus doses, 0.3 to 0.5 mg/kg, or as a low-dose continuous infusion, 10–50 mg/kg/hr. The potential advantages of using dexmedetomidine, an alpha$_2$-agonist, include supplemental sedation, modest analgesia, minimal respiratory depression, and preserved cognitive function. Careful attention is necessary during administration to avoid hemodynamic instability (i.e., transient hypertension, hypotension, and bradycardia).

5. Equipment should be immediately available to convert to a general anesthetic if intraoperative conditions warrant.

6. Advantages of regional anesthesia include the following:
   a. Superior neurologic monitoring associated with an awake patient
   b. Potential to minimize interventions such as shunt insertion based on the presence or absence of neurologic symptoms at cross-clamping
   c. Less expensive
   d. Reports of more rapid recovery and shorter hospitalization

7. Disadvantages of regional anesthesia include the following:
   a. Requirement of an operating room staff committed to working with patients under regional anesthesia, which necessitates patience, gentle technique, and reinforcement of the block as needed
   b. Lack of airway and ventilatory control
   c. Potential need to deal with complications in an awake patient: stroke or transient cerebral ischemia, cross-clamp intolerance, seizure, airway obstruction, hypoventilation, confusion, agitation, and angina
   d. Complications associated with cervical plexus blocks: local anesthetic toxicity, inadvertent injection into either the subarachnoid space or the vertebral artery, and phrenic or recurrent laryngeal nerve block

B. **General anesthesia**
   1. General anesthesia represents the most common anesthetic technique for CEA.
   2. Intraoperative monitors are the same as for regional anesthesia.
      a. Monitoring central venous and pulmonary artery pressure is used infrequently. A central venous catheter facilitates the management of intraoperative fluid administration and provides central access for drug administration or resuscitation. A pulmonary artery catheter may be helpful in patients who have high-risk cardiovascular disease (e.g., unstable angina, poor left ventricular function, recent myocardial infarction). Care should be exercised to avoid carotid puncture when inserting these catheters into the jugular vein.
   3. The key consideration during the induction of anesthesia is the maintenance of stable

hemodynamic conditions during intubation, positioning, and draping.

4. Thiopental, midazolam, propofol, and etomidate are all appropriate induction drugs and should be supplemented with opioid.

5. All of the nondepolarizing neuromuscular-blocking drugs facilitate tracheal intubation. Succinylcholine is a reasonable alternative. However, its use is contraindicated in patients who have had a recent paretic cerebral infarct.

6. General anesthesia is usually maintained with a combination of volatile anesthetic (typically isoflurane, desflurane, or sevoflurane) and opioid. Neuromuscular blockade is maintained throughout the procedure. Propofol infusion is a reasonable alternative. The use of remifentanil, an ultrashort-acting opioid, has also become popular as an adjunct to general anesthesia for CEA. Its short duration of action facilitates titration of anesthesia and promotes early emergence, particularly when used in combination with short-acting volatile anesthetic drugs such as desflurane and sevoflurane.

7. The administration of nitrous oxide is controversial as a result of reports of potential adverse effects on cerebral metabolism and increased risk of postoperative vomiting.

8. Blood pressure is maintained at preoperative levels. Small bolus doses of vasopressor (e.g., phenylephrine, 40 to 60 mcg, or ephedrine, 5 to 7.5 mg) can be administered to support blood pressure if necessary. Some anesthesiologists use infusions of phenylephrine to maintain or increase blood pressure, especially during cross-clamping. However, evidence suggests that this practice may be associated with an increased risk of myocardial ischemia.

9. Ventilation is adjusted to maintain normocapnia.

10. Advantages of general anesthesia include the following:
    a. Is potentially more comfortable for patients and operating room staff
    b. Facilitates intraoperative control of ventilation, airway, and sympathetic responses
    c. Facilitates management of complications (e.g., cross-clamp intolerance and transient cerebral ischemia) through the use of induced hypertension or pharmacologic suppression of electroencephalographic (EEG) activity
    d. Reduces the need for expedience in performing surgery because patient tolerance is not a factor
    e. May provide some cerebral protection

    11. Disadvantages of general anesthesia include the following:

        a. There is the need for an alternate method for monitoring cerebral function.

        b. In the absence of a completely reliable cerebral function monitor, it is possible that some remediable complications will not be detected before the occurrence of irreversible neuronal injury (e.g., cross-clamp intolerance, kink in carotid shunt).

        c. Prolonged emergence might confuse postoperative evaluation.

        d. It is more expensive.

C. Carotid cross-clamping

    1. Before cross-clamping, heparin, 75 to 100 U/kg, is administered intravenously.

    2. Carotid cross-clamping is often associated with an increase in blood pressure of up to approximately 20% above preoperative levels. Excessive increases can reflect cerebral ischemia. This should be considered before controlling the increase in blood pressure pharmacologically.

    3. Neurologic monitoring

        a. The purpose of neurologic monitoring is to identify patients at risk for adverse neurologic outcome owing to the development of cerebral ischemia, particularly during carotid cross-clamping.

        b. An awake patient represents the least expensive and most sensitive neurologic function monitoring during CEA.

        c. Because patients are not awake during general anesthesia, various other techniques are available to monitor neurologic function. EEG, carotid stump pressure measurements, transcranial Doppler (TCD), cerebral oximetry, and CBF measurements are used most commonly, either individually or in combination (i.e., EEG and TCD).

        d. Each of these techniques can identify significant reductions in cerebral perfusion. However, controversy continues regarding the reliability of these techniques, individually or in combination, to predict outcome accurately.

        e. Interventions available but unproven in clinical trials in response to evidence of cerebral ischemia include the following:

            (1) Increasing CPP by administering systemic vasopressor drugs (e.g., phenylephrine)

            (2) Reducing the risk of ischemia by pharmacologic suppression of cerebral metabolic requirements (e.g., thiopental, propofol)

        (3) Restoring internal carotid artery blood flow by inserting a carotid shunt

D. Emergence
1. Emergence should be designed to avoid excessive coughing or straining and surges in systemic blood pressure, which might open the freshly closed arteriotomy.
2. Heparin is usually partially reversed at the time of wound closure.
3. Many surgeons prefer patients to be awake and their tracheas extubated at the conclusion of the procedure to facilitate neurologic examination in the early postoperative period.

V. Postanesthetic management
A. The intra-arterial cannula is maintained during the initial postoperative period to permit continuous blood pressure monitoring.
B. All patients receive supplemental oxygen postoperatively. Pulse oximetry monitors the adequacy of oxygenation. Bilateral CEA is associated with the abolition of the ventilatory and cardiovascular responses to hypoxemia. Providing supplemental oxygen and closely monitoring ventilatory status are particularly important in these patients.
C. Postoperative hemodynamic instability occurs in >40% of patients after CEA and is postulated to be related to carotid baroreceptor dysfunction.
1. CEA performed using a carotid sinus nerve-sparing technique is associated with a higher incidence of postoperative hypotension, most likely because of increased exposure of the carotid sinus after removal of the atheromatous plaque. Associated with a marked decrease in systemic vascular resistance, hypotension can be prevented or treated with local anesthetic blockade of the carotid sinus nerve, the administration of intravenous fluid or, if necessary, the administration of vasopressor drugs such as phenylephrine.
2. Hypertension after CEA is less well understood and has been reported to be more common in patients who have preoperative hypertension and in patients who undergo CEA with denervation of the carotid sinus. Mild increases in postoperative blood pressure of up to 20% above preoperative levels are acceptable, but marked increases are treated with antihypertensive drugs.
3. Other causes of hemodynamic instability after CEA include myocardial ischemia or infarction, arrhythmias such as atrial fibrillation, hypoxia, hypercarbia, pneumothorax, pain, confusion, and distention of the urinary bladder.
D. In most hospitals, patients are discharged from the postanesthetic care unit to an environment in which intensive neurologic and cardiovascular monitoring

is available (e.g., intensive care unit or neurosurgical observation unit).

VI. **Complications.** Major postoperative complications after CEA include stroke, myocardial infarction, and hyperperfusion syndrome.

A. **Stroke**

1. Approximately two-thirds of strokes associated with CEA occur in the postoperative period. Most of these appear to be related to surgical factors resulting in either carotid occlusion (e.g., thrombosis, intimal flap) or emboli originating at the surgical site.

2. Intraoperative strokes represent approximately one-third of strokes that occur in the perioperative period. Most intraoperative strokes happen at the time of carotid cross-clamping and are either technical (i.e., shunt malfunction) or embolic, rather than hemodynamic, in origin.

3. Monitoring intraoperative neurophysiologic function is directed to identifying a relatively small group of patients who develop hemodynamically induced ischemia, which is potentially reversible with early recognition and intervention.

4. It is likely that, beyond using current anesthetic and monitoring techniques and meticulously manipulating hemodynamic and ventilatory parameters, the anesthesiologist has little ability, at present, to affect the incidence of stroke—and the outcome—during CEA.

B. **Myocardial infarction**

1. Myocardial infarction represents the major cause of mortality after CEA. The incidence of fatal postoperative myocardial infarction is 0.5% to 4%, and the proportion of total perioperative mortality (within 30 days of operation) attributed to cardiac causes is estimated to be at least 40%.

2. On the basis of the high incidence of coronary artery disease among patients undergoing CEA, routine coronary angiography has been advocated. However, little evidence supports the premise that routine preoperative coronary angiography improves cardiac outcome after CEA. It seems more reasonable to assume that all patients presenting for CEA have atherosclerotic disease involving the coronary arteries and to gauge perioperative risk in relation to the patient's functional status.

3. High-risk patients including those who have unstable angina, recent myocardial infarction, or recent heart failure may be considered more appropriate candidates for CEA staged or combined with a coronary artery bypass graft (CABG) procedure.

4. Existing evidence is insufficient to formulate firm recommendations regarding the staging of CEA

with CABG surgery. The risk of stroke is similar if CEA precedes or is combined with CABG. This risk is lower than when CABG is performed before CEA. However, the incidence of myocardial infarction and death is higher when CEA precedes CABG. Pending results from well-designed prospective studies, recommendations from the Canadian Neurosurgical Society suggest that CEA should precede CABG if possible. When the patient's cardiac condition is too unstable to permit a prior CEA, combined surgery should be considered.

C. **Death**
   1. Stroke and myocardial infarction represent the major causes of perioperative mortality associated with CEA.
   2. Patient selection, the experience of the surgeon, and the institution where the surgery is performed affect operative risk.
   3. On the basis of these considerations, the American Heart Association Stroke Council has recommended that the combined risk for either death or stroke associated with CEA should not exceed 3% for asymptomatic patients, 5% for symptomatic (transient cerebral ischemia) patients, 7% for patients who have suffered a previous stroke, and 10% for patients undergoing reoperation for recurrent carotid stenosis.

D. **Hyperperfusion syndrome**
   1. An increase in CBF occurs frequently after CEA. Typically the magnitude of this increase is relatively small ($<35\%$). However, in severe cases, increases in CBF can exceed 200% of preoperative levels and are associated with an increase in morbidity and mortality.
   2. Clinical features of this hyperperfusion syndrome include headache (usually unilateral), face and eye pain, cerebral edema, seizures, and intracerebral hemorrhage.
   3. Patients at greatest risk include those who already have a preoperative reduction in hemispheric CBF owing to bilateral high-grade carotid stenoses, unilateral high-grade carotid stenosis with poor collateral cross-flow, or unilateral carotid occlusion with contralateral high-grade stenosis.
   4. The syndrome is thought to result from restoration of perfusion to an area of the brain that has lost its ability to autoregulate as the result of a chronic decrease in CBF. The restoration of CBF leads to a state of hyperperfusion that persists until autoregulation is reestablished, usually over a period of days.
   5. Patients at risk for this syndrome should be monitored closely in the perioperative period,

and blood pressure should be meticulously controlled.

E. **Other complications.** Other complications associated with CEA include hematoma formation and cranial nerve palsies. Hematoma formation can lead to airway compromise owing to mass effect, which might require opening the wound acutely to reestablish the airway before emergent reoperation. Cranial nerve palsies are typically temporary and could manifest themselves as vocal cord paralysis and altered gag reflex.

VII. **Neuroradiology—CAS**

A. **General considerations**

1. Carotid angioplasty with or without the use of endovascular stenting is a relatively new technique for the treatment of carotid stenosis. Its safety and efficacy relative to CEA, particularly with respect to perioperative and long-term neurologic outcome, are currently the subject of several multicenter studies.

2. CAS techniques have been progressively modified as new technologies become available to include self-expanding stents and cerebral-protection devices.

3. Advocates suggest that the technique offers advantages in patients who have high-risk medical conditions and those who have surgically inaccessible carotid disease (e.g., previous neck irradiation, intracranial stenosis).

B. **Anesthetic technique**

1. CAS can be performed under either general anesthesia or sedation. No evidence is available to recommend one technique over the other.

a. Advantages of general anesthesia include the following:

(1) Provides better airway control

(2) Provides better quality of the images

(3) Facilitates control of blood pressure, $Paco_2$

(4) Facilitates treatment of neurologic emergencies

b. Advantages of an awake, sedated patient include the following:

(1) Awake cerebral function monitoring

(2) Identification of intraoperative complications

(3) Rapid emergence and postoperative neurologic assessment

(4) Less expensive

C. **Anesthetic considerations**

1. Preoperative assessment is the same as for patients scheduled for CEA.

2. For patients undergoing CAS, factors affecting the selection of the awake (sedation) technique

include the presence of gastroesophageal reflux and evidence of orthopnea.

3. Monitoring should be consistent with operating room standards including intra-arterial blood pressure measurement, pulse oximetry, ECG, and capnography. Central venous access is optional depending on the patient's medical condition.

4. Hemodynamic changes typically associated with carotid distension at the time of angioplasty or stent expansion, especially bradycardia and asystole, can be profound. A small dose of atropine or glycopyrrolate is often administered to attenuate this response. The immediate availability of external pacing equipment is prudent.

VIII. Summary. This chapter focuses on the anesthetic management of patients undergoing CEA. It also includes a brief overview of the current status of CAS. Physiologic concepts that form the basis for current recommendations regarding the choice of anesthetic technique, drugs, monitoring, and hemodynamic and ventilatory management are discussed. Newer anesthetic drugs facilitate the titration of anesthesia in relation to the patient's responses to changing intraoperative conditions and promote rapid emergence and early assessment after CEA. Expanded criteria defining appropriate candidates for CEA suggest that the anesthesiologist will increasingly be called upon to care for patients who are older and present with significant complex needs. The management of coexisting disease, particularly the risk of cardiac complications, continues to represent important perioperative challenges for the anesthesiologist.

SUGGESTED READINGS

Barnett HJM, Meldrum HE, Eliasziw M. The appropriate use of carotid endarterectomy. *Can Med Assoc J* 2002;166:1169–1179.

Bond R, Warlow CP, Naylor AR, et al. Variation in surgical and anesthetic technique and associations with operative risk in the European carotid surgery trial: implications for trials of ancillary techniques. *Eur J Vasc Endovasc Surg* 2002;23:117–126.

Coward LJ, Featherstone RL, Brown MM. Safety and efficacy of endovascular treatment of carotid artery stenosis compared with carotid endarterectomy: a Cochrane systematic review of the randomized evidence. *Stroke* 2005;36(4):905–911.

Findlay JM, Marchak BE, Pelz DM, et al. Carotid endarterectomy: a review. *Can J Neurol Sci* 2004;31(1):22–36.

Findlay JM, Tucker WS, Ferguson GG, et al. Guidelines for the use of carotid endarterectomy: current recommendations from the Canadian Neurosurgical Society. *Can Med Assoc J* 1997;157:653–659.

Herrick IA. Cerebrovascular disease. *Curr Opin Anaesthesiol* 2003; 16:337–342.

Herrick IA, Gelb AW. Occlusive cerebrovascular disease: anesthetic considerations. In: Cottrell JE, Smith DS, eds. *Anesthesia and Neurosurgery*, 4th ed. St. Louis, MO: Mosby, 2001:459–472.

Moore WS, Barnett HJM, Beebe HG, et al. Guidelines for carotid endarterectomy. A multidisciplinary consensus statement from the ad hoc committee, American Heart Association. *Stroke* 1995;26: 188–201.

Sundt TM Jr, Sandok BA, Whisnant JP. Carotid endarterectomy. Complications and preoperative assessment of risk. *Mayo Clin Proc* 1975;50:301.

Yadav JS, Wholey MH, Kuntz RE, et al. Protected carotid-artery stenting versus endarterectomy in high-risk patients. *N Engl J Med* 2004;351:1493–1501.

Neuroendocrine Tumors: Pathophysiology

David L. Schreibman and M. Jane Matjasko

I. **Anatomy**
   A. **Intracranial mass.** Many neuroendocrine tumors are microadenomas (<10 mm in size) and require routine induction and maintenance of anesthesia for their surgical extirpation. Some tumors are very large and require attention to blood pressure (BP), airway dynamics, and other factors affecting intracranial pressure (ICP) during induction of anesthesia, maintenance, and emergence.
   B. **Pituitary gland and stalk** are very close to the optic chiasm, intracranial carotid arteries, cavernous sinuses, and cranial nerves.
   C. **Pituitary adenomas** may be either intrasellar or extracranial and may extend laterally into the cavernous sinuses.
      1. **Cavernous sinus** contains the intrasphenoid carotid artery and cranial nerves III, IV, V_1, V_2, and VI (Figure 11-1).
      2. **Magnetic resonance imaging (MRI)** appearance and extension of the tumor are important for planning anesthetic management and neurophysiologic monitoring.
   D. **Pituitary tumors** can extend out of the sella into the intracranial space and involve the optic chiasm and carotid arteries.
II. **Endocrine physiology: anterior pituitary**
   A. The hypothalamus secretes hormone-releasing factor (RF), which is transported to the median eminence of the hypothalamus by axonal flow. The RF is then transported via the hypothalamo-hypophyseal portal system to the anterior pituitary. Hormones are secreted into the systemic circulation in response to a variety of stimuli. Target organs respond to stimuli and send negative feedback to the pituitary and the hypothalamus to turn off the secretion of RF and stop the release of the hormone. The incidence of asymptomatic microadenomas on autopsy is up to 27%. The peak age of occurrence is 40 years. Prolactinomas account for approximately 40% of all microadenomas.
   B. **Anterior pituitary hormones** (adrenocorticotropic hormone [ACTH], growth hormone [GH], prolactin [PRL], thyroid-stimulating hormone [TSH], luteinizing hormone [LH], melanocyte-stimulating hormone [MSH], and follicle-stimulating hormone [FSH]) may all be produced by microadenomas. ACTH, GH, and

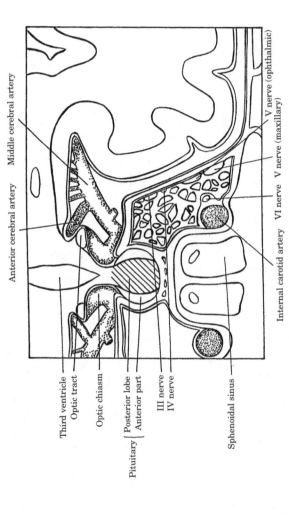

Figure 11-1. Coronal section through pituitary gland demonstrating perisellar structures and sphenoid sinuses. Cranial nerves: ocular nerve (III), trochlear nerve (IV), trigeminal nerve (V), abducens nerve (VI).

PRL are produced most commonly. All have inhibiting factors and RFs, and all can be accurately measured in the blood using radioimmunoassay techniques.

C. **Cushing's disease** is caused by an ACTH-secreting pituitary tumor.
  1. **Cushing's syndrome** occurs when there is an ACTH-dependent (ACTH administration, ectopic ACTH syndrome) or ACTH-independent (adrenal adenoma, carcinoma, or exogenous cortisol administration) excess secretion of cortisol.
  2. **Ectopic ACTH** is associated with a primary oat cell carcinoma of the lung.
    a. The tumor produces ACTH- and corticotropin-releasing factor (CRF)-like peptides.
    b. Plasma cortisol is >50 mcg/dL.
    c. Explosive hypercortisolism may occur with the following:
      (1) Hypertension
      (2) Glucose intolerance
      (3) Hyperaldosteronism (hypokalemic alkalosis)
      (4) Marked hyperpigmentation
  3. **Cushing's disease**
    a. **Truncal obesity,** posterior cervical fat pads, osteoporosis, and moon facies are characteristics.
    b. **Hypertension** and glucose intolerance can occur.
    c. **Adrenal hyperplasia.** In the past, many patients had bilateral adrenalectomy to treat what was thought to be a primary adrenal condition (Nelson's syndrome). These patients may then come for surgery later to remove what was actually a primary pituitary tumor.
    d. **CRF** is stimulated by acetylcholine and serotonin and inhibited by norepinephrine.
    e. **Cortisol secretion** is 16 mcg/day, 75% of which is bound to transcortin protein.
    f. **Normal diurnal variation** is 4 AM to 8 AM: 25 mcg/dL; 4 PM to 8 PM: <10 mcg/dL. Normal diurnal variation increases with stress and pregnancy.
    g. **Diagnosis** is based on loss of diurnal variation, increased ACTH, and probable MRI evidence of sellar adenoma.
D. **Acromegaly,** a GH-producing tumor, leads to the following:
  1. **Signs and symptoms**
    a. Bony and soft tissue enlargement (frontal bossing, prognathism, increased ring, glove, and shoe size)
    b. Hypertension
    c. Glucose intolerance
    d. Visual loss if tumor is large and involves chiasm

   e. Hoarseness (soft tissue stretching of cranial nerve X)
   f. Dyspnea (narrow glottis from soft tissue overgrowth)
   g. Cardiomyopathy from lymphocytic infiltration, a common cause of death, if untreated
   h. Carpal tunnel syndrome from soft tissue overgrowth
   i. Lumbar spinal stenosis and cervical compression from bony overgrowth

2. **Hypoglycemia** is the most potent stimulus to the secretion of GH. Somatostatin inhibits the release of GH.
3. **Diagnosis** includes random blood GH of >10 ng/mL (2 to 5 ng/mL normally) and elevation of somatomedin C (produced in the liver in response to GH stimulation so that high levels occur only with acromegaly).
4. **Acromegaly and the airway**
   a. Hypertrophy of the mandible, nasal turbinates, soft palate, tonsils, epiglottis, arytenoids, tongue, lips, and nose may occur.
   b. The glottis might be narrow.
   c. Vocal cord paralysis can be present from soft tissue overgrowth.
   d. Most often routine intubation techniques are successful, but the ready availability of extra-long blades, smaller endotracheal tubes, laryngeal masks, and fiberoptic intubation equipment is essential.
   e. Anticipate difficult mask fit and potential postextubation stridor.
   f. Patients frequently have a consultation with an otolaryngologist before an operation. A report of the indirect laryngoscopy performed by that consultant is obtained to facilitate anticipation of and preparation for airway difficulty.

E. **PRL-secreting tumors** may be larger in men than women because women tend to seek medical attention earlier because of infertility. Other signs and symptoms include amenorrhea, galactorrhea, anovulation, decreased libido, gynecomastia, and osteoporosis.
   1. **PRL secretion** is primarily regulated by dopamine, which functions as an inhibitory factor. PRL is released by thyrotropin-releasing hormone, serotonin, and the stress of anesthesia and surgery. The secretion of PRL is increased by pituitary stalk section (which interrupts dopaminergic fibers), serotonin, phenothiazines, alpha-methyldopa, and menopause.
   2. **Normal PRL** is 15 to 25 ng/mL.
   3. **Diagnosis.** PRL >25 ng/mL is present. Eighty percent of patients whose PRL exceeds 200 ng/mL

have adenomas even if their presence is not demonstrated neuroradiologically. When PRL exceeds 2,000 ng/mL, invasion of the cavernous sinus is likely. This may warrant additional intravenous access and monitoring with electroencephalogram (EEG) and evoked potentials.

4. **Amenorrhea.** PRL >30 ng/mL is present.
   Loss of libido. PRL of >300 ng/mL is present.
   Menopause. PRL is increased, and estrogen is decreased.

F. **Nonfunctioning pituitary tumors** include adenomas, craniopharyngiomas, meningiomas, and aneurysms. These tend to be large and involve perisellar structures.

III. **Endocrine physiology: posterior pituitary**

A. **Antidiuretic hormone (ADH)**
   1. Produced in the supraoptic and paraventricular nuclei of the hypothalamus
   2. Stored in the median eminence of the hypothalamus
   3. Transported with a carrier protein, neurophysin, along the hypothalamic hypophyseal tract to the posterior pituitary
   4. Released into the systemic circulation after appropriate stimulus: increased serum osmolality, pain, opiates, and decreased circulating blood volume, which causes the greatest ADH release and concurrent vasoconstriction
   5. Secretion inhibited by decreased serum osmolality, alcohol ingestion, increased blood volume, phenytoin

B. **ADH** attaches to an adenyl cyclase receptor on the medullary interstitial surface of the renal collecting duct epithelium. This causes an increase in cyclic adenosine monophosphate, which increases the permeability of the collecting ducts to water, and water is reabsorbed. In the absence of ADH, pure water is lost.

C. **Diabetes insipidus (DI)** can be present preoperatively, may also occur intraoperatively, and may be temporary or permanent in the postoperative period.
   1. **Signs and symptoms** include polyuria (3 to 15 L/day), polydipsia, serum hyperosmolality (>320 mosmol/mL), dilute urine (specific gravity 1.001 to 1.005, osmolality 50 to 150 mosmol/mL), and urine/serum osmolality <1.
   2. **Administration of salt-containing solutions** causes the patient to develop severe hypernatremia and hyperosmolality. Oral intake is initiated as soon as possible.
   3. **Administration of glucose-containing solutions** causes the patient to develop hyperglycemia and osmotic diuresis. Oral intake is initiated as soon as possible.

4. **Total body water deficit calculation** in a 70-kg patient:

Normal serum sodium (Na) = 140 mEq/L

Total body water = 60% of total body weight = 42 L

Normal body sodium = 42 L × 140 mEq/L

$$= 5,880 \text{ mEq Na}$$

Patient's Na = 160 mEq/L

Patient's body water = 5,880 mEq/160 mEq/L

$$= 36.7 \text{ L}$$

Water deficit = 42 L − 36.7 L = 5.3 L

5. **Drug therapy** indicated in patients who cannot drink the necessary volume, are not taking anything by mouth, or are anesthetized includes:
    a. **1-Deamino-8-D-arginine vasopressin (DD-AVP),** 10 to 40 mcg intranasally. This daily dose may be divided into 2 or 3 doses beginning with 10 mcg at bedtime and increased by 2.5 mcg/day up to a total dose of 40 mcg/day. DDAVP, 0.01 to 0.03 ng/kg every 12 hours, may also be given intravenously.
    b. **Lysine vasopressin,** 5 to 10 units administered subcutaneously or intramuscularly 2, 3, or 4 times a day, or 0.5 to 2 microunits/kg/hour administered intravenously (i.v.).
    c. **Other drugs** include vasopressin tannate-in-oil, which is used less commonly. Its effect lasts up to 36 hours after a single dose.
    d. **Overdose** of drugs leads to an iatrogenic syndrome of inappropriate antidiuretic hormone (SIADH) secretion.

IV. **Pituitary tumors**
  A. **Signs and symptoms**
    1. **Headaches** are bitemporal or bifrontal.
    2. **Bitemporal hemianopsia** is classic but its presence depends on the relationship of the pituitary stalk to the optic chiasm.
    3. **Ophthalmoplegia** involving cranial nerves III, IV, and VI and **facial paralysis** involving cranial nerve VII occur. **Corneal anesthesia** involving cranial nerve V is related to invasion or compression of the cavernous sinus.
    4. **Seizures** may be related to the extension of the tumor into the temporal lobe but are rare.
    5. **Hypothalamic dysfunction** includes abnormal temperature regulation, thirst, and appetite changes, all of which are rare.
    6. **DI may occur.**
    7. **Endocrinopathies.** Syndrome of multiple endocrine neoplasia may include parathyroid

dysfunction with hypercalcemia and TSH-, ACTH-, LH-, and FSH-producing adenomas.

B. **Diagnosis**. **MRI** is the gold standard for diagnosing micro- versus macroadenoma (T1-hypointensity; T2-hyperintensity) but is poor for visualizing bony changes and identifying cavernous sinus invasion. Angiography facilitates hormone sampling from the petrosal vein.

C. **Panhypopituitarism** is a clinical diagnosis confirmed by assaying specific hormones.

   1. Most patients who have microadenomas are clinically normal and do not demonstrate any signs of panhypopituitarism.

   2. Nonetheless, in some institutions, it is customary to administer **hydrocortisone**, 50 to 100 mg i.v., before induction of anesthesia and then 10 mg/hour by infusion until the patient's postoperative course indicates that the drug is no longer necessary.

   3. Thyroid replacement may be administered orally as **levothyroxine** sodium (Synthroid) and very rarely as an intravenous infusion.

   4. DI is treated with **DDAVP** and appropriate fluids. If panhypopituitarism has been diagnosed preoperatively, the patient may already be receiving replacement steroids and DDAVP.

D. **Intraoperative management**

   1. **Monitoring** is appropriate for the patient's physiologic status.

      a. Consider either EEG or evoked potential monitoring if there is marked involvement of the cavernous sinus or perisellar area.

      b. In some institutions, pituitary operations are performed in a head-elevated position. Venous air embolism (VAE) could occur, so end-tidal gas monitoring is recommended. If VAE occurs, the head can be lowered rapidly to treat the air embolism. The need for central venous access is determined by the size and location of the tumor and/or by the patient's medical condition. However, careful monitoring of fluid intake and output is indicated in every patient.

      c. Visual evoked responses are not monitored in most institutions and are not indicated for patients who have microadenomas.

   2. **Anesthetic technique** is selected to permit early postoperative assessment of vision, ocular movements, pupil size, and motor strength.

   3. **Antibiotic prophylaxis** is typically cefazolin, 1 g i.v. every 3 to 4 hours.

   4. **Topical cocaine 4% and injected lidocaine 1%** with epinephrine; if both are used, severe hypertension might occur from the unopposed alpha sympathetic effect.

   5. **Valsalva maneuvers** advance the pituitary gland toward the surgeon to facilitate excision of the

tumor and examination for trans-sellar cerebrospinal fluid (CSF) leak.

6. **Avoid** hyperventilation, insertion of nasogastric tubes, incentive spirometry, and the use of drinking straws. Hypoventilation (Pa_{CO_2} 42 mm Hg, ICP up to 20 mm Hg) is successful in producing the descent of the suprasellar portion of the tumor.

E. **Postoperative management**

1. **Careful fluid and electrolyte management** and treatment of DI, SIADH, and cerebral salt wasting are necessary.

2. **Steroid maintenance and tapering.** Patients who have Cushing's disease may have prolonged adrenal insufficiency and require steroid replacement for several months.

3. **Acromegalics and patients with Cushing's disease** have excess body water and will diurese postoperatively.

4. **Patients who have had previous adrenalectomies** (Nelson's syndrome) require mineralocorticoid replacement such as fludrocortisone acetate (Florinef), 0.1 to 0.2 mg/day by mouth.

5. **Deep vein thrombosis** and pulmonary emboli are not uncommon. Prophylaxis is recommended with heparin, intermittently inflating antithromboembolism stockings, and early mobilization.

6. **Lumbar drains** may be used postoperatively to treat CSF leaks.

V. **Pituitary apoplexy**

A. This syndrome is related to the **sudden enlargement of a pituitary tumor** because of hemorrhage or necrosis.

B. **Symptoms and signs** include acute loss of consciousness, hypertension, meningismus, eye pain, blindness, ophthalmoplegia, panhypopituitarism. It is important to differentiate this condition from subarachnoid hemorrhage from the rupture of an intracranial aneurysm.

C. **Diagnosis is made on clinical grounds** and with radiologic evidence of a pituitary tumor.

D. **Treatment is urgent:** surgical decompression of the optic system, systemic steroid replacement, and other hormone replacement as necessary. Some recommend bromocriptine therapy in lieu of surgery.

VI. **Treatment of pituitary tumors**

A. **Radiation therapy** is rarely used now because of the high incidence of panhypopituitarism and the long lag time for clinical effect.

B. **Medical therapy**

1. **ACTH (Cushing's disease).** Because there is no effective medical therapy, operative removal is recommended.

2. **GH (acromegaly).** Octreotide, a somatostatin inhibitor, is an expensive drug ($7,800 annually) that requires multiple daily subcutaneous injections. Octreotide reduces headaches and improves

cardiomyopathy and can be used to treat patients in whom surgical results have been less than optimal. However, operative removal is preferred.
3. **PRL.** Bromocriptine or similar drugs such as pergolide are the first-line treatment.
    a. They reduce tumor size and PRL levels.
    b. They restore fertility. The risks of pregnancy in the presence of a pituitary tumor include its enlargement during pregnancy, which may necessitate operative removal. Perhaps tumor resection should precede pregnancy.
    c. If patients are intolerant of the drug's side effects (nausea, dizziness, orthostatic hypotension), surgery is indicated.
    d. Medical therapy must be continued long term to indefinitely when surgery is not performed.
C. **Surgical therapy**
    1. **Transsphenoidal:** Approach to the floor of the sella is midline, transnasal, transsphenoidal.
        a. **Advantages** include less damage to frontal lobes and olfactory apparatus, no external scar, direct visualization of microadenomas, minimal damage to normal pituitary, lower incidence of temporary and (rarely) permanent DI, less blood loss, and shorter hospitalization. Endoscopic transseptal approach to the sphenoid sinus has been found to be easy, time saving, and without complications.
        b. **Disadvantages** include the potential for CSF leak and meningitis, lack of direct visualization of the optic apparatus, inaccessibility of large tumors, and blood loss that is more difficult to control. Bleeding may require packing the cavernous sinus with resultant compression of the cranial nerves and carotid artery, which could lead to contralateral neurologic deficit.
    2. **Transfrontal: bifrontal or unilateral craniotomy**
        a. **Advantages** include the ability to access suprasellar tumor extension and visualize optic system and other perisellar structures.
        b. **Disadvantages** are higher morbidity than with transsphenoidal, increased likelihood of temporary and permanent DI, possible optic system and vascular injury, cerebral edema, and longer hospitalization.

SUGGESTED READINGS

Ciric I, Ragin A, Baumgartner C, et al. Complications of transsphenoidal surgery: results of a national survey, review of the literature, and personal experience. *Neurosurgery* 1997;40:225.

Inder WJ, Hunt PJ. Glucocorticoid replacement in pituitary surgery: guidelines for perioperative assessment and management. *J Clin Endocrinol Metab* 2002;97:2745–2750.

Korula G, George SP, Rajshekhar V, et al. Effect of controlled hyper-capnia on cerebrospinal fluid pressure and operating conditions during transsphenoidal operations for pituitary macroadenoma. *J Neurosurg Anesthesiol* 2001;13:255–259.

Matjasko MJ. Anesthetic considerations in patients with neuroen-docrine disease. In: Cottrell JE and Smith DS, eds. *Anesthesia and Neurosurgery.* St Louis: Mosby, 2001:591–607.

Rappaport H, Yaniv E. Endoscopic transseptal transsphenoidal surgery for pituitary tumors. *Neurosurgery* 1997;40:944–946.

Shimon I, Melmed S. Management of pituitary tumors. *Ann Intern Med* 1998;129(suppl 6) 472–483.

12

Epilepsy, Epilepsy Surgery, Awake Craniotomy for Tumor Surgery, and Intraoperative Magnetic Resonance Imaging

Pirjo Hellen Manninen and Jee Jian See

I. **Epilepsy**
   A. **Definitions**
      1. **Epileptic seizures** are the clinical manifestations (signs and symptoms) of excessive and/or hyper-synchronous abnormal activity of neurons in the cerebral cortex. This activity is usually self-limited. The features of the seizure reflect the functions of the cortical areas from which the abnormal activity originates and to which it spreads. Epileptic seizures have electrophysiologic correlates that are recorded on a scalp electroencephalogram (EEG).
      2. **Epilepsy** is a chronic disorder caused by a variety of pathologic processes in the brain and is characterized by epileptic seizures. The incidence of epilepsy ranges from 0.5% to 2% of the total population; 25% to 30% of persons who have epilepsy experience more than one seizure a month.
   B. **Classification of epileptic seizures**
      1. **Partial seizures** have an onset that is localized or focal within the brain.
         a. **Simple partial.** Alteration in consciousness does not occur during these seizures. They are classified according to symptoms: motor, sensory, autonomic, and psychic. **Auras** are the sensory, autonomic, or psychic symptoms that precede a progression to impaired consciousness or motor seizure.
         b. **Complex partial.** These seizures spread into multiple areas of the brain and alter consciousness; they are also called **psychomotor** or **temporal lobe** seizures. A simple partial seizure can progress to become complex.
         c. **Convulsive.** These seizures have a partial onset but then spread to involve most areas of the brain and brain stem. They are not easily distinguishable from generalized seizures.
      2. We speak of **generalized seizures** when the EEG shows simultaneous involvement of both cerebral hemispheres and consciousness is impaired. These seizures are the following:
         a. Inhibitory or nonconvulsive, such as atonic or absence seizures (petit mal)

   b. Excitatory or convulsive, which produce myoclonic, tonic, or clonic seizures
   3. Unclassified seizures
C. Mechanisms of epilepsy are diverse and include abnormalities in the regulation of neural circuits and
   the balance of neural excitation and inhibition. Factors
   that influence the appearance of epilepsy can be genetic,
   environmental, or physiologic.
D. Associated medical problems include the following:
   1. Psychiatric disorders
   2. Rare syndromes: tuberous sclerosis, neurofibroma-
      tosis, multiple endocrine adenomatosis
   3. History of trauma
   4. Sleep deprivation
E. Treatment of epilepsy
   1. Medical therapy involves the following:
      a. Various antiepileptic drugs are used: pheny-
         toin, phenobarbital, primidone, carbamazepine,
         clonazepam, valproic acid, and diazepam. Some
         of the newer drugs are gabapentin, lamotrigine,
         and topiramate.
      b. Treatment consists of either a single medication
         or multiple drug therapy.
      c. The choice depends on considerations of the
         pharmacokinetics, clinical toxicity, efficacy, and
         type of epilepsy.
   2. Adverse effects of antiepileptic drugs are dose
      dependent and are usually associated with long-
      term therapy. Newer drugs claim to have fewer
      side effects.
      a. Many drugs have neurologic side effects includ-
         ing sedation, confusion, learning impairment,
         and ataxia as well as gastrointestinal problems
         such as nausea and vomiting.
      b. Most anticonvulsants are metabolized by the
         liver. Therefore, long-term usage may cause
         induction of liver enzymes, which increases the
         rate of metabolism of other drugs, particularly
         anesthetics.
      c. Long-term therapy with phenytoin causes gin-
         gival hyperplasia with poor dentition and, po-
         tentially, difficulties with airway management.
      d. Carbamazepine can depress the hemopoietic
         system and, in rare cases, causes cardiac toxic-
         ity.
      e. Valproic acid may occasionally lead to throm-
         bocytopenia and platelet dysfunction.
   3. Surgical treatment. Epilepsy is deemed refrac-
      tory if unacceptable side effects associated with
      antiepileptic drugs preclude adequate seizure con-
      trol. This occurs in **5%** to **30%** of patients. Approxi-
      mately **15%** to **20%** of patients who have intractable
      epilepsy are candidates for surgical resection of the
      epileptogenic focus.

F. Status epilepticus

1. Status epilepticus is defined as epileptic seizures that are so frequently repeated or so long in duration that they create a fixed and lasting epileptic condition, either convulsive or nonconvulsive. This is considered a neurologic emergency.

2. **Treatment.** To prevent brain damage, seizures must be stopped as quickly as possible. Approaches for treatment are as follows:

   a. Secure the airway, provide oxygen, and maintain circulation.

   b. Protect the patient from traumatic injury secondary to involuntary motor movements.

   c. If hypoglycemia is present or cannot be ruled out, 50% glucose, 50 mL intravenously (i.v.), and thiamine, 100 mg i.v., should be given.

   d. There are different approaches, but the initial drug choices usually include phenobarbital, phenytoin, and benzodiazepines; an example is diazepam, 0.2 mg/kg i.v., or lorazepam, 0.1 mg/kg i.v., followed by phenytoin, 15 to 20 mg/kg, given slowly at a rate of no >50 mg/minute.

   e. Seizures that continue to be refractory might require barbiturate coma titrated to EEG effect.

   f. Other anesthetic drugs that have been used include etomidate, ketamine, propofol, halothane, enflurane, isoflurane, and desflurane.

G. Pro- and anticonvulsant effects of anesthetic drugs. Numerous reports describe how anesthetic agents can paradoxically exhibit convulsant and anticonvulsant properties with different doses, under different physiologic situations, and with different species.

1. The inhalation drugs isoflurane and desflurane are effective anticonvulsants. Although controversial, sevoflurane has also been shown to produce epileptiform activity. Nitrous oxide (N_2O) does not have any anticonvulsant properties, nor does it produce seizure activity on EEG.

2. Barbiturates are anticonvulsants, but when given in small doses, thiopental and methohexital activate the epileptiform activity from a seizure focus, as indicated by EEG monitoring. Etomidate and ketamine can activate the epileptogenic focus and have also been used to treat status epilepticus. Benzodiazepines are effective anticonvulsants. Propofol is an anticonvulsant but there have been controversial reports of seizure and seizure-like activity after its use in patients who have and do not have epilepsy.

3. Opioids (e.g., fentanyl, alfentanil, and remifentanil) can activate the epileptiform activity from a seizure focus in patients who have epilepsy.

4. Local anesthetic drugs are anticonvulsant in low doses but, at higher serum concentrations, can produce central nervous system excitation.

H. Interaction between anesthetic and antiepileptic drugs
  1. The requirements for muscle relaxants, opioids, and barbiturates increase in patients taking most anticonvulsants, particularly phenytoin and phenobarbital, on a long-term basis owing to the enhanced activity of hepatic microsomal enzymes, which accelerates hepatic biotransformation.
  2. Interactions with endogenous neurotransmitters and changes in the number of receptors, including opioid, may occur.

I. Anesthetic management of an epileptic patient for nonepilepsy surgery
  1. **Preoperative assessment** focuses on the following:
     a. General assessment and preparation
     b. Specific concerns with an epileptic patient
        (1) Medical problems including psychiatric disorders associated with epilepsy
        (2) Complications from anticonvulsant therapy
        (3) Continuation of anticonvulsant therapy
  2. **Anesthetic management and monitoring** depend on the needs of the patient and the procedure.
     a. Drugs that potentiate seizure activity should not be used.
     b. The requirement for anesthetic drugs may increase.
     c. Consideration should be given to the administration of additional doses of antiepileptic drugs during prolonged procedures.
     d. Hyperventilation might potentiate seizure activity and should be avoided unless necessary for surgery.
     e. Seizures can occur postoperatively because anesthetic drugs and changes in body physiology during the operation can significantly affect blood levels of anticonvulsants.

II. Epilepsy surgery
  A. Procedure
  1. Surgery for partial seizure disorders involves the resection of a specific epileptogenic focus that may show either sclerosis or gliosis. This is frequently accomplished by some form of a temporal lobectomy.
  2. Generalized seizures are treated by interrupting the seizure circuits by a corpus callosotomy or a hemispherectomy.
  3. A patient who either remains seizure free or has a significant reduction in seizure frequency is considered a surgical cure. This occurs in 50% to 80% of patients.
  4. Cognitive improvement also results because the doses of anticonvulsive drugs are either reduced or eliminated.

B. **Patient suitability for epilepsy surgery.** A complete multidisciplinary evaluation is needed to assess whether the patient is a candidate for epilepsy surgery. Invasive and noninvasive investigations are needed to identify the origin of seizure activity and to evaluate the feasibility of performing surgery safely with minimal risk of neurologic and cognitive injury. Advances in neuroimaging techniques have reduced the need for invasive evaluation.

1. **Noninvasive evaluation** includes medical history; assessment of the frequency, severity, and type of seizures; physical examination; and psychosocial and neuropsychiatric testing. Surface-electrode monitoring of EEG activity may also be combined with video-camera monitoring of the seizures.

2. **Radiologic imaging** can supplement EEG data. Computed tomographic (CT) scanning and magnetic resonance imaging (MRI) can help identify areas of sclerosis and low-grade intracranial neoplasms.

3. **Functional imaging** is accomplished with positron emission tomography, single-photon emission CT scan, and functional MRI and spectroscopy to assess brain activity, cerebral blood flow, and the metabolic effects of resection of the seizure focus.

4. **Thiopental testing** may be performed to assist in EEG localization of the seizure focus. The technique is accomplished by producing a gradual increase in the blood level of thiopental during EEG recording. This causes an increase in beta activity in normally functioning neural tissue but not in the seizure focus.

5. **Intracarotid sodium amytal injection (Wada test)** is used to test for lateralization of language and memory.

6. **Invasive evaluation** is accomplished by the insertion of intracranial electrodes. Epidural electrodes are inserted through multiple burr holes; subdural grids or strip electrodes are inserted through a full craniotomy. Stereotactic techniques can also be used. These electrodes are inserted several weeks before the definitive operation to monitor the patient for an adequate period of time. The patient's behavior and EEG are continuously recorded and displayed on a television monitor in specialized units.

   Placement of intracranial electrodes or grids is usually performed under general anesthesia. The anesthetic plan should consider the concerns of a patient who has epilepsy and the precautions that apply to any craniotomy. Routine noninvasive monitoring is required with the addition of intra-arterial blood pressure measurement as indicated. The anesthetic drugs used are not specific because there is no EEG recording. Electrode plates and large grids are quite bulky and might require brain shrinkage through the use of mannitol and hyperventilation. These patients may develop postoperative problems with brain edema and require urgent removal of the grid because of the development of intracranial hypertension.

C. **Intraoperative localization of epileptogenic focus**

1. **Electrocorticography (ECoG) is performed** during surgery after opening of the dura by placing electrodes directly on the cortex over the area predetermined to be epileptogenic as well as on adjacent cortex. Additional recordings can be obtained from microelectrodes inserted into the cortex or depth electrodes into the amygdala and hippocampal gyrus.

2. **Stimulation of epileptogenic focus is possible** pharmacologically, if insufficient information is obtained to define the seizure focus adequately during routine ECoG. Drugs used in adults include a small dose of methohexital, 10 to 50 mg; thiopental, 25 to 50 mg; propofol, 10 to 20 mg; or etomidate, 2 to 4 mg. If the patient is under general anesthesia, other drugs such as alfentanil, 20 to 50 mcg/kg, and enflurane can be used with or without hypocarbia.

3. Direct electrical stimulation of the cortex **delineates eloquent areas** of brain function, such as speech, memory, and sensory and motor function. This allows these areas to be preserved during resection of the seizure focus. Only motor testing can be done when the patient is under general anesthesia.

D. **Preoperative preparation for epilepsy surgery.** Communication among all members of the team, including the neurologist, neurosurgeon, and anesthesiologist, is vital to the successful management of the patient throughout the perioperative period.

1. Routine and specific epilepsy assessment is carried out.

2. Appropriate preparation of the patient for the anesthetic technique selected is carried out.

3. Anticonvulsant agents are administered before surgery in consultation with the neurologist and surgeon.

4. Premedication for the purpose of sedation is rarely required because these patients are usually well informed; all drugs that might influence EEG, such as benzodiazepines, should be avoided.

E. **Techniques of anesthesia.** Historically, epilepsy surgery was performed with the patient awake for at least some part of the procedure. These procedures are now performed with the use of either conscious sedation (neurolept anesthesia) or general anesthesia. The neurosurgeon usually makes the decision, which depends on the location of the seizure focus, the need for testing of eloquent function, and the patient's ability to withstand an awake procedure.

1. **Conscious sedation/neurolept anesthesia**
    a. **The reasons** for having an awake patient are as follows:
        (1) Better ECoG localization of the seizure focus without the influence of general anesthetic drugs
        (2) Availability of immediate responses from the patient to direct electrical stimulation of the cerebral cortex to delineate eloquent areas of brain function to preserve them during surgical resection
        (3) Continuous clinical neurologic monitoring of the patient throughout the procedure
    b. **The challenge** is to have the patient comfortable enough to remain immobile through a long procedure but sufficiently alert and cooperative to comply with testing. The analgesic and sedative drugs employed must have minimal interference with ECoG and stimulation testing.
    c. **Specific preoperative preparation**
        (1) The patient is prepared psychologically and informed about the complexities and demands of an awake craniotomy.
        (2) The establishment of good rapport between the anesthesiologist and the patient is absolutely essential.
        (3) The anesthesiologist should be aware of the signs and symptoms that may indicate that the patient is experiencing the onset of a seizure.
    d. **Preparation of the operating room.** An awake craniotomy adds additional stress to the patient and the entire team. All preparations should be complete before the patient arrives in the room so that the patient can receive the full attention of all team members.
        (1) Anesthetic drugs and equipment for conscious sedation, induction of general anesthesia, and the treatment of complications are available.
        (2) Routine monitoring equipment is ready to connect to the patient.
        (3) Extra pillows, soft mattress, and soft headrest or fixed head frame are available for positioning the patient.

(4) Room environment is at normal room temperature with a quiet, reassuring atmosphere. It is essential to prevent unnecessary traffic by placing a sign on the door advising people of the procedure within.

e. **Patient management**

(1) Positioning is usually in the lateral decubitus, which is most comfortable for the patient and allows better access to the patient.

(a) Pillows are placed behind patient's back, between the legs, and under the arms.

(b) Extra blankets may be needed at the beginning.

(c) Patients should be positioned in such a way as to have some freedom of movement of the extremities.

(d) The patient's head is positioned on a pillow of appropriate size and shape. However, neuronavigation for imaging is now frequently used, which necessitates the placement of the patient's head in a rigid skull pin-fixation system. Pins are inserted with the use of local anesthesia under conscious sedation.

(e) The placement of the surgical drapes should allow for maximum visibility of the patient's face by the anesthesiologist and for the patient to see the anesthesiologist continuously.

(2) The neurosurgeon usually performs **scalp block**.

(a) Long-acting local anesthetic agents, such as bupivacaine with the addition of epinephrine, are used.

(b) Lidocaine, which has a fast onset, may be added and used to infiltrate areas that are still painful during the procedure, such as dura.

(c) The maximum dose for bupivacaine is 3 mg/kg and for lidocaine, 5 to 7 mg/kg.

(d) The scalp block is painful. The patient might need analgesia and sedation.

(3) **Monitors**

(a) Electrocardiogram (ECG), noninvasive blood pressure cuff, pulse oximeter, and end-tidal carbon dioxide (CO_2) via nasal prongs used to deliver supplemental oxygen.

Invasive monitoring is not routinely required for all patients.

(b) The intravenous catheter should be inserted in the arm not involved in seizure activity.

(c) Fluids should be kept to a minimum; therefore, a urinary catheter is not routinely needed.

(d) Dextrose-containing fluids should be avoided.

(4) **Anesthetic drugs**

(a) The techniques of drug administration and dosage requirements vary greatly and need to be titrated to each patient.

(b) The drugs may be administered by intermittent bolus, continuous infusion, target-controlled infusion, patient-controlled analgesia, or a combination.

(c) Short-acting anesthetic drugs provide good conditions and ensure that the patient is alert for assessments.

(d) Traditionally, intermittent boluses of fentanyl and droperidol were used. Now the most common combination is an infusion of propofol (25 to 100 mcg/kg/minute) with either intermittent boluses of fentanyl (0.5 to 1 mcg/kg) or an infusion of remifentanil (starting at 0.0125 mcg/kg/minute). Other opioids (e.g., sufentanil and alfentanil) have also been used.

(e) The infusion of propofol has to be discontinued at least 20 minutes before the start of ECoG recording.

(f) Dexmedetomidine, a new $alpha_2$-adrenoreceptor agonist, has been used as an adjunct for sedation and analgesia with minimal risk of respiratory depression.

(g) Antiemetic drugs including dimenhydrinate, prochlorperazine, metoclopramide, odansetron, dolasetron, and granisetron, may also be needed and do not affect the ECoG.

(5) **Nonpharmacologic measures** are very useful to help the patient through the procedure. These include frequent reassurance, allowing the patient to move intermittently, warning the patient in advance about loud noises (drilling and rongeuring bone) and painful interventions, providing ice chips and a cold cloth

to the face, and just holding the patient's hand.

f. Intraoperative complications

(1) **Pain/discomfort.** At certain times, patients might feel either pain or discomfort and should be warned about this (e.g., the scalp block) in advance. Patients may also experience pain during the bone work if dural vessels come in contact with instruments and during the manipulation of the dura mater and major vessels within brain tissue. The loud noises of drills and rongeurs can be frightening if not actually painful.

(2) **Nausea/vomiting.** Many factors may be responsible for the high incidence of nausea and vomiting including anxiety, medications, and surgical stimulation, especially the stripping of the dura and manipulation of the temporal lobe and meningeal vessels.

(3) **Seizures** can occur at any time.

  (a) Short, mild seizures may not require any treatment. Convulsive or generalized seizures need to be treated immediately.

  (b) The patient should be protected from injury.

  (c) A patent airway, adequate oxygenation, and circulatory stability must be ensured.

  (d) Before ECoG recording, seizures can be treated with a small dose of either thiopental, 25 to 50 mg, or propofol, 10 to 20 mg.

  (e) After all recordings have been completed, benzodiazepines may be used.

  (f) If repeated treatments are required, the patient may become very drowsy and need airway support.

(4) **Respiratory.** Oxygen desaturation and airway obstruction may result from oversedation, seizures, mechanical obstruction, or loss of consciousness from an intracranial event. Treatment needs to be immediate and includes decreasing sedation and jaw thrust, or the insertion of an oral airway, laryngeal mask, or endotracheal tube.

(5) **Induction of anesthesia.** If a patient either becomes uncooperative or complications such as hemorrhage or continuous seizures develop, the induction of general anesthesia may be required. To do

this safely a plan of action is necessary. Airway assessment determines the best approach.

- (a) The laryngeal mask airway may be used temporarily or for completion of the procedure.
- (b) Occasionally, endotracheal intubation will be required. This can be accomplished with the patient either on his or her side or supine. With adequate assistance, the anesthesiologist comes to the patient's head while the surgeon protects the sterile brain field. After preoxygenation, anesthesia can be induced if necessary with a small dose of propofol (with or without opioids and muscle relaxant). Intubation may be accomplished with any airway device with which the anesthesiologist is comfortable, such as direct or fiberoptic laryngoscopy or the intubating laryngeal mask.
- (c) If any difficulty in securing the airway is anticipated, an awake intubation with local anesthesia should be performed.
- **(6)** Other less common complications include excessive blood loss and a tight brain.
- **g. Closure.** During closure of the wound, the patient may be sedated with other drugs, such as benzodiazepines, that were not used up to this point.
- **h. Recovery of the patient takes place** in an intensive care or specialized observation unit. Postoperative complications are the same as for any patient after a craniotomy. Seizures might still occur and may require treatment.
2. **Asleep-awake-asleep** is a modified technique of conscious sedation that may also be used.
   - **a.** General anesthesia is used for the craniotomy and closure. Either inhalation or intravenous anesthetic drugs with or without controlled ventilation may be used.
   - **b.** Appropriate airway devices include endotracheal tube, special oral airway, or, most commonly, the laryngeal mask airway.
   - **c.** The advantages of the laryngeal mask airway are easier placement and decreased coughing and laryngospasm.
   - **d.** The patient is awakened completely and the airway device removed for the period of intraoperative neurologic evaluation.

      e. For resection of the lesion and for closure, general anesthesia is again induced with reinsertion of the airway device.

      f. This technique requires complex intraoperative airway manipulation after neurologic testing while the head is fixed.

      g. Advantages include increased patient comfort and tolerance during craniotomy and a secured airway with ability to control ventilation and prevent hypercapnia.

3. **General anesthesia**

    a. **The reason for choosing general** anesthesia depends on the preference of the neurosurgeon, or the patient's inability to tolerate an awake craniotomy, or both.

    b. **The advances** in preoperative neuroimaging, functional testing, and the use of frameless stereotactic surgery for localization of the epileptic focus have lessened the need for the patient to be awake during the procedure.

    c. **The challenge** to general anesthesia, if intraoperative localization is needed, is to provide good conditions for EEG, ECoG, and motor testing. The influence of the anesthetic drugs needs to be kept at a minimum while avoiding long periods of potential awareness on the part of the patient.

    d. **Specific preoperative preparation** involves informing patients of the possibility that awareness might occur at the time of ECoG recording and testing but reassuring them that it will be brief and painless.

    e. **Preparation** of the operating room, anesthetic equipment and drugs, and positioning supplies are as for any craniotomy. In addition to routine monitors, intra-arterial and urinary catheters are frequently used.

    f. **Anesthetic management**

      (1) **Specific concerns** include the increased dosage requirements for opioids and neuromuscular blocking drugs effected by long-term anticonvulsant therapy.

      (2) **N_2O.** If the patient has had a recent craniotomy or burr holes for electrode placement, intracranial air might still be present. N_2O should be avoided to prevent complications from an expanding pneumocephalus.

      (3) **Anesthetic drugs**

         (a) Drugs should be short acting with minimal influence on EEG and ECoG and nonseizure-producing activity.

         (b) A balanced technique *may be used* with opioids, muscle relaxant, N_2O, and low concentrations of inhalation drugs.

(c) Total intravenous anesthesia with propofol may also be used.

(d) Inhalation drugs and propofol must be eliminated at least 20 minutes before ECoG recording. N_2O may also have to be eliminated.

(4) **Motor testing** is possible during general anesthesia by discontinuing all inhalation drugs and propofol and either reversing or allowing the muscle paralysis to wear off. This testing demands very careful planning and care of the patient. Either additional opioids or lidocaine might decrease the chance of the patient's coughing.

g. **Complications**

(1) Craniotomy-related complications

(2) The possibility of awareness

(3) Movement from seizures, especially during any stimulation testing

h. **Recovery** is the same as for awake patients

F. **Pediatric surgery.** The considerations for epilepsy surgery in pediatric patients are similar to those for adults, except that most children are not able to tolerate an awake craniotomy.

1. **General anesthesia** is used for most procedures.

2. **Awake craniotomy** may be tolerated by an older child.

3. **Asleep-awake-asleep** technique with the use of a laryngeal mask airway is an alternative.

4. **Coexisting conditions** with multiple organ system involvement and significant psychological and behavior problems may be present.

5. **Parents** may be very actively involved in the patient's management and also require consideration and education.

G. **Cerebral hemispherectomy and corpus callosotomy.** Treatment of diffuse generalized seizures might require either resection of substantial portions of the entire cerebral hemisphere or section of the corpus callosum. These procedures are usually performed under general anesthesia because they involve a large craniotomy and most of the patients are children. The major concern with these lengthy procedures is the possibility of extensive blood loss and air emboli because the surgical site is close to major vessels and sinuses.

III. **Awake craniotomy for tumor.** The awake craniotomy has been adapted for the resection of tumors located either in or close to areas of eloquent brain function, especially those involving speech, motor, and sensory pathways.

A. **Reasons for awake craniotomy**
   1. The accurate localization of eloquent brain function through intraoperative mapping allows for optimal tumor resection and minimization of the risk of neurologic injury.
   2. This technique facilitates more efficient use of high-dependency facilities and earlier discharge from the hospital.

B. **Patient selection**
   1. Cooperative and alert patients who are able to understand the demands of the procedure are ideal candidates.
   2. Confused, demented, or agitated patients are poor candidates.
   3. Tumor size and location also influence selection. Supratentorial tumors with minimal dural involvement are amenable to resection under awake craniotomy.

C. **Anesthesia.** The aim is to provide adequate sedation and analgesia with stable respiratory and hemodynamic control during craniotomy but an awake and cooperative patient for the period of neurologic testing.
   1. **Preoperative management**
      a. The management is similar to that of the patient who has epilepsy.
      b. The establishment of good rapport between the anesthesiologist and patient is crucial.
      c. The patient is prepared psychologically and informed about the complexities of an awake craniotomy.
      d. The preoperative assessment and management of all patients who have intracranial tumors are instituted.
      e. Medications such as dexamethasone and anticonvulsant drugs are reviewed and continued because some patients may present with seizures.
      f. Obese patients and those who have either a known difficult airway or a large vascular tumor may pose additional challenges.
   2. **Operating room preparation**
      a. This is similar to the preparation and setup for epilepsy surgery.
      b. Positioning may be lateral, supine, or semisitting.
      c. Neuronavigation for imaging is usually used, necessitating rigid three-point pin fixation of the head.
      d. Monitoring depends on the needs of the patient. Routine invasive monitoring is not required for all patients.

3. **Anesthetic techniques**
   a. **Scalp anesthesia for craniotomy**
      (1) Local anesthetic drugs, such as long-acting bupivacaine with the addition of epinephrine, are used. Lidocaine is helpful for areas that are still painful during the procedure.
      (2) Local infiltration of the craniotomy site with a "ring block" is frequently used.
      (3) Scalp nerve blocks of the auriculotemporal, occipital, zygomaticotemporal, supraorbital, and supratrochlear nerves may be used.
   b. **Sedation techniques** are similar to those discussed for epilepsy surgery, but, because EEG and ECoG are not performed, the choice of anesthetic drugs is more flexible.
      (1) **Conscious sedation**
         (a) Commonly used drugs include midazolam, propofol, fentanyl, and remifentanil.
         (b) The drugs may be administered as either bolus injections or infusions.
         (c) Dexmedetomidine, a new alpha$_2$-adrenoreceptor agonist, has been used as an adjunct for sedation and analgesia with minimal respiratory depression.
         (d) Nonpharmacologic measures including frequent reassurance, warning the patient in advance about loud noise (drilling bone) and painful areas, and holding the patient's hand are also useful.
      (2) **Asleep-awake-asleep** is a technique commonly used for tumor surgery.
         (a) General anesthesia with some technique for securing the airway is used for the craniotomy, tumor resection, and closure. Either inhalation or intravenous anesthetic drugs may be used with or without controlled ventilation.
         (b) Airway management may be performed with an endotracheal tube, oral or nasal airway, or, most commonly, the laryngeal mask airway.
         (c) The patient is fully awakened for the cortical mapping.
         (d) Advantages include increased patient comfort and tolerance during craniotomy, especially for longer

procedures, and a secured airway with the ability to use hyperventilation.

4. **Intraoperative cortical mapping** for speech, motor, and sensory functions is accomplished by placing a stimulating electrode directly on the cortex. The patient needs to be alert and cooperative during this time. For some patients, continuous monitoring is also helpful during tumor resection.

5. **Postoperative care** is the same as for any craniotomy for tumor surgery. However, shorter hospital stays are often possible.

6. **Common problems**
   a. **Airway complications**
      (1) Oxygen desaturation and airway obstruction may result from oversedation, seizures, mechanical obstruction, or loss of consciousness from an intracranial event.
      (2) Treatment needs to be immediate and can include stopping or decreasing sedation or jaw thrust or securing of the airway with an oral or nasal airway, laryngeal mask, or endotracheal tube.
   b. **Pain** may occur during pin fixation, dissection of the temporalis muscle, traction on the dura, and manipulation of the intracerebral blood vessels.
   c. **Seizures** may occur in patients who have or do not have preoperative seizures, most commonly during cortical stimulation.
   d. **Other** less common problems are an uncooperative or disinhibited patient, a tight brain, and nausea and vomiting (less frequent during tumor surgery).
   e. **Induction of general anesthesia** may be required for the management of ongoing complications and catastrophic intracranial events including loss of consciousness and bleeding.

IV. **Intraoperative MRI.** The merger of an MRI and an operating room to provide intraoperative real-time imaging during surgery is steadily gaining acceptance. Intracranial anatomy changes constantly during neurosurgical procedures with shifts and compression of the brain and its structures. The advantage of intraoperative MRI is the ability to assess brain parenchyma immediately before, during, and after the operation; to determine the extent of surgical removal of the tumor; and to avoid the transfer of the patient to another suite if imaging is needed.

A. **Preparation and safety considerations**
   1. **Safety** concerns are the same as in any MRI unit.
   2. **The intraoperative MRI unit** is frequently situated in a location in the hospital remote from the main operating rooms.

3. **The intraoperative MRI unit provides a new and unique work environment** for the anesthesiologists, neurosurgeons, radiologists, nurses, and technologists.
4. **Personnel** training and education are necessary before the inception of the program.
5. **A magnetic field** is constantly present and extends beyond the magnet.
6. **The greatest hazard** of the magnetic field is that any ferromagnetic object brought close to the magnet can be sucked into the magnetic field, which can cause serious injury to patients and health care personnel.
7. **Patient selection** and screening are critical. Patients who have ferromagnetic implants such as older cerebral aneurysm clips, defibrillators, and pacemakers are not candidates for MRI.

B. **Intraoperative MRI systems.** The specifications and layout of each intraoperative MRI system vary greatly. Each system has its own particular set of anesthetic concerns.
1. The strength of the MRI ranges from 0.2 to 3 Tesla.
2. The MRI scanner can be fixed in place or mobile.
3. The site of the operating field affects the anesthetic plan.
   a. Within the magnet itself
      (1) Real-time imaging is possible.
      (2) Minimal patient transport is needed.
      (3) All equipment, anesthetic and surgical, must be MRI compatible.
      (4) Disadvantages include space constraints for the surgeons and limited access to the patients for the anesthesiologist.
   b. In close proximity to a fixed MRI scanner
      (1) Allows the use of equipment and technologies (e.g., surgical instruments and the operating microscope) that are not MRI compatible
      (2) Requires transfer of the patient to the scanner
      (3) Still requires all anesthesia equipment to be MRI compatible
      (4) Must shield equipment that is not MRI compatible
      (5) Limits the number of images taken
   c. In close proximity to a mobile MRI scanner
      (1) A mobile ceiling-mounted scanner is placed over the patient when scanning is needed.
      (2) A mobile, compact, low field-strength MRI system is positioned and shielded under the operating room table.

C. **Equipment considerations**
1. MRI-compatible anesthetic, surgical, monitoring, and imaging equipment should ideally be available,

but the equipment actually used depends on the strength of the magnet and the proximity to the magnetic system with which that equipment will be used.

  a. The magnetic field decreases in strength from the core of the magnet outward. Safety zones and gauss lines should be marked on the floor.

  b. All equipment must be tested before use.

2. Physiologic monitors, anesthesia machines, and ventilators need to be fully MRI compatible. They also must not distort the images.

3. The location of the patient and the need for movement within the room may require extra-long circuits, intravenous lines, and monitoring cables.

4. Conventional ECG monitors will not function properly in the MRI suite. There is currently no capability for monitoring the ST segment.

5. Because they are potential sources of skin burns, wires and loops of cable must not have direct contact with the skin. Procedures to prevent this must be set.

6. Visual as well as audio alarms should be in place because the loud noise generated by the scanner may mask the sound of the audio alarms.

D. Anesthetic management

1. Advanced planning by and communication among all members of team are crucial.

2. Preoperative evaluation involves thorough assessment of the patient for the surgical procedure and eligibility for the MRI.

3. Anesthetic management includes considerations for the patient and the surgical procedure as well as for MRI scanning.

4. Induction of anesthesia.

  a. Induction in a separate room adjacent to the MRI operating room allows the use of non-MRI–compatible equipment such as the fiberoptic bronchoscope and facilitates management of anticipated and unanticipated difficult airway.

  b. When anesthesia is induced in the MRI suite itself, it is essential to use only MRI-compatible equipment.

5. The anesthesiologist has limited access to and visualization of the patient during operation and scanning.

6. The patient and health care personnel need protection from the MRI's noise to prevent damage to hearing.

7. Anesthesiologists need to interact not only with the surgical team but also with the radiologist and the MRI technologist.

8. At the completion of the procedure, safe transfer to a recovery or intensive care unit must be planned. Because this may involve travel over a relatively

long distance, the use of appropriate monitoring during the transfer is indicated.
  E. **Anesthetic techniques.** The choice of the anesthetic technique depends on the procedure, the patient, and the preference of the surgeon and the anesthesiologist.
    1. **Conscious sedation** has these characteristics:
      a. It is similar to the technique for awake craniotomy for tumor
      b. It has problems.
        (1) Visibility of and access to the patient are limited.
        (2) Monitoring and communication are more difficult.
        (3) Sedation may be unacceptable to the patient because of the scanner's confined nature and noise.
        (4) Transfers may be uncomfortable for the patient.
    2. **General anesthesia** has these characteristics:
      a. Principles and concerns are similar to those for any patient undergoing a neurosurgical procedure.
      b. Working around the MRI constrains equipment and access.
      c. It has no best techniques or drugs.

SUGGESTED READINGS

Davidson AJ. Anesthesia for paediatric epilepsy surgery. *J Clin Neurosci* 2004;11:280–282.

Eldredge EA, Soriano SG, Rockoff MA. Surgical treatment of epilepsy in children: neuroanesthesia. *Neurosurg Clin N Am* 1995;6:505.

Engel J Jr. *Seizures and Epilepsy.* Philadelphia, PA: FA Davis Co, 1989.

Gooden CK. Anesthesia for magnetic resonance imaging. *Curr Opin Anaesthesiol* 2004;17:339.

Herrick IA, Gelb AW. Anesthesia for temporal lobe epilepsy surgery. *Can J Neurol Sci* 2000;27(Suppl 1):S64–S67.

Kofke WA, Tempelhoff R, Dasheiff RM. Anesthetic implications of epilepsy, status epilepticus, and epilepsy surgery. *J Neurosurg Anesthesiol* 1997;9:349.

Manninen PH, Contreras J. Anesthetic considerations for craniotomy in awake patients. *Int Anesthesiol Clin* 1986;24:157.

Modica PA, Tempelhoff R, White PF. Pro- and anticonvulsant effects of anesthetics, Parts 1 and 2. *Anesth Analg* 1990;70:303–433.

Sarang A, Dinsmore J. Anesthesia for awake craniotomy—evolution of a technique that facilitates neurological testing. *Br J Anaesth* 2003;90:161.

Spinal Cord: Injury and Procedures

Gary R. Stier, Joseph P. Giffin, Daniel J. Cole,
Stephen Onesti, and Elie Fried

I. General considerations

A. Spinal anatomy and physiology

1. **Structure**

   a. The vertebral column consists of 33 superimposed vertebrae that are divided into 7 cervical (C), 12 thoracic (T), 5 lumbar (L), 5 sacral (fused), and 4 coccygeal (fused) bones. Each individual vertebra (Figure 13-1) is composed of a ventral vertebral body and a dorsal bony neural arch formed from a pedicle on either side of the vertebral body, both of which join with the lamina posteriorly to form the spinous process. The posterior vertebral body, pedicles, and lamina form the vertebral foramen. The neural laminar arches bear lateral transverse processes and superior and inferior articular facets.

   b. The vertebral column is stabilized (from posterior to anterior) by the supraspinous, interspinal, ligamentum flavum, posterior longitudinal, and anterior longitudinal ligaments (Figure 13-1). The ligaments provide flexibility and limit excessive movement that could damage the spinal cord.

   c. The spinal cord begins at the foramen magnum and terminates at the conus medullaris (L2 in adults). Below the termination of the spinal cord, the lumbar and sacral roots form the cauda equina. The spinal cord is surrounded by the meninges, layers of tissue including the dura mater and arachnoid membranes which have cerebrospinal fluid (CSF) between them. This provides additional protection for the spinal cord. The anterior portion of the cord gives rise to the motor nerves. Nerves that originate posteriorly are sensory in function.

2. **Blood supply**

   a. **Anterior spinal artery.** A single vessel, formed from the union of the two anterior spinal branches of the vertebral arteries, descends down the entire length of the anterior portion of the spinal cord. This artery supplies perfusion to the anterior 75% of the cord including the anterior column and most of the lateral column.

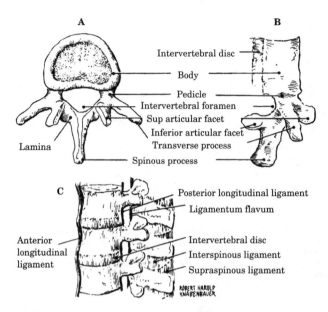

A **A:** View of a typical vertebra from above; B: Lateral view; C: Ligaments of the spine. (Used with permission: Stier GR, Schell RM, Cole DJ. Spinal Cord Injury. In: Cottrell JE and Smith DS, eds. *Anesthesia and Neurosurgery.* 4th ed. St. Louis, MO: Mosby, 2001.)

Figure 13-1.   **A:** View of a typical vertebra from above; B: Lateral view; C: Ligaments of the spine. (Used with permission: Stier GR, Schell RM, Cole DJ. Spinal Cord Injury. In: Cottrell JE and Smith DS, eds. *Anesthesia and Neurosurgery.* 4th ed. St. Louis, MO: Mosby, 2001.)

  b. **Posterior spinal arteries.** Two vessels originating from the posterior inferior cerebellar arteries supply the posterior 25% of the cord including the entire posterior column and the balance of the lateral column.
  c. **Radicular arteries.** These vessels originate from branches of the vertebral, deep cervical, intercostal, and lumbar arteries. They anastomose with the anterior and posterior spinal arteries. The artery of Adamkiewicz (arteria radicularis magna), the major radicular artery, is most commonly located in the lower thoracic or upper lumbar region and provides most of the blood supply to the lower cord.
 3. **Regulation of blood flow** (Figure 13-2). Autoregulation maintains spinal cord blood flow (SCBF) by altering vascular resistance in response to changes in mean arterial pressure (MAP).
  a. Normal autoregulation exists for a MAP between 50 and 150 mm Hg.
  b. Failure of autoregulation at a MAP of <50 mm Hg leads to ischemia.

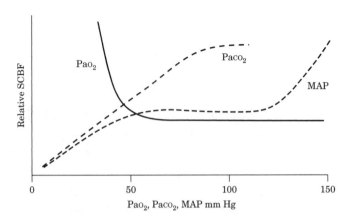

Figure 13-2. Illustration of effect of changes in Paco₂, Pao₂, and mean arterial pressure (MAP) on spinal cord blood flow (SCBF). (Used with permission: Stier GR, Schell RM, Cole DJ. Spinal Cord Injury. In: Cottrell JE and Smith DS, eds. *Anesthesia and Neurosurgery.* 4th ed. St. Louis, MO: Mosby, 2001.)

    c. At a MAP of >150 mm Hg, the increased flow leads to tissue edema and disruption.

    d. The autoregulatory range of individuals who have chronic hypertension is shifted to the right (higher range of MAP).

    e. Alterations in the partial pressure of carbon dioxide ($Paco_2$) and oxygen (Pao_2) disrupt autoregulation in the spinal cord much as they do in the brain. Between 20 and 80 mm Hg, SCBF is linearly related to $Paco_2$. SCBF is well maintained at varying degrees of oxygenation until Pao_2 falls to 50 mm Hg; below this value, SCBF increases as oxygenation decreases further.

II. Spinal cord injury (SCI)

  A. Introduction. In the United States, 11,000 new cases of SCI occur each year. The annual incidence of traumatic SCI is approximately 40 cases per million population, with an estimated prevalence approaching 250,000 cases. SCI in the United States remains more common in males than in females by a 4:1 ratio. Early mortality is around 50% with <10% of survivors experiencing neurologic improvement. Accordingly, the perioperative care of patients during the acute phase of injury is extremely important. Perioperative strategies that prevent further injury, limit the extension of the existing injury, or salvage even a few dermatomal levels can have a significant influence on morbidity, mortality, long-term disability, quality of life, and health care costs.

The distribution of SCI consists of incomplete tetra-plegia, 29.5%; complete paraplegia, 27.9%; incomplete paraplegia, 21.3%; and complete tetraplegia, 18.5%. Common causes of SCI include motor vehicle accidents (40% to 56%), falls (15% to 20%), violence (5% to 20%), sports injuries (5% to 16%), and other causes (5% to 10%). Most injuries occur at the mid-cervical (C4-6, C5 most common) or thoracolumbar (T12) region and are often associated with concomitant injuries. Surgical treatment for SCI is aimed at immobilization, medical stabilization, spinal alignment, operative decompression, and spinal stabilization. This section focuses on the perioperative care of the patient who has acute SCI or is at risk for it. It also discusses specific issues pertaining to the intermediate or chronic phase of injury.

B. **Pathogenic correlates of SCI**
   1. **Primary SCI,** caused by the mechanical forces of the trauma, results in direct neuronal disruption and destruction, petechial hemorrhages, and hematomyelia. Histologic changes consist of hemorrhage and protein extravasation into the central gray matter, which spread to the adjacent white matter. The traumatized areas then undergo cavitating necrosis and ultimately glial scar formation. Spinal cord edema is maximal at 3 days and can persist for 2 weeks. Rarely does physical transection of the spinal cord occur.
   2. **Secondary SCI** is caused by the activation of biochemical, enzymatic, and microvascular processes in proportion to the severity of the initial lesion. Damage results from progressive hemorrhagic necrosis, loss of cellular membrane integrity, edema, inflammation, arachidonic acid release, lipid peroxidation, and loss of vascular autoregulation. These processes lead to vascular stasis, decreased blood flow, ischemia, and cell death.

C. **Anatomical correlates of SCI** (Table 13-1). Flexion injuries cause anterior subluxation or fracture-dislocations of the vertebral bodies. Hyperextension is associated with transverse fractures of the vertebra, disruption of the anterior longitudinal ligaments, and posterior dislocations. Vertical compression produces burst fractures and ligamentous rupture. Rotational injuries result in fractures of the vertebral peduncles and facets. The designation of a SCI as stable or unstable considers the potential for furthering spinal injury or failure to heal properly if left untreated.

D. **Clinical correlates of SCI.** SCI can result in either complete (total loss of sensory and motor function distal to the injury) or incomplete (presence of any nonreflex function distal to the injury; see Table 13-2) loss of neurologic function. Complete SCI has less than a 10% chance of total return of normal neurologic function. Incomplete SCI has a 59% to 75% chance of recovering

Table 13-1. Spinal injury, clinical finding, and indicated treatment

Spinal Injury	Clinical Finding	Treatment
Atlanto-occipital dislocation	Usually unstable; commonly fatal	Reduction, immobilization, fusion
Atlantoaxial injury		
Isolated atlas fracture	Usually stable/no neurologic injury	Philadelphia collar
Isolated odontoid fracture	Usually neurologically intact	Immobilization
Displaced fracture C1-2	Commonly fatal or quadriplegic	Immobilization and reduction
Posterior subluxation C1-2	Usually neurologically intact	Immobilization
Axis pedicle fracture	Can be neurologically intact	Immobilization
Hyperflexion dislocation C3-T1	Any subluxation is unstable	If neurologic deficit, decompression
Dislocated facets	Neurologically variable	Traction and surgery
Flexion-rotation injuries	Neurologically variable	Surgical reduction and fusion if anterior subluxation and jumped facet

Compression fractures C3-T1		
Wedge compression/burst fractures	Frequent neurologic damage	Surgical decompression
Teardrop fractures (vertebra dislocated anteriorly with inferior vertebral fracture)	Usually unstable	Posterior fusion
Hyperextension injuries	Geriatric patients with spondylosis producing central cord syndrome	Immobilization; if significant spinal canal narrowing, decompression
Thoracic spine injuries	Incomplete neurologic injury most common	Realignment and stabilization
Thoracolumbar injuries	Neurologic deficits complex	Decompression and fusion
Lumbar injuries	Incomplete neurologic injury	Realignment and decompression
Penetrating injuries	Neurologic deficit variable	Decompression/foreign body removal

Table 13-2. Incomplete spinal cord injury syndromes

Syndrome	Clinical Findings
Anterior cord syndrome	Motor, sensory, temperature and pain lost; vibration/position intact
Central cord syndrome	Motor impairment of upper more than lower extremities
Posterior cord syndrome	Loss of fine, vibratory, and position sensation; preserved motor function
Brown-Séquard (hemicord) syndrome	Ipsilateral paralysis, loss of proprioception, touch, and vibration; contralateral loss of pain and temperature
Conus medullaris syndrome	Areflexic bladder, bowel, and lower extremities; sacral reflexes can be preserved; reduced rectal tone and perirectal sensation
Cauda equina syndrome	Sensory loss with flaccid weakness; sacral reflexes abnormal or absent

lost function. Table 13-3 details the range of cardiac and respiratory dysfunction, depending on the site of acute SCI. Medical problems include these:

Cardiovascular
- Spinal shock
- Bradycardia
- ↓ Myocardial contractility
- Deep venous thrombosis
- Hypothermia

Respiratory
- Respiratory impairment
- Poor cough
- Viscous mucous

Gastrointestinal
- Atony
- Prone to aspiration

Genitourinary
- Bladder distension
- Infection

Electrolytes
- Hypercalcemia
- Hyperphosphatemia
- Hyponatremia
- Hyperkalemia

The effect of SCI on the cardiovascular system depends on the level of injury (Table 13-3). For levels of SCI below T6, the major problem involves varying degrees of hypotension resulting from the functional sympathectomy. With complete SCI above T6, more significant cardiovascular abnormalities including bradycardia, hypotension, ventricular dysfunction, and dysrhythmias are encountered.
1. **Spinal shock,** seen most commonly with physiologic or anatomic transection of the spinal cord

Table 13-3. Level of spinal cord injury and pulmonary/cardiac function

Level of Spinal Cord Injury	Pulmonary Function Ventilatory Function	Cough	Cardiovascular Function Sympathetic Function	Cardiovascular Reserve
C1-2	0	0	Minimal	Minimal
C3-4	0	0	Minimal	Minimal
C5-6	+	+	Minimal	Minimal
C7	+ to ++	+ to ++	Minimal	+
High thoracic	++	++	+ to ++	++
Low thoracic	++ to +++	++ to +++	++ to +++	++ to +++
Lumbar	+++	+++	+++	+++
Sacral	+++	+++	+++	+++

Scale is 0 (no function) to + + + (normal).

above C7, results from a total loss of impulses from higher centers as an immediate consequence of the injury.

a. Spinal shock is characterized by flaccid paralysis, loss of reflexes below the level of the lesion, paralytic ileus, and loss of visceral and somatic sensation, vascular tone, and the vasopressor reflex.

b. This syndrome of autonomic dysfunction and loss of sensory and motor function lasts from days to weeks and is prolonged by serious infection.

c. Neurogenic shock is manifest by hypotension, bradycardia, and hypothermia. The higher the spinal level of injury, the more severe the physiologic derangements. Shock occurs from the disruption of the sympathetic outflow from T1-L2, which results in unopposed vagal tone and vasodilatation with pooling of blood in the peripheral vascular beds. The most common cardiovascular abnormalities encountered after an acute cervical SCI and the associated incidence are listed in the following table.

Marked bradycardia (<45 beats/ minute)	71%
Episodic hypotension	68%
Need for intravenous pressors	35%
Use of atropine or temporary transvenous pacemaker	29%
Primary cardiac arrest	16%

These cardiovascular derangements remain most problematic during the first 2 weeks after acute cervical SCI.

(1) **Bradycardia,** universal with acute complete cervical SCI, results from a functional sympathectomy with interruption of cardiac accelerator nerves (T1-4) and unopposed vagal innervation. Bradycardia usually resolves over a 2- to 6-week period. More profound degrees of bradycardia, as well as cardiac arrest, can occur during stimulation of the patient (e.g., turning the patient, performing tracheal suctioning). Familiarity with the factors precipitating bradycardia lead to the use of preventive interventions (sedation, anticholinergics, 100% oxygen before suctioning, and limiting the time allowed for suctioning). Although the bradycardia is effectively treated with atropine in most cases, a temporary pacemaker can be required.

(2) **Hypotension,** defined as a systolic blood pressure (BP) below 90 mm Hg or 30%

below baseline, is seen in 60% to 80% of patients after acute cervical SCI. Early intervention to maintain the MAP at 85 mm Hg for the first 7 days after injury is recommended to preserve neurologic function while autoregulation is impaired. The heart rate is useful in differentiating between neurogenic shock, manifest by the triad of bradycardia, hypotension, and hypothermia, and hemorrhagic shock as the cause of tachycardia. Hypovolemia from coexisting hemorrhagic shock in patients who also have spinal shock is treated with prompt blood replacement and administration of isotonic crystalloid. The total volume of fluid administered is limited because pulmonary edema and cardiac decompensation can occur, especially in the setting of high SCI.

(a) If hypotension persists despite adequate fluid administration, vasopressor therapy should be instituted. The vasopressor should have beta-agonist properties (e.g., dopamine or dobutamine). Supplementation with an alpha-agonist such as phenylephrine could be necessary. However, care is indicated when choosing a more potent alpha-agonist, such as norepinephrine, which can substantially increase cardiac afterload, impair cardiac output, and precipitate frank left ventricular failure.

(b) Invasive central hemodynamic monitoring is recommended in high SCI as an aid in guiding the clinical management of hypotension. A pulmonary artery occlusion pressure of 14 to 18 mm Hg appears to optimize spinal cord perfusion. In patients who have suffered multiple trauma, hypotension and bradycardia secondary to neurogenic shock can conceal hemorrhagic shock. Operative intervention for spinal injury should be postponed until the patient's hemodynamic status has been optimized.

2. **Disturbances of cardiac rhythm** are commonly observed in SCI and include bradycardia, primary asystole, supraventricular dysrhythmias (atrial fibrillation, reentry supraventricular tachycardia), and ventricular dysrhythmias. An acute autonomic imbalance resulting from a disruption

of sympathetic pathways in the cervical cord is causative. The arrhythmias usually resolve within 14 days of injury.

3. **Left ventricular impairment** has been noted in complete cervical SCI and is attributed to the functional sympathectomy with resulting autonomic imbalance.

4. **Autonomic hyperreflexia** occurs in 85% of patients who have spinal cord transections above T6. This clinical constellation is secondary to autonomic vascular reflexes, which usually begin to appear approximately 1 to 3 weeks after injury (when spinal shock has resolved).

   a. Afferent impulses originating from cutaneous, proprioceptive, and visceral stimuli (bladder or bowel distention, childbirth, manipulations of the urinary tract, or surgical stimulation) are transmitted to the isolated spinal cord. They, in turn, elicit a massive sympathetic response from the adrenal medulla and sympathetic nervous system, which is no longer modulated by the normal inhibitory impulses from the brain stem and hypothalamus. Vasoconstriction occurs below the level of the spinal cord lesion. Reflex activity of carotid and aortic baroreceptors produces vasodilatation above the lesion, which is often accompanied by bradycardia, ventricular dysrhythmias, and even complete heart block.

   b. Common signs and symptoms include hypertension, bradycardia, hyperreflexia, muscle rigidity and spasticity, diaphoresis, pallor, flushing above the lesion, and headache. Horner's syndrome, pupillary changes, anxiety, and nausea occur less frequently. Systolic pressures in excess of 260 mm Hg and diastolic pressures of 220 mm Hg have been reported.

   c. Adverse sequelae include myocardial ischemia, intracranial hemorrhage, pulmonary edema, seizures, coma, and death.

   d. Treatment involves cessation of the offending stimulus and a change to the upright position (pooling of blood in the lower extremities). Pharmacologic intervention includes direct-acting vasodilators (e.g., sodium nitroprusside), beta-blocking drugs (e.g., esmolol), combination alpha- and beta-blocking drugs (e.g., labetalol), calcium-channel blocking drugs, and ganglionic blocking drugs. Because the attacks are often paroxysmal, drugs of rapid onset and short duration are preferred.

E. **Acute care of the patient after SCI.** Preservation of spinal cord function involves maintaining oxygen delivery, stabilizing the spine, and decreasing spinal cord edema and the secondary biochemical processes that exacerbate the neurologic injury. The initial care of the patient after SCI can be considered in the following areas:

1. **External splinting and immobilization.** The spine is immobilized in the field by placing the patient on a spine board with sandbags on either side of the head to prevent rotation.

2. **Medical management.** Identification of associated injuries is crucial. These include the following:

Cervical Spine Injury	*Thoracic Spine Injury*
• Head	• Myocardial
• Airway	• Pulmonary
• Esophagus	• Ribs
Lumbar Spine Injury	• Major vascular
• Abdominal	
• Pelvic	

a. **Airway**

   (1) SCI presents several problems in airway management. Many maneuvers used for intubation can cause displacement and worsening of the injury, especially at the level of the cervical spine (C-spine). For this reason, all patients who have head trauma, multiple trauma, or decreased level of consciousness should be considered as having a spinal injury until proved otherwise radiographically (see Figure 13-3 for the algorithm for airway management for suspected C-spine injury).

   (2) Patients who have a normal level of consciousness, an intact "gag reflex," and a patent airway can be managed conservatively with supplemental oxygen. However, these patients should be observed closely to detect progressive loss of ventilatory ability as a result of developing diaphragmatic or intercostal paralysis. Because profound reductions in forced vital capacity (FVC) and expiratory flow rates are observed immediately after injury, nearly all patients who have an acute cervical SCI require mechanical ventilation within 24 to 48 hours of hospital admission.

   (3) The initial airway management of the C-spine injured patient includes consideration of the following issues:
      (a) The urgency of airway intervention
      (b) The presence of associated facial, neck, or soft tissue injuries

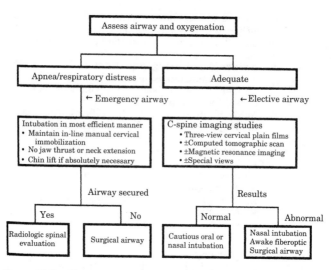

Figure 13-3. Airway management algorithm for the patient who has suspected C-spine injury.

      (c) The presence of basilar skull fracture or midface fractures that contraindicate nasal intubation

      (d) The status of the patient, whether awake or not

      (e) The skill of the operator in using different airway techniques

    (4) Direct laryngoscopy remains the method of choice for emergent airway control in patients who have confirmed or possible C-spine injuries. Mouth opening for laryngoscopy can be facilitated by removing the cervical collar, and neck movement can be minimized by manual in-line stabilization without axial traction. Manual in-line stabilization can in fact result in more movement of unstable structures lower in the neck. Manual in-line stabilization can sometimes make a difficult intubation more difficult. Cricoid pressure can be utilized to reduce the risk of pulmonary aspiration of gastric contents.

    (5) Blind nasal intubation is commonly recommended for airway management. The benefit of this technique is minimal head movement. Potential disadvantages include an extended period of time to perform and trauma to the nasal passage. Nasotracheal intubation is contraindicated in the presence of a basilar skull fracture or extensive facial trauma.

(6) Fiberoptic intubation is appropriate in nonemergent situations in which the airway is free of blood and stomach contents. This technique can facilitate intubation of the larynx with the least amount of neck movement.

(7) In patients who have particularly difficult airways, a catheter passed through a needle inserted into the cricothyroid membrane ("retrograde intubation") and directed out the nose or mouth can also serve as a guide for intubation. Cricothyroidotomy is also an appropriate choice for an anatomically abnormal airway in an emergent situation.

(8) Flexion and extension of the neck during maintenance of the airway and intubation could lead to catastrophic exacerbation of the SCI. Therefore, in-line manual stabilization should be carefully utilized when traditional laryngoscopy proves necessary. This is accomplished by having an assistant hold the sides of the neck and the mastoid process, preventing any movement of the neck. The airway can be opened with a "jaw thrust" technique while the head is maintained in a neutral position without either flexion or extension.

(9) Because of gastric atony and paralytic ileus, SCI patients are considered to have "full stomachs" and are at increased risk for aspiration. Therefore, airway adjuncts such as the laryngeal mask, although helpful in maintaining oxygenation in a situation in which intubation has proven difficult, should not be relied on as a long-term solution. Cricoid pressure is administered with minimum force to avoid inadvertent further injury to the cord. As the application of cricoid pressure can cause neck displacement of up to 9 mm, the risk of causing or exacerbating C-spine injury should be weighed against the risk of pulmonary aspiration. Although excessive movement of the spine is to be avoided, hypoxia secondary to a failure to intubate worsens the prognosis even more so that intubation should be

accomplished as expeditiously as possible.

(10) A brief neurologic examination after intubation reveals any further deterioration in the patient's neurologic condition related to manipulation of the airway or positioning in preparation for intubation.

b. **Pulmonary system.** SCI can have a profound effect on the respiratory system, depending on the level and degree of injury, because of paralysis of the abdominal, intercostal, diaphragmatic, and accessory muscles. Problems include respiratory failure, recurrent lobar atelectasis, hypoventilation, ventilation-perfusion mismatching, pulmonary edema (neurogenic, cardiogenic), bacterial pneumonia, aspiration pneumonitis, and coexisting blunt chest trauma.

(1) Respiratory failure is present in nearly all patients with SCI above C7. The resultant abnormality in respiratory mechanics leads to a reduction in lung volume (tidal volume, expiratory reserve volume, functional residual capacity), impairment of respiratory function (decreased FVC, forced expiratory volume in 1 second [FEV_1], peak forces, peak flows), and retention of pulmonary secretions with progressive hypoxemia and CO_2 retention. In addition, patients can have abdominal distention secondary to gastric atony, which further impairs pulmonary function. Even patients whose weakness does not extend above the abdominal muscles are at risk for abnormal respiratory function because of their inability to clear secretions.

(2) Patients require frequent assessment of respiratory function because significant declines in pulmonary reserve can occur before overt clinical signs of respiratory failure are seen. It is particularly important to perform serial measurements of vital capacity (VC) and negative inspiratory force. When the VC decreases to <50% of predicted, more frequent serial determinations of VC must be made (i.e., every 6 hours). When the VC decreases to <1 L, especially if the patient is dyspneic and hypoxemic, endotracheal intubation should be performed.

(3) The aim of mechanical ventilation in this scenario is to incorporate spontaneous patient effort into the respiratory dynamic

so as to maintain diaphragmatic muscle mass. The combination of synchronized intermittent mandatory ventilation with pressure support will achieve this goal.

(a) Positive end-expiratory pressure is added, beginning with 5 cm H_2O, to recruit collapsed alveoli and prevent further atelectasis. Choosing intermittent "sigh" breaths (e.g., 1 to 2 "sigh" breaths per minute at 10 mL/kg) can also enhance alveolar recruitment.

(b) Weaning from mechanical ventilation after cervical SCI is facilitated by the respiratory muscles' development of spasticity at approximately 3 weeks. Spasticity of the respiratory muscles stabilizes the chest wall sufficiently to improve lung volume and overall ventilatory ability. The VC doubles in volume within 5 weeks of injury in patients whose injuries are at the C4-5 level. Respiratory dynamics in the supine position improve owing to the more cephalad position of the diaphragm. This position is therefore used when weaning.

(4) Lobar atelectasis, common in SCI above C7, requires aggressive pulmonary therapy emphasizing the prevention, recognition, and treatment of secretion retention. Instituted at the time of hospitalization, this regimen includes frequent nasotracheal suctioning, frequent repositioning or rotational beds (i.e., continuous lateral rotation to $\geq 45°$), chest percussion, bronchodilator therapy, deep breathing exercises, incentive spirometry, and assisted coughing. Even with the most aggressive pulmonary care and management, retained secretions result in repeated lobar collapse during the first 2 weeks of hospitalization. Therapeutic bronchoscopy is frequently required during this period.

(5) Pulmonary edema is observed in patients who have acute SCI. Neurogenic causes include intracranial hypertension with high cervical cord injury and increases in extravascular lung water secondary to autonomic dysfunction with sympathetic discharge at the time of injury. Cardiogenic pulmonary edema could also occur because of reduced myocardial inotropy and overzealous fluid administration.

Meticulous fluid management guided by central monitoring is essential in limiting pulmonary complications.

(6) Pneumonia is observed in 70% of cervical and high thoracic spinal cord injuries. Pneumonia can develop from aspiration of gastric contents at the time of the initial injury or can occur later from nosocomial bacterial infection.

(7) Chest trauma resulting in hemothorax, pulmonary contusions, pneumothorax, and rib fractures could be present in patients who have sustained SCI. These injuries often necessitate prolonged mechanical ventilation with difficulty in weaning and delayed operative intervention to stabilize the spine.

c. **Cardiovascular support.** For the first few minutes after SCI, a brief and substantial autonomic discharge from direct compression of sympathetic nerves occurs. This results in severe hypertension and arrhythmias and can cause left ventricular failure, myocardial infarction, and pulmonary capillary leak. This transient phase is usually no longer evident by the time the patient reaches the hospital when hypotension from neurogenic shock and traumatic hypovolemia is commonly seen.

d. **Gastrointestinal (GI) tract.** During the acute stages of SCI, the GI tract loses autonomic neural input and becomes atonic. Intestinal ileus (especially after thoracic and lumbar SCI) and gastric atony can cause gastric distention and place the patient at risk for aspiration. Moreover, the dilatation can also cause upward pressure on the diaphragm, adversely affecting ventilation. Insertion of a nasogastric tube limits distention and reduces the risk of regurgitation.

(1) Because hypochloremic metabolic alkalosis can occur with excessive gastric suctioning, careful monitoring of fluid and electrolyte balance must be provided.

(2) Gastritis and gastric ulceration and hemorrhage can occur after SCI, especially in patients requiring mechanical ventilation or as a result of administration of corticosteroids. Preventive techniques include monitoring gastric pH and the use of antacids or H_2 blocking drugs.

(3) Other diseases occurring in critically ill patients after SCI include pancreatitis, acalculous cholecystitis, and gastric perforation (especially in those receiving high-dose steroids).

(4) Patients who have acute SCI are characteristically catabolic. Therefore, the initiation of nutritional supplementation within the first few days after injury is advised.

e. **Genitourinary.** During the acute stages of SCI, the bladder is flaccid. Insertion of a latex-free (to prevent the development of latex allergy) indwelling urinary catheter is often necessary. Adequate hydration is likely if urinary volume is >0.5 mL/kg/hour in the absence of renal dysfunction.

(1) Bladder flaccidity is followed by bladder spasticity. The abnormalities of bladder emptying predispose the patient to recurrent urinary tract infections, bladder stones, nephrocalcinosis, and recurrent urosepsis.

(2) Although an indwelling drainage catheter is required during the initial 2 to 3 weeks after injury to prevent urinary retention and reflex vagal responses, intermittent straight catheterization of the bladder with latex-free catheters should be instituted as soon as feasible.

(3) Acute renal failure is uncommon but can occur as a result of hypotension, dehydration, sepsis, or associated trauma.

f. **Temperature control.** The body temperature of patients who have injuries above C7 tends to approach that of the environment (poikilothermia) owing to the inability to conserve heat in cold environments through vasoconstriction and the inability to sweat in hot ambient conditions. Consequently, these patients are prone to hypothermia if the ambient temperature is lower than normal body temperature. While hypothermia can provide some degree of spinal cord protection, it can also increase the incidence of arrhythmias and prolong the effects of anesthesia. Delayed awakening is problematic because it interferes with prompt neurologic examination.

g. **Deep venous thrombosis (DVT).** Without prophylaxis against DVT after acute SCI, patients have an incidence of asymptomatic DVT of 60% to 100%. Venograms become positive within 6 to 8 days after injury. Despite an increased awareness of DVT as a complication of SCI, pulmonary embolism (PE) occurs in 10% to 13% of SCI patients and ranks as the third leading cause of death. Given the high risk of DVT and PE after SCI, a multimodal prophylactic medical management plan is recommended. With effective treatment, the occurrence of DVT can be decreased to 5%. A recent consensus statement on the prevention of DVT in the SCI patient has been published to guide therapy. It includes the following:

(1) Thromboprophylaxis should be provided for all patients after acute SCI.

(2) Single prophylactic modalities such as low-dose unfractionated heparin (LDUH), graduated compression stockings (GCS), and intermittent pneumatic compression (IPC) should be avoided.

(3) Prophylaxis should be instituted as soon as feasible after primary hemostasis has been ensured. The combination of IPC and either LDUH or low-molecular-weight heparin (LMWH) should be used.

(4) In patients who have an incomplete SCI and evidence of a perispinal hematoma on computed tomographic (CT) scan or magnetic resonance imaging (MRI), the administration of LMWH should be delayed for 1 to 3 days.

(5) IPC and/or GCS should be used when prophylaxis with an anticoagulant is contraindicated.

(6) An inferior vena caval filter should not be used as primary thromboprophylaxis against PE, but should be used when anticoagulation is contraindicated or after a documented PE in a patient already receiving anticoagulant therapy.

(7) During the rehabilitation phase after acute SCI, either LMWH prophylaxis should be continued or the patient should be converted to an oral vitamin K antagonist to achieve an international normalized ratio (INR) of 2 to 3.

(8) DVT prophylaxis should be continued for 3 months.

3. **Neurologic examination.** The neurologic examination determines areas that need radiologic evaluation and establishes a baseline for subsequent assessment. The following neurologic examination can be performed quickly and efficiently. A more thorough examination can be performed if indicated.

a. **Consciousness.** Is the patient alert, oriented, and responsive?

b. **Motor system.** Function and strength of the major muscle groups are graded with reference to the normal segmental innervation. If possible, cerebellar function can be assessed by having the patient touch finger to nose.

c. **Sensory system.** This examination includes an assessment of proprioception and the patient's response to light touch and pinprick. Perirectal sensation and the presence of either the bulbocavernosus reflex or the anal-cutaneous reflex are important indicators of the preservation of distal function (sacral sparing), which can mean a more favorable prognosis. A rectal examination is performed to assess voluntary contraction of the anal sphincter. The most caudad level with normal motor and sensory function is designated as the level of injury (Table 13-4).

d. **Cranial nerves.** The specific nerves evaluated depend on the patient's level of injury, associated injury, and level of consciousness. The responses most often evaluated include the pupillary reflex, ocular movement, tongue movement, and function of the trigeminal and facial nerves.

e. **Reflexes.** Commonly tested reflexes include the biceps, triceps, patellar, Achilles, abdominal, cremasteric, and Babinski.

4. **Radiologic evaluation**

a. The incidence of cervical spinal injury in comatose trauma patients is 7%. Therefore, radiologic assessment of the spine is essential after traumatic injuries, particularly in those individuals who are either comatose or have signs and symptoms referable to a SCI.

b. Assessment begins with plain X-ray films. The three-view cervical spine series, composed of lateral, anteroposterior, and open-mouth odontoid views, detect most cervical spinal injuries. For C-spine injuries, a useful method of analysis of the plain films addresses the following:

(1) *Adequacy* and quality of the occipital-cervical junction (C1-2), C3-7, and the C7-T1 junction.

(2) *Alignment* of the anterior edge of the vertebral body, the posterior edge of the vertebral body, the spinolaminar junction, and the tips of the spinous process (Figure 13-4).

(3) *Bones* should be assessed for fractures of the vertebral body, pedicle, lamina, and spinous process.

(4) *Cartilage* assessment includes analysis of the disk space and the facet joints.

(5) *Soft tissue* space should be observed for edema and other abnormalities.

c. As many as 15% to 20% of patients with a C-spine injury do not have an abnormality on

Table 13-4. Muscle group with corresponding level of innervation

Injury Level	Sensory Deficit	Affected Muscle Group
C4	Acromioclavicular joint	Diaphragm
C5	Antecubital fossa (lateral)	Shoulder rotators and abductors, elbow flexors
C6	Thumb	Supinators, pronators, wrist extensors
C7	Middle finger	Elbow extensors, wrist flexors
C8	Little finger	Finger flexors, distal phalanx
T1	Antecubital fossa (medial)	Intrinsic hand muscles
L2	Upper anterior thigh	Hip flexors
L3	Medial femoral condyle	Knee extensors
L4	Medial malleolus	Ankle dorsiflexors
L5	Dorsum of foot	Toe extensors
S1	Lateral heel	Plantar flexors
S2-5	Popliteal fossa, ischial tuberosity, perianal area	Sphincter ani, bulbocavernosus reflex

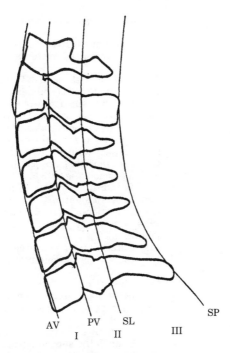

Figure 13-4.   The lateral cervical spine. Spinal column stability after traumatic injury is often based on a system that divides the spine into four longitudinal lines from anterior to posterior, starting with the anterior edge of the vertebral body (AV), the posterior edge of the vertebral body (PV), the spinolaminar junction (SL), and the tips of the spinous process (SP). Each line provides the border for three columns (I, II, and III). Disruption of two or more of these columns indicates spinal instability.

the plain film. A more comprehensive radiologic evaluation can be indicated.

(1)   CT scan is helpful to do the following:

   (a)   Define bony and soft tissue abnormalities
   (b)   Evaluate the lower C-spine
   (c)   Measure spinal canal and neuroforaminal diameter
   (d)   Provide detailed anatomy of the facet joints
   (e)   Detect hematoma formation
   (f)   Determine compression of the spinal canal and spinal stability
   (g)   Detect a unilateral jumped facet or bone fragments in the canal or root foramen

- **(h)** Confirm complete reduction of a dislocation
- **(i)** Demonstrate hyperdense acute blood or retropulsed vertebral body fragments
- **(2)** Axial CT scan through C1 and C2 and through the lower C-spine is indicated in situations in which poorly visualized or suspicious areas are noted on plain films. The negative predictive value of the combination of a normal three-view cervical spine series supplemented with CT scan through areas that are poorly visualized and "suspicious" is 98% to 100%.
- **(3)** MRI is indicated within 48 hours of injury for symptomatic SCI and in comatose trauma patients who can have a cervical spinal injury. MRI is helpful for the following:
  - **(a)** Determining the degree of injury to the soft tissue contents of the spinal canal
  - **(b)** Identifying ligamentous injury, nerve root compression, and pathologic signals from the spinal cord itself
  - **(c)** Predicting functional neurologic outcome in the subacute stage of SCI
  - **(d)** Visualizing the epidural and subarachnoid spaces
  - **(e)** Detecting elevation of the anterior or posterior longitudinal ligaments
- **(4)** Flexion–extension films performed under fluoroscopic guidance are recommended as an alternative to MRI to evaluate the degree of ligamentous stability in awake patients who have symptoms of cervical spinal injury and in comatose trauma patients.

5. Neuroprotective strategies

   a. Spinal alignment

- **(1)** Studies have shown that movement of the injured segment results in exacerbation of the initial injury. Therefore, an important neuroprotective strategy is to relieve cord compression and ischemia and prevent further neurologic compromise by immediate and effective immobilization of the spine with either tongs or halo traction devices. Failure to accomplish this can lead to either loss of residual neurologic function or even ascension of the patient's level of neurologic injury.
- **(2)** Patients who have unstable injuries are placed in traction to align and immobilize

the spine, decompress neural structures, and prevent further injury. Diminished pressure on the cord improves microvascular circulation, which could reduce spinal cord edema. If there is no bony instability, traction is not usually needed for patients who have sustained penetrating injuries.

   (3) Thoracic and lumbar fractures and dislocations can initially be stabilized by restricting the patient to bed rest and turning him or her in a log-roll fashion to preserve spinal alignment. Surgical intervention usually stabilizes subluxations in these regions.

b. **Surgical reduction** and stabilization could be necessary for dislocations that cannot be reduced by traction and/or manipulation because of the nature of the injury. **Surgical decompression** within the first 2 hours of injury can increase the chances of recovery. The decision as to the timing of surgery after spinal injury depends on these factors:

   (1) Assessment of the underlying injury
   (2) Failure of medical, manipulative, and bracing procedures to achieve adequate alignment
   (3) The documented benefit of early decompression or stabilization of the spine
   (4) The presence of progressive neurologic deficits and/or refractory pain
   (5) The severity of any coexisting illnesses, infections, or trauma
   (6) The documented benefit of earlier patient mobilization and rehabilitation from early surgical intervention (within 8 to 72 hours after injury)

c. **Physiologic therapy**

   (1) Cooling has been shown to be effective in the treatment of SCI. The limitations of the clinical studies are small cohorts and lack of controls. The high mortality is also of concern. The effect of modest hypothermia on spinal recovery after trauma continues to be evaluated, but clinical efficacy in human SCI has demonstrated little benefit thus far. Conversely, hyperthermia is deleterious. Aggressive measures to prevent hyperthermia should be taken to minimize the propagation of secondary neuronal damage after traumatic SCI.
   (2) Some advocate hypertension to improve perfusion in the posttraumatic patient who has evidence of impaired

autoregulation and hypoperfusion of the spinal cord. Definitive human data are not available. The MAP is maintained in the normal to high-normal range (85 mm Hg) by either volume replacement (nondextrose-containing crystalloid, colloid, or blood products) if hemorrhagic shock predominates or inotropes and vasopressors if neurologic shock is the cause of hypotension. More aggressive achievement of hypertension carries the risk of intramedullary hemorrhage and edema.

(3) Glucose-containing solutions are avoided. Studies in experimental models have shown that even minimally increased blood glucose levels worsen neurologic outcome.

d. Pharmacologic therapy

(1) **Corticosteroids** administered after acute SCI are currently considered the standard of care. Previous studies have shown that steroids have the potential to stabilize membrane structures, maintain the blood-spinal cord barrier, enhance SCBF, alter electrolyte concentrations at the site of injury, inhibit endorphin release, scavenge damaging free radicals, and limit the inflammatory response after injury.

The current use and dosage of corticosteroids are based on the National Acute Spinal Cord Injury II Study (NASCIS) reported in 1990. This prospective, randomized, placebo-controlled study compared high-dose methylprednisolone (MP) with naloxone and placebo in patients who had complete and incomplete acute SCI. MP, administered within 8 hours of injury as a 30 mg/kg bolus over the first hour and then infused at 5.4 mg/kg/hour for 23 hours, was associated with improvement in motor function and in sensation at 6 months of follow-up as compared to both naloxone and placebo.

The National Acute Spinal Cord Injury III Study, published in 1997, showed that if MP is given within 3 hours of SCI, the steroid infusion need be continued for only 24 hours. If therapy is initiated within 3 and 8 hours of injury, however, the steroid infusion should be administered for 48 hours. Both studies demonstrated an increase in medical complications in steroid-treated patients: longer hospitalizations, increased wound infections, and an increased incidence of pneumonia, GI bleeding, and severe sepsis.

(2) **Mannitol,** 0.25 to 1 g/kg, can be used to treat cord edema. The ensuing osmotic diuresis necessitates close attention to the patient's intravascular volume.

(3) **Hypertonic saline (HS)** use in experimental models of acute SCI has suggested that it can enhance the delivery of MP and prevent immunosuppression, leading to improvements in overall neurologic function and survival rates after SCI. No conclusive evidence has yet been published demonstrating similar benefits in human SCI. The use of HS in the setting of acute SCI, therefore, remains largely experimental.

(4) Other pharmacologic agents have been studied in acute SCI as treatment modalities either to limit secondary injury or enhance neurologic recovery. Such agents have included GM_1 ganglioside, tirilazad, naloxone, thyrotropin-releasing hormone, and nimodipine. None of these agents has clearly demonstrated an improvement in outcome after acute SCI, and their use is therefore not currently recommended.

F. Anesthetic management of acute SCI

1. **Preoperative evaluation.** The SCI patient frequently has multiple medical complications that can impact the anesthetic plan.

   a. **Indicated studies** include complete blood count, serum electrolytes, blood urea nitrogen, creatinine, glucose, liver function tests, and a urinalysis. A preoperative electrocardiogram (ECG), arterial blood gas, chest x-ray, and pulmonary function tests can also be indicated.

   b. **Airway evaluation** is necessary. Examination of the airway must include the oropharynx with a Mallampati classification and range of motion of the neck with particular attention to any limitation from either pain or neurologic symptoms. If movement elicits any abnormality, the offending position is avoided. Airway problems are most frequently encountered in patients who have atlantoaxial subluxations, traumatic C-spine injuries in combination with facial trauma, severe kyphoscoliosis or spinal deformities, and spinal stabilization devices. When the patient is in a halo brace or other cervical fixation device, plans for either an awake tracheal intubation or other technique to secure the airway should be made.

    c. Neurologic evaluation is performed preoperatively to document any preexisting neurologic deficits. Regional anesthesia is chosen only after careful evaluation and review of all preexisting deficits.

    d. Pulmonary evaluation must consider the level of SCI. For instance, patients who have a C-spine injury have restrictive pulmonary defects and marked reductions in lung volumes that predispose them to hypoxemia. Injuries of the cervical and high thoracic spine engender difficulties with clearance of secretions, which could also predispose patients to hypoxemia and hypercarbia.

    e. Cardiac evaluation is essential to elicit evidence of cardiovascular dysfunction from either the acute SCI or preexisting abnormalities. In addition, an assessment of the degree of orthostatic hypotension and the risk of autonomic hyperreflexia should be made.

2. Monitoring. Decisions regarding the utilization of advanced monitoring are based on the level of injury and neurologic deficit, the complexity and length of the surgical procedure, and any preexisting underlying medical diseases.

    a. Neurophysiologic monitoring is often indicated for patients who have no neurologic injuries but are at high risk owing to the instability of their spinal abnormalities and for patients who have incomplete neurologic injuries and are undergoing operations for spinal stabilization. Neurophysiologic monitoring could consist of an intraoperative wake-up test, somatosensory evoked potential (SSEP) monitoring, or motor evoked potential monitoring. SSEPs monitor the posterior columns of the spinal cord, whereas motor evoked potentials monitor the anterior portion of the spinal cord. For a more comprehensive description of spinal cord monitoring, see Chapter 3.

    b. Intracranial pressure monitoring can be necessary for patients who also have head injuries.

    c. Routine monitors (ECG, pulse oximetry, capnography, noninvasive BP, temperature) are employed for every procedure. A latex-free urinary catheter is used to monitor the patient's volume status.

    d. In patients who have spinal shock, the institution of **direct BP** monitoring is indicated, ideally before induction of anesthesia. The arterial catheter is also useful for blood gas measurements and other laboratory determinations that can be necessary intraoperatively.

e. Early use of **pulmonary artery catheters** during spinal shock is appropriate. Measurement of intracardiac pressures (central venous pressure [CVP], pulmonary capillary wedge pressure [PCWP], left ventricular end diastolic pressure [LVEDP]) in conjunction with cardiac output and BP is necessary to differentiate hypovolemia from low systemic vascular resistance (SVR). The information obtained is helpful in determining the appropriate form of management (fluid versus vasopressors) and in monitoring the response to therapy.

   (1) Patients who have low SVR can be treated with titrated infusions of a direct-acting alpha-agonist, as above.

   (2) Patients who are hypovolemic can receive fluid boluses of 250 to 500 mL. A Starling curve, identifying the optimal fluid filling pressure, can be derived from the changes in intracardiac pressures (CVP, PCWP, LVEDP), cardiac output, and BP in response to the fluids.

3. **Anesthetic technique**

   a. **Securing the airway** without causing or exacerbating SCI is the principal concern.

   (1) **An awake intubation** has the advantage that the patient acts as a monitor to avoid worsening the SCI. In addition, a neurologic evaluation can document the absence of any new changes. An awake intubation also avoids the use of succinylcholine and the attendant risk of hyperkalemia.

   (2) **A *blind* nasal endotracheal intubation** is often recommended as one of the best means to avoid spinal manipulation during intubation. This approach is contraindicated with facial trauma or a basilar skull fracture. Topical application of 0.2% phenylephrine hydrochloride in 4% lidocaine is essential to shrink nasal tissues and limit bleeding. Anesthesia of the tongue can be achieved using 2% lidocaine ointment or local anesthetic sprays. Anesthesia of the vocal cords and larynx is achieved by using the combination of a transtracheal injection of 4% lidocaine via a percutaneous puncture of the cricothyroid membrane and superior laryngeal nerve blocks with the bilateral injection of lidocaine 1%, 2 mL, into the thyrohyoid membrane just above the lateral wings of the thyroid cartilage. An alternative technique uses nebulized lidocaine 4% to a maximum dose of no >4 to 5 mg/kg.

Calculations of toxicity must include all topical and injected local anesthetics.

(3) **Fiberoptic endotracheal intubation** can be used in a nonemergent situation after anesthetizing the airway as detailed in the preceding text. With the oral route, the use of either a bite block or large oral airway containing a central passageway for the fiberoptic scope is essential. In addition, oral intubation often mandates the use of mild sedation to facilitate patient acceptance. Blood, debris, and vomitus in the airway mitigate against fiberoptic intubation.

(4) **Direct laryngoscopy** can be appropriate if the previous methods do not seem feasible. Neutrality of the neck must be maintained to prevent further SCI. Extension or flexion during intubation can cause displacement and worsening of the original SCI. In-line manual cervical immobilization appears to be the safest method to minimize spinal column motion.

(5) When either severe facial trauma or neck instability exists or the airway is lost, a **surgical airway** via cricothyrotomy or tracheotomy can be necessary. The method selected for intubation depends on perceived airway difficulties, coexisting disease and trauma, and other factors including facial trauma and soft tissue swelling.

b. **Induction**

(1) The sympathetic function of SCI patients is unpredictable. Because they are also frequently hypovolemic, the induction should proceed slowly in an elective situation. When the patient has a full stomach, a rapid-sequence induction is indicated after adequate volume replacement has been accomplished.

(a) Ketamine, 1 to 2 mg/kg i.v., provides a more stable hemodynamic profile during induction. It has the added advantage of amplifying the electrophysiologic monitor's signal amplitude, but its use is not generally recommended in the presence of intracranial hypertension.

(b) Etomidate provides cardiovascular stability during induction.

(2) During the induction of general anesthesia, the maintenance of a spinal cord perfusion pressure of at least 60 mm Hg (ideally 80 to 90 mm Hg) is essential. The

patient in the early phase of spinal shock after a high cord injury is at risk of developing bradycardia or asystole. Accordingly, some have advocated the use of a prophylactic anticholinergic to avoid this complication.

(3) Excessive fluctuations of cardiovascular parameters should be treated with direct-acting agonists and antagonists. These drugs should preferably be short acting and delivered via intravenous infusion. Sympathetic agonists and antagonists that release catecholamines indirectly are avoided.

c. **Muscle relaxants.** The SCI patient whose injury involves skeletal muscles develops a supersensitivity to depolarizing muscle relaxants. With muscle denervation, the number of postsynaptic acetylcholine receptors increases greatly and amplifies any small neuromuscular signal that can be present. When depolarized by succinylcholine, pores on the neuromuscular junction open maximally, allowing massive egress of stored intracellular potassium. The occurrence of succinylcholine-induced ventricular fibrillation secondary to this acute hyperkalemic response has been reported.

Because the time course for the development of the extrajunctional receptors is not known precisely (but can be as short as 24 hours), succinylcholine is best avoided even in recently injured patients. It is also important to realize that the magnitude of the potassium release is more a function of the amount of muscle mass affected than of the dose of depolarizing drug given. Even small doses of succinylcholine have triggered significant hyperkalemia. The administration of succinylcholine should be avoided in patients who have SCI.

d. **Positioning.** Spinal operations are most often performed in the **prone** position. Patients can be anesthetized on the bed or stretcher and then log rolled onto the operating table. Important goals include maintaining the head and neck in a neutral position; providing adequate padding to the chest, abdomen, head, and extremities; and avoiding excessive neck flexion or extension. Special attention should be given to the endotracheal tube because significant movement or obstruction can occur with changes of position. Sudden changes of position should also be avoided because they can have significant hemodynamic consequences owing to the lack of adequate compensatory vasoconstrictor and cardiac reflexes to maintain venous return and cardiac output.

The head is positioned so that the bony prominences support its weight without pressure on the eyes, ears, or nose. The position of the head can be adjusted slightly every 15 minutes or so throughout the procedure to ensure adequate perfusion under the weight-bearing area.

When an awake intubation is employed, the use of nerve blocks instead of sedatives enables the patients to position themselves. This allows a neurologic examination to be performed after positioning and helps ensure that the operative position does not aggravate the injury. Information gleaned from the preoperative neurologic examination (range of motion, motions that worsen symptoms) also helps to prevent the positioning from exacerbating the neurologic injury.

e. **Maintenance.** The choice of anesthetic drugs is guided by the patient's underlying condition. The anesthetic drugs selected should maintain optimal SCBF. The use of neurologic monitors necessitates the avoidance of drugs (e.g., volatile anesthetics) that either suppress the monitored responses or cause fluctuations in the anesthetic depth, which can confuse the interpretation of the evoked responses.

In general, drug regimens that utilize opiate infusions serve this purpose. Regional techniques can be considered, but the high incidence of coexisting injury and the frequency of hemodynamic and respiratory compromise virtually guarantee that general anesthesia is preferable.

Some evidence indicates that hypocapnia decreases SCI from ischemia. However, because hypocapnia could also compromise perfusion, normocapnia is recommended.

4. **Fluid management.** Fluid administration is based on the estimated preoperative fluid deficits, intraoperative blood and fluid losses, and a knowledge of the effect of the level of SCI on cardiac and pulmonary function. Meticulous fluid management is essential because patients who have high thoracic and cervical spine injuries have an increased propensity for developing pulmonary edema. In addition, cervical spine injury can cause cardiac dysfunction with decreased inotropy and chronotropy (from reduced sympathetic neural input to the heart). Whether to use either crystalloid or colloid for volume resuscitation is of less importance than the need to avoid glucose-containing solutions, which are known to exacerbate SCI.

5. **Temperature regulation.** SCI patients have impaired thermoregulation below the level of the injury. Prophylactic measures to prevent intraoperative hypothermia should be aggressively instituted. These include a warm ambient environment, warming of intravenous fluids, standard warming mattresses, humidification of the respiratory circuit, and forced hot-air blankets. Keep in mind, however, that hyperthermia exacerbates neurologic injury.

6. **Postoperative care.** Even patients who had adequate respiratory function before surgery could require a weaning period postoperatively before extubation owing to the residual effects of the anesthetics. Because of the potential difficulty in reintubating the trachea of the SCI patient, determination of the appropriate time for extubation should be extremely conservative. Critical care weaning parameters are used in place of routine extubation criteria after most operative procedures. Once the trachea has been extubated, the patient is monitored for several hours to ensure that the respiratory status does not deteriorate.

   Extubation criteria include the following:

   a. **Blood gases**
      (1) pH >7.3
      (2) Pa_{O_2} >60 mm Hg
      (3) Pa_{CO_2} <50 mm Hg
      (4) Ratio of partial pressure of arterial oxygen to inspired fraction of oxygen (Pa_{O_2}/fraction of inspired oxygen [F_{IO_2}]) >200

   b. **Pulmonary functions**
      (1) Maximal negative inspiratory forces <-25 cm H_2O
      (2) VC >15 mL/kg
      (3) Respiratory rate <25/minute
      (4) Dead space-to-tidal volume ratio <0.6

   c. **Other**
      (1) Patient conscious and oriented
      (2) Unlabored, or minimally labored, breathing
      (3) Ability to generate a cough
      (4) Minimal volume of tracheal secretions
      (5) Stable cardiac function
      (6) Optimal intravascular fluid volume and electrolyte status
      (7) Absence of infection

G. **Chronic SCI.** As improved emergency medical care increases the survival of patients who have high-level spinal cord injuries, one is more likely to encounter patients who now have chronic SCIs scheduled for surgical procedures for spinal and other indications. Many issues raised regarding acute SCIs apply equally to patients who have chronic injury. There are, however, a number of additional medical problems (Table 13-5).

Table 13-5. Medical problems of the patient who has chronic spinal cord injury

System	Abnormality	Relevant Comment
Cardiovascular	• Autonomic hyperreflexia • ↓ Blood volume • Orthostatic hypotension	Susceptible to hypertensive crisis if SCI level is above T6. Positional changes and intrathoracic pressure can cause hypotension.
Respiratory	• Muscle weakness • ↓ Respiratory drive • ↓ Cough	SCI patient is susceptible to postoperative pneumonia and can be difficult to wean from mechanical ventilation.
Muscular	• Proliferation of acetylcholine receptors • Spasticity	Hyperkalemia from succinylcholine.
Genitourinary	• Recurrent urinary tract infections • Altered bladder emptying	Can lead to renal insufficiency, pyelonephritis, sepsis, or amyloidosis. Frequent catheterization can cause latex allergy.

Gastrointestinal	• Gastroparesis	Susceptible to aspiration.
	• Ileus	
Immunologic	• Urinary tract infection	Watch for subtle signs of infection and sepsis. Questionable risk of seeding an infection from invasive monitoring.
	• Pneumonia	
	• Decubitus ulcers	
Skin	• Decubitus ulcers	Prevention.
Hematologic	• Anemia	DVT prophylaxis.
	• Risk of DVT	
Bone	• ↓ Bone density	Osteoporosis, hypercalcemia, heterotopic ossification, muscle calcification, pathologic fractures.
Nervous system	• Chronic pain	Perioperative pain can be difficult to control.

SCI, spinal cord injury; DVT, deep vein thrombosis.

1. **Preoperative.** Respiratory complications are the most common cause of morbidity in SCI patients. Pneumonia is second only to anoxia at the time of injury as the cause of death. Any fever with a leukocytosis or physical or radiographic evidence of pneumonitis should be treated aggressively.

   Patients who have chronic injury are more prone to episodes of hypertension secondary to autonomic hyperreflexia, especially with lesions above T6. Muscle spasms also occur because of hyperactive spinal reflexes without the modulating effect of cortical, brain stem, and cerebellar centers. This "mass reflex" could require the therapeutic use of skeletal muscle relaxants in the awake patient.

2. **Intraoperative**

   a. Regional anesthesia can offer some advantage for patients who still have instability of the cervical spine or whose initial repair limits their cervical range of motion. Should general anesthesia prove necessary for this subset of patients, all precautions for airway manipulation should be employed.

   b. General anesthesia and regional anesthesia are equally effective in preventing autonomic hyperreflexia. Techniques based on the use of oxygen/nitrous oxide/narcotics seem to be less efficacious in this regard. When deciding on the appropriateness of a regional technique, one should consider the site of injury as well as the site of surgery. The patient's underlying hemodynamic status should also be considered. Regardless of the technique, direct-acting vasodilators (e.g., nitroprusside), alpha-adrenergic blocking drugs (e.g., phentolamine), antiarrhythmics (e.g., lidocaine, esmolol), atropine, and other antihypertensives (e.g., labetalol) should be readily available.

   c. Chronic SCI puts all patients at risk for a hyperkalemic response to depolarizing muscle relaxants. Decreasing the dose does not reliably prevent the response. Therefore, succinylcholine is to be avoided.

      As the receptors at the neuromuscular junction of denervated muscle are upregulated, basing the dose of nondepolarizing muscle relaxants on twitch response from a denervated limb leads to a relative overdose of muscle relaxant. This should be considered when giving the initial dose, when reversing the relaxation at the end of the procedure, and when judging readiness for extubation.

   d. Urinary retention and urinary tract infections are persistent problems. A distended bladder can trigger the hypertensive response of autonomic hyperreflexia. Therefore, in addition to routine monitors, these patients should have a latex-free urinary catheter inserted for most procedures.

3. **Postoperative.** Postoperative management, including when to extubate the trachea, should be guided primarily by the requirements of the surgical procedure and the patient's underlying medical condition.

III. **Spinal cord tumors.** Spinal tumors can be primary or metastatic in origin. The medical problems associated with the patient are determined by the location of the spinal lesion and by the location of the primary tumor in metastatic lesions. Depending on the length of time since the presentation of the spinal lesion and its associated signs and symptoms, these patients could have many of the same complications seen in patients after traumatic injury to the spinal cord.

A. **Preoperative management**

1. Lesions of the upper spinal cord are the most damaging physiologically. Respiratory impairment secondary to loss of activity of the intercostal muscles and/or diaphragmatic is common. A blood gas measurement is indicated to determine the patient's baseline respiratory status. In addition, the decreased ability to clear secretions can frequently result in pneumonitis, which can require further intervention. Such infections are not always associated with elevated temperature, nor does elevated temperature always point to an infection because temperature regulation is frequently impaired as well.

2. Cardiovascular tone could be diminished with resulting hypotension. This also occurs in patients with acute SCI. One must differentiate neurogenic hypotension from the hypotension resulting from dehydration and malnutrition, commonly associated with patients who have cancer. Such dehydration could be exacerbated in patients who have recently undergone diagnostic radiographic tests that involved the use of contrast dyes because these usually act as diuretics.

3. In addition to the basic chemistries, preoperative blood determinations should include liver function tests to identify the presence, if any, of metastasis to the liver. The possibility of pituitary and adrenal insufficiency should also be considered because these are frequent sites of metastatic lesions.

4. Premedication should be kept to a minimum because it is useful to be able to reassess neurologic function immediately before operation. In particular, sedatives are avoided in situations in which the respiratory status is already impaired.

B. Intraoperative management

1. The planned procedure and the location of the lesion dictate the choice of monitors beyond the routine. Patients who exhibit signs of spinal shock are managed more effectively with the cardiovascular information provided by a pulmonary artery catheter and an arterial line. Those patients at risk for autonomic hyperreflexia can also require the "beat-to-beat" BP monitoring provided by an arterial line.

2. The positioning of these patients for the procedures frequently places the surgical site above the level of the heart. This increases the risk for pulmonary air embolism. The anesthetic plan should incorporate a monitor for the detection of air embolism (e.g., precordial Doppler, transesophageal echocardiography, pulmonary artery pressure) as well as an appropriately positioned CVP line to aspirate air.

3. The risk of hyperkalemia with the use of succinylcholine is increased as it was for the patient who has SCI. The use of nondepolarizing relaxants is recommended to ensure a quiet surgical field. However, because of upregulation of receptors in the neuromuscular junction secondary to denervation, care should be taken to select an appropriate site for monitoring twitch suppression via the nerve stimulator.

4. Maintenance of anesthesia can be accomplished with any general anesthetic technique. However, in procedures in which the use of SSEPs is anticipated, drugs that suppress the monitored potentials are avoided. In such circumstances, a nitrous oxide/oxygen/narcotic technique is more appropriate. Frequent changes of anesthetic depth are avoided because they interfere with the interpretation of the SSEPs.

C. Postoperative management. The decision regarding early extubation of these patients is made on a case-by-case basis. Early extubation in a fully awake patient facilitates postoperative neurologic examination. The appropriateness of early extubation depends on the patient's baseline respiratory function, location and size of the tumor, and duration and degree of difficulty of surgical dissection. Patients who were operated for high-level lesions require close monitoring for as long as 48 to 72 hours postoperatively. During this time, edema at the surgical site can cause renewed compression of the spinal cord and lead to progressive respiratory compromise and loss of protective gag reflexes. Reintubation, when necessary, should be done early in the course of respiratory deterioration. This allows accomplishing control of the airway in a patient who has a potentially unstable neck in as nonemergent an environment as possible.

IV. Scoliosis
  A. General
    1. Scoliosis is a structural disease of the vertebral column causing lateral curvature of the spine with rotation of the vertebra.
    2. Scoliosis most frequently involves the thoracic and lumbar regions.
    3. The severity of the disease is expressed in "degrees of lateral angulation." A larger degree of angulation represents more severe disease. The side of the convexity of the curve designates it as a right or left curvature.
    4. Idiopathic scoliosis, accounting for almost 75% of cases, occurs most frequently in adolescent girls. Other types are classified as *nonstructural* (caused by gait/posture), *congenital, neuromuscular*, and *traumatic*.
    5. The degree of severity of scoliosis correlates directly with the degree of respiratory dysfunction. Curvatures of <60° are not usually associated with significant pulmonary involvement, whereas patients who have curvatures of >100° are typically severely impaired.
    6. Pulmonary function testing typically reveals a restrictive pattern owing to the reduction in chest wall compliance with reductions in all measures of lung capacity and volume. The greatest decrease is noted in the VC. Blood gas analysis reveals a lower Pao_2, which is primarily because of the ventilation-perfusion mismatch that occurs. $Paco_2$ is not usually altered unless an obstructive pulmonary component has also developed, a condition more common in the elderly.
    7. In patients who have more severe thoracic disease, rib cage deformities lead to the underdevelopment of the pulmonary vasculature. This is exacerbated by hypoxic pulmonary vasoconstriction and can result in potentially significant elevations in pulmonary vascular resistance. Right ventricular hypertrophy and right atrial enlargement can occur as a result of these changes in pulmonary vascular resistance. Eventually patients develop irreversible pulmonary hypertension and cor pulmonale.
  B. Preoperative management
    1. The preoperative assessment should include information about the location and degree of scoliosis as well as its etiology. Both location and degree of disease play a role in determining the amount of pulmonary/cardiac involvement one can expect to find. Scoliosis owing to concurrent neurologic motor deficits can alter the choice of muscle relaxants.
    2. Physical examination indicates necessary testing. Patients who have limited exercise tolerance

require further pulmonary function testing to ascertain the extent of their pulmonary insufficiency. Patients who have vital capacities below 25 mL/kg are high operative risks.

   3. Preoperative sedation is avoided in patients who have significant pulmonary compromise.

C. **Intraoperative management**
   1. Decisions regarding monitoring are guided by the extent of pulmonary and cardiac involvement. One should consider an arterial line for blood gas measurement in any patient who has even moderately reduced pulmonary reserve. An arterial line is also necessary for closer monitoring of BP when "deliberate hypotension" is employed to reduce intraoperative blood loss.
   2. Pulmonary artery catheter monitoring should be reserved for those patients who have either pulmonary hypertension or significantly diminished right ventricular output.
   3. No advantage can be demonstrated for any particular anesthetic induction or maintenance regimen. The underlying hemodynamic condition of the patient should be used to guide the choice and dose of drugs.
   4. Placement of spinal instrumentation involves traction to correct the curvature. SSEPs are frequently utilized to monitor the sensory component of the spinal cord. However, SSEPs monitor only the posterior cord. Anterior cord elements could be damaged despite normal SSEPs. When SSEP monitoring is utilized, one should limit either the use or the concentration of inhalation anesthetics, which interferes with signal interpretation (see preceding text).
   5. A wake-up test definitively confirms adequate blood flow to, and therefore the function of, the anterior motor portion of the spinal cord. This is accomplished by having the patient awaken and move the lower extremities in response to verbal command. With a multitude of short-acting muscle relaxants and maintenance anesthetics, it has become relatively simple to maintain a deep level of anesthesia until the time of the wake-up test yet to allow for a quick awakening at the appropriate time during the procedure.

D. **Postoperative management.** The spinal fusion and rodding procedure prevents further deterioration of pulmonary and cardiac parameters. These abnormalities are not typically corrected by the procedure. Careful consideration of the patient's baseline status helps to determine which patients are suitable candidates for early extubation.

SUGGESTED READINGS

Atkinson PP, Atkinson JLD. Spinal shock. *Mayo Clin Proc* 1996;71: 384–389.

Chiles BW, Cooper PR. Acute spinal injury. *N Engl J Med* 1996;334: 514–520.

Eltorai IM, Wong DH, Lacerna M, et al. Surgical aspects of autonomic dysreflexia. *J Spinal Cord Med* 1997;20:361–364.

Geerts WH, Pineo GF, Heit J, et al. Prevention of venous thromboembolism: the seventh ACCP conference on antithrombotic and thrombolytic therapy. *Chest* 2004;126:338S–400S.

Grande CM, Barton RB, Stene JK. Appropriate techniques for airway management of emergency patients with suspected spinal cord injury. *Anesth Analg* 1988;67:714–715.

Hadley MN, Walters BC, Grabb PA, et al. Guidelines for the management of acute cervical spine and spinal cord injuries. *Clin Neurosurg* 2002;49:407–498.

Hastings RH, Marks JD. Airway management for trauma patients with potential cervical spine injuries. *Anesth Analg* 1991;73: 471–482.

Kwon BK, Tetzlaff W, Grauer JN, et al. Pathophysiology and pharmacologic treatment of acute spinal cord injury. *Spine J* 2004; 4:451–464.

Pediatric Neuroanesthesia

Philippa Newfield, Lawrence H. Feld,
and Rukaiya K. A. Hamid

I. **Intracranial physiology.** The development of the central nervous system (CNS) is incomplete at birth; maturation continues until the end of the first year of life. Cerebral blood flow (CBF) affects cerebral blood volume (CBV), intracranial volume, and, in turn, intracranial pressure (ICP). In children from 3 to 12 years of age, the CBF is 100 mL/100 g/minute and is higher than in adults. The CBF in children from 6 to 40 months is 90 mL/100 g/minute and in newborns and premature infants, it is approximately 40 to 42 mL/100 g/minute.

Autoregulation in the newborn is easily impaired or abolished. This can lead to intraventricular hemorrhage (IVH) with grave consequences. Recent studies have demonstrated that hyperventilation restores autoregulation in the neonate and that CBF velocity changes logarithmically and directly with end-tidal carbon dioxide tension (ET_{CO_2}) in infants and children. Under normal conditions, ICP depends more on CBF and CBV than on cerebrospinal fluid (CSF) production. All inhalational anesthetics must therefore be used with care because they increase CBF and CBV by producing vasodilatation.

II. **Anesthetic requirements.** The anesthetic requirements in pediatric patients vary with age and maturity. Neonates and premature infants have decreased anesthetic requirements relative to older children. The reasons for the lower requirements in babies are the immaturity of the newborn's nervous system, the presence of maternal progesterone, and elevated levels of endorphins, along with the immaturity of the blood-brain barrier. Neonates do sense pain and can develop a stress response to surgical stimulation. They therefore require adequate levels of anesthesia to blunt the stress response. Because the neonate's immature organ systems are sensitive to anesthetic drugs, a narcotic-based anesthetic offers more hemodynamic stability, but emergence may be delayed because the liver and kidneys are not fully developed. Induction of anesthesia in infants is more rapid, however, because of the following:

A. The ratio of alveolar ventilation to functional residual capacity (FRC) is 5:1 in the infant and 1.5:1 in the adult.

B. The neonate has a greater cardiac output per kilogram of body weight than the adult.

C. More of the neonate's cardiac output goes to the vessel-rich group of organs including the brain (up to 25%) and the heart.

D. The infant has a lower blood-gas partition coefficient for volatile anesthetics and a lower anesthetic requirement.

- The rapid induction of anesthesia occurring with most volatile anesthetics may be hazardous in the premature, small for gestational age, or unstable patient.
- Whatever the choice of anesthetic drugs, sick neonates require resuscitation and normalization of fluid and electrolyte balance before the induction of anesthesia.

The common denominator of neonatal surgery is that the operations are frequently performed emergently. This contributes significantly to the >10-fold increase in perioperative morbidity and mortality in neonates compared to other pediatric age groups. Additional difficulties can arise because intraoperative hypoxia and hemodynamic instability can be the first indication of previously unrecognized congenital cardiac and pulmonary anomalies. Regression to fetal circulation may also occur intraoperatively in neonates because of hypercarbia, hypoxia, hypothermia, and acidosis. In addition, respiratory complications are not uncommon in neonates owing to the small size of their airway, laryngotracheal lesions, craniofacial anomalies, and acute (e.g., respiratory distress syndrome, transient tachypnea of the newborn) or chronic (e.g., bronchopulmonary dysplasia) lung disorders.

III. Anatomy of the airway. The newborn period is defined as the first 24 hours of life. The neonatal period is the first 30 days of extrauterine life and includes the newborn period. The infant is an obligate nose breather in part because of the immaturity in the coordination between respiratory efforts and the oropharyngeal motor and sensory input. Conditions such as congenital choanal atresia or simple nasal congestion can cause respiratory distress and asphyxia in the infant.

The oxygen demand in the infant is high: 7 to 9 mL/kg as compared to 3 mL/kg in the mature state. Infants have a high closing volume, high minute ventilation-to-FRC ratio, and soft pliable ribs. Therefore, even some degree of airway obstruction can have a major impact on the oxygen supply in the neonate.

IV. Anesthetic considerations

A. Preoperative assessment. The preoperative assessment of a pediatric patient who has neurologic dysfunction involves establishing the degree of change in the cerebral compliance. The clinical presentation varies with the age of the patient as well as the rapidity and degree of change in the intracranial contents. Infants might present with a history of irritability, lethargy, and failure to feed. They may have an enlarging head circumference, bulging fontanelle, or lower extremity motor deficits. Older children might have headache, nausea, vomiting, or change in the level of alertness. Funduscopic examination might reveal papilledema. This can be a late sign in neonates owing to the presence of an open fontanelle. Some children, especially neonates, might need further evaluation by pediatric cardiologists and other subspecialists because of the presence of cardiopulmonary disorders and other coexisting diseases.

B. **Fluid balance.** The evaluation also includes assessing any fluid and electrolyte imbalance from lack of intake or active vomiting because of changes in the ICP. Furthermore, fluid restriction and the combination of hyperosmolar (e.g., mannitol) and diuretic (e.g., furosemide) therapy may result in hemodynamic instability and shock when coupled with intraoperative blood loss. It is therefore necessary to establish and maintain normovolemia throughout the perioperative period. Normal saline (or other nonglucose-containing solution) may be used as the maintenance fluid because it is slightly hyperosmolar to plasma. Enough glucose is administered to prevent hypoglycemia (*vide infra*). It is imperative to secure excellent intravenous access for fluid and blood replacement and drug delivery before the start of the operation because the opportunities to do so will be limited once the operation is in progress. Two large-bore intravenous catheters are necessary for children undergoing craniotomy, craniofacial reconstruction, or extensive spine procedures.

C. **Administration of glucose.** The administration of glucose-containing fluids during neurosurgical procedures is determined by the intraoperative measurement of blood glucose. The automatic addition of glucose to intraoperative maintenance fluid is unnecessary because hypoglycemia may not be a common occurrence in fasting pediatric patients, even in infants <1 year of age. This is especially true because the stress response to surgery itself results in hyperglycemia from increased sympathoadrenal activity with decreased glucose tolerance, decreased glucose utilization, and increased gluconeogenesis. Furthermore, the hyperglycemia caused by excessive glucose administration can be detrimental in pediatric patients at risk for hypoxic-ischemic insults.

Solutions containing 1% to 2.5% glucose are less likely to cause hyperglycemia than are 5% solutions, especially when administered at a rate of 120 mg/kg/hour (2 to 5 mg/kg/minute), which is sufficient to maintain an acceptable blood glucose level and prevent lipid mobilization in infants and children. The monitoring of intraoperative blood glucose and the continual adjustment of glucose administration may be necessary during long procedures, after prolonged preoperative fasting, and for neonates and small infants, infants of diabetic mothers, infants who have intrauterine growth retardation, children who are small for their age, children receiving extensive transfusion (because the preservative solution in blood products contains glucose), and children who have Beckwith-Wiedemann syndrome, hypopituitarism, adrenal insufficiency, pancreatic islet cell adenoma or carcinoma, large hepatoma, fibroma, or sarcoma, and pheochromocytoma.

The rate of delivery of hyperalimentation may need to be reduced owing to a decrease in the glucose requirement of children receiving hyperalimentation. Alternatively, they may receive a continuous infusion of dextrose 10% in water (D10W), but still require intraoperative glucose monitoring. Other patients who may require the intraoperative monitoring and administration of glucose include neonates under the age of 48 hours, children fasted during the daytime, patients who have poor nutritional status, and patients under regional anesthesia (especially subarachnoid block) which attenuates the stress response to surgery and lowers blood glucose concomitantly.

D. **Premedication.** Sedative premedication should be avoided in all patients suspected of increases in ICP because these drugs might further embarrass respiration, cause hypercarbia and cerebral vasodilatation, and lead to tonsillar herniation. Patients scheduled for the repair of vascular lesions whose ICP is normal may be sedated to control preoperative anxiety and avoid hypertension and rupture of the vascular abnormality.

E. **Inhalational anesthetics.** Inhalational anesthetics affect mean arterial pressure (MAP), ICP, and cerebral perfusion pressure (CPP) in children. At 0.5 and 1 minimum alveolar concentration, sevoflurane, isoflurane, and desflurane in 60% nitrous oxide (N_2O) increase ICP and decrease MAP and CPP in a dose-dependent manner. There is no relationship between the patient's baseline ICP and the ICP elevation after exposure to sevoflurane and isoflurane. Desflurane, however, may increase ICP to a greater extent in children whose ICP is elevated preoperatively. Because the effect of a change in MAP on CPP is 3 to 4 times greater than the effect of a change in ICP, maintaining MAP is the more important factor in preserving CPP. For children who have a known increase in ICP, intravenous anesthesia may be the better alternative.

F. **Monitoring.** Monitoring depends on the patient's age and condition and the planned surgical procedure. Routine monitoring includes the use of the precordial stethoscope, electrocardiogram (ECG), oxygen saturation (Sao_2) by pulse oximeter, $ETco_2$, noninvasive blood pressure (NIBP) measurement, esophageal stethoscope and temperature probe, and a peripheral nerve stimulator to monitor the degree of neuro-muscular blockade. Direct arterial blood pressure monitoring, at least two good peripheral intravenous catheters, and a urinary catheter are recommended for extensive and invasive surgical procedures. Measurement of central venous pressure (CVP) may not reflect intravascular volume accurately, especially in patients in the prone position, so that the risk of inserting a CVP catheter may exceed the benefits.

G. **Venous air embolism (VAE).** VAE occurs commonly during craniotomy in infants because of the head position and surgical approach. The head of a small child is large in relation to the rest of the body, causing it to lie above the heart, even in the supine position. In addition, the head of the bed is often elevated to facilitate drainage of blood and CSF during operation. Pressure within the superior sagittal sinus decreases as the head is elevated, increasing the likelihood of VAE. Patients who have a patent ductus arteriosus or foramen ovale are also at risk for paradoxical air embolism through these defects. Consequently, precordial Doppler ultrasonography is used in conjunction with $ETCO_2$ sampling and direct measurement of arterial blood pressure for detecting and assessing treatment of VAE. The optimal position for the Doppler probe is on the anterior chest just to the right of the sternum in the fourth intercostal space. The probe may also be positioned on the posterior chest in infants weighing <6 kg. The anesthesiologist may also elect to monitor for the presence of nitrogen in the end-tidal gas mixture. Because the risk of VAE is present- and VAE has occurred- in the sitting, prone, *and* supine positions, the use of N_2O should be avoided to prevent an increase in the size of entrained air bubbles.

H. **Neurophysiologic monitoring.** Electrocorticography and electroencephalography (EEG) necessitate low concentrations of inhalational anesthetics. Inhalational anesthetics and N_2O depress somatosensory evoked potentials for operations on the spine and brain stem; a narcotic technique may be preferable. The use of electromyography and motor evoked potentials requires that muscle relaxation be reversed during electromyography and monitoring of muscle movement.

I. **ICP monitoring.** ICP monitoring has seen increased utilization in the management of pediatric head injury because it facilitates the achievement of preset physiologic and biochemical goals and the assessment of patients' response to therapy. ICP after traumatic brain injury is controlled by maintaining normal colloid osmotic pressure and decreasing hydrostatic capillary pressure. Microcirculation around contusions is enhanced by maintaining normovolemia and decreasing sympathetic discharge by maintaining adequate levels of anesthesia. This approach has been correlated with an improvement in outcome from traumatic brain injury over the past 10 years.

J. **Temperature regulation.** Because hypothermia is an issue in infants and small children, they require active heating in the operating room by elevating room temperature, using warm-air blankets, radiant warming lights, and humidification of inspired gases, and warming intravenous fluids.

K. **Positioning.** The extended duration of neurosurgical procedures and the unusual access requirements necessitate paying close attention to the positioning of the patient before placing surgical drapes through the use of padding potential pressure points, checking peripheral pulses, and avoiding stretching of peripheral nerves. For patients operated in the prone position, there must be free movement of the abdominal wall without undue flexion of the head. Excessive neck flexion may cause the endotracheal tube to kink, exert excessive pressure on the tongue, or advance the tube into a mainstem bronchus. The resultant hypoxia and hypercarbia will increase ICP, causing upper spinal cord and lower brain stem ischemia. Patients who already have posterior fossa abnormalities such as a mass lesion or Arnold-Chiari malformation are especially at risk for this complication. Patients may also experience flexion-induced swelling of the head and tongue from obstruction of venous and lymphatic drainage and resultant postextubation obstruction of the airway or croup. Extreme rotation of the head can also limit venous return through the jugular veins, increasing ICP, impairing cerebral perfusion, and causing bleeding from cerebral veins.

L. **Emergence.** The goals for emergence include prompt awakening to aid early assessment of neurologic function, hemodynamic stability, and minimal coughing or straining on the endotracheal tube to avoid intracranial hypertension and bleeding. Patients may receive fentanyl before emergence; arterial hypertension is treated with vasoactive drugs such as esmolol and labetalol. Naloxone is avoided because its use has been associated with uncontrolled hypertension and coughing when the endotracheal tube is in place.

The trachea is extubated after the patient responds to commands or when infants and toddlers open their eyes. Alternatively, some anesthesiologists prefer to extubate the trachea when the patient is still deeply anesthetized if there is no contraindication (e.g., intraoperative catastrophe, loss of airway reflexes, poor preoperative condition). If the patient's awakening is delayed and no anesthetic cause can be determined, the presence of a neurologic issue can be revealed by a computed tomographic (CT) scan before tracheal extubation.

M. Postoperative intubation. In several circumstances, the patient's trachea remains intubated into the postoperative period. Operations that interfere with cranial nerve nuclei or brain stem function with resultant impairment of airway reflexes and respiratory drive require ongoing airway protection and ventilation until these functions can be assessed. The loss of several blood volumes, even with replacement, may necessitate continued maintenance of an artificial airway and protection of the airway reflexes. Also, prolonged operation in the prone position may lead to edema of the face and airway with the possibility of airway obstruction after extubation.

N. Postoperative care. Complications in the postoperative period involve a number of organ systems. Respiratory dysfunction occurs frequently after posterior fossa craniectomy. There may also be airway obstruction secondary to either edema or cranial nerve injury and apnea from injury to the respiratory control center in the brain stem. Operative injury to either the hypothalamus or the pituitary gland can lead to the syndrome of inappropriate secretion of antidiuretic hormone (SIADH) or diabetes insipidus (DI) with seizures, changes in the level of consciousness, and abnormalities of fluid and electrolyte (especially sodium) balance. When children require sedation for endotracheal intubation postoperatively, the administration of propofol is not recommended for long-term sedation because there have been reports of children who have developed metabolic acidosis, lactic academia, and bradyarrhythmias after prolonged administration. The guideline is to limit the infusion of propofol to a period of not longer than 5 days.

V. Neuroanesthetic management
A. Hydrocephalus
1. **Definition.** Hydrocephalus is the enlargement of the ventricles from increased production of CSF, decreased absorption by the arachnoid villi, or obstruction of the CSF pathways. Hydrocephalus is classified as communicating (nonobstructive) or noncommunicating (obstructive). The causes of the increased CSF collection can be congenital or acquired.
   a. **Etiology**
      (1) **Congenital.** Aqueductal stenosis, myelomeningocele, Arnold-Chiari malformation, spina bifida, Dandy-Walker syndrome, mucopolysaccharidoses (with obliteration of the subarachnoid space), achondroplasia (with occipital bone overgrowth).
      (2) **Acquired.** IVH, space-occupying lesions, infections (abscess and meningitis).

Hydrocephalus causes an increase in the head circumference. Prevention of any further increase in intracranial contents is vital as this increase may precipitate herniation. Drainage of CSF can also be a problem because ventricular arrhythmias may be associated with the rapid removal of CSF. In some circumstances, epidural or subdural hemorrhage can result from a sudden reduction in the ICP. This sudden change in ICP from the hemorrhage can cause a change in the level of consciousness of the child, although the shunt may still be functioning.

2. **Surgical procedures** include ventriculoperitoneal shunt, ventriculoatrial shunt, ventriculopleural shunt, ventriculojugular shunt, and ventriculostomy.

3. **Preoperative management.** Assess the patient for any effects of increased ICP such as nausea, vomiting, changes in the ventilatory pattern, irritability, decreased level of consciousness, bradycardia, or hypertension. A CT scan might demonstrate increase in the size of the ventricles. Sudden neurologic deterioration in the pediatric patient must be treated quickly with emergency endotracheal intubation, muscle relaxation, hyperventilation with $ETCO_2$ monitoring, and administration of cerebral vasoconstricting drugs (e.g., barbiturates) and diuretics (e.g., mannitol, furosemide) until emergency surgical reduction of the ICP is achieved. Control of the ICP is sometimes accomplished by a direct needle puncture of the lateral ventricle and aspiration of CSF.

4. **Premedication.** Sedation is contraindicated because the resulting hypoventilation may increase ICP. EMLA cream (eutectic mixture of local anesthetics: lidocaine and prilocaine) may be used whenever possible to achieve intravenous access without causing distress to young patients.

5. **Anesthesia.** An inhalation induction is usually not attempted because all inhalational anesthetics are cerebral vasodilators and can increase ICP. A modified rapid-sequence intravenous induction is preferred to minimize the risk of aspiration from either gastric hypotonia secondary to the effects of increased ICP or a recent meal. Preoxygenation is followed by intravenous induction with a sedative-hypnotic (e.g., barbiturate, propofol) and a fast-acting nondepolarizing muscle relaxant such as rocuronium for intubation. Muscle relaxation is maintained throughout the procedure along with total intravenous anesthesia (TIVA) with propofol and fentanyl. Intravenous fluid is given at a maintenance level, and either intravenous ceftriaxone or vancomycin is

given (after checking sensitivity) slowly (over 60 minutes) and in a diluted solution to prevent histamine release. At the end of the procedure, the stomach is suctioned and the trachea is extubated when the patient is fully awake. This is usually not a problem as long as the shunt is functioning well.

B. Craniosynostosis. Craniosynostosis is a congenital anomaly resulting from premature fusion of the cranial sutures. It can cause severe cranial deformity, depending on the involved sutures, and, rarely, intracranial hypertension and psychomotor retardation from abnormal brain growth. Males are more often affected than females. Sagittal synostosis accounts for nearly half of all cases of craniosynostosis. Surgery is usually performed in the first 6 months of life for best results.

1. **Preoperative assessment.** Patients are otherwise healthy but require assessment for any evidence of increased ICP. Hemoglobin is determined preoperatively, and blood is made available for surgery. The surgeons work in close proximity to major venous sinuses, so sudden and massive blood loss is a possibility. Blood loss also increases as the number of involved sutures increases.

2. **Monitoring.** Monitoring includes ECG, SaO_2, $ETCO_2$, NIBP, and esophageal temperature as well as an arterial catheter for direct blood pressure and arterial blood gas (ABG) measurement and a precordial Doppler to monitor for VAE. The patient must have at least two good lines for adequate intravenous access and a urinary catheter to monitor urinary output.

3. **Anesthesia.** Induction of anesthesia is either inhalational or intravenous if a catheter is already in place. The endotracheal tube is well secured so that ventilation is undisturbed with head movements. Anesthesia is maintained with an inhalational agent, air/oxygen, an intermediate-acting nondepolarizing relaxant, and a narcotic (fentanyl or morphine) for analgesia.

A key point in the procedure occurs when the surgeons manipulate the sagittal sutures due to the possibility of VAE or massive bleeding. The possibility of VAE may be decreased by maintaining intravascular blood volume and entrainment of air attenuated by continuous monitoring with Doppler ultrasonography. If evidence of VAE exists, alerting the surgical team enables members to irrigate the entire field with saline, which, along with assumption of the head-down position, prevents further entrainment of intravenous air and enhances hemodynamic stability. If a central venous catheter is in place, the anesthesiologist attempts to aspirate air from the central circulation.

4. **Postoperative management.** At the conclusion of the procedure, the patient is first awakened and then the trachea is extubated. The hematocrit is measured during the recovery period because blood loss continues from the surgical incision, and patients may need either blood or blood products to counteract oozing. Maintaining adequate urine output throughout the procedure indicates the adequacy of regional organ perfusion.

C. **Tumors.** Intracranial tumors are the most common solid tumors of childhood and the second most common pediatric cancer after the leukemias. Supratentorial tumors account for approximately half of all intracranial malignancies and arise from midline structures. Two-thirds of the infratentorial tumors are in the posterior fossa. The pathologic distribution includes gliomas (30%), medulloblastomas (30%), astrocytomas (30%), ependymomas (7%), and others (3%: acoustic neuromas, meningiomas, etc.). All intracranial tumors increase intracranial volume. Infratentorial lesions produce signs and symptoms of brain stem compression and intracranial hypertension from hydrocephalus secondary to obstruction of flow of CSF. Craniopharyngioma, the most common tumor of the hypothalamic-pituitary area, may cause disorders of the neuroendocrine system including DI.

1. **Preoperative considerations.** Signs and symptoms of increased ICP are noted, and the need for performing either a ventriculostomy or a shunt before the definitive operation is determined. Patients most commonly present with headache and vomiting for several days and sometimes weeks. Neonates and infants may have a history of poor feeding, irritability, or lethargy. The anterior fontanelle may bulge, eyes may exhibit a "sunset sign," or the cranium may be enlarged. There may be obvious engorgement of the scalp veins, and some patients may show changes in the level of consciousness or focal neurologic deficits, depending on the area of brain compression. Posterior fossa tumors may cause cranial nerve dysfunction along with signs and symptoms of increased ICP. An endocrine evaluation may also be indicated if a craniopharyngioma is suspected along with a plan for steroid replacement to compensate for damage to the hypothalamic-pituitary axis. The hypovolemia and electrolyte imbalance caused by DI are corrected before surgery is undertaken.

2. **Anesthetic considerations**

   a. The history is reviewed, including the presence of seizures and measures to control them, and documented. A complete physical examination to identify any neurologic deficits is also performed and noted.

b. The anesthesiologist assesses the patient for signs and symptoms of increased ICP and DI and reviews the results of investigative procedures such as CT scan and magnetic resonance imaging (MRI).

c. Measures to control ICP including insertion of either a ventriculostomy or shunt before the definitive operation are noted. Elevated ICP can also be decreased by the use of dexamethasone (to reduce peritumoral edema), furosemide (which also reduces CSF production), or hypertonic saline. The routine use of mannitol is not advised when the presence of a craniopharyngioma is suspected because it may interfere with the intraoperative identification of DI.

d. Patients who have increased ICP may have either altered gastric emptying or dehydration and electrolyte imbalance from poor feeding, vomiting, and SIADH.

e. The patient's position is discussed with the surgeon, and the head is positioned to avoid any obstruction to venous return. The Mayfield horseshoe headrest is used for prone positioning because pins may cause skull fractures, dural tears, and intracranial hematomas. Blood is typed and crossmatched and immediately available in the operating room. Intraoperative DI, although more common in the postoperative period, is treated with intravenous aqueous vasopressin and administration of intravenous fluid.

f. Monitoring for the operation to remove an intracranial tumor includes the use of all routine monitors and a urinary catheter. In addition, an arterial catheter for direct hemodynamic monitoring and determination of blood chemistry is necessary for pediatric patients undergoing craniotomy. A central venous catheter is recommended when blood loss is expected, when there is a concern about DI and SIADH, or when the head position and the surgical approach increase the risk of VAE. The femoral vein is recommended for central venous access in small children because of the ease of entry and lack of interference with cerebral venous drainage as may occur when the jugular veins are cannulated.

3. Anesthesia. Induction is focused on measures to reduce the ICP. The recommended sequence is intravenous induction, hyperventilation, and gentle, brief laryngoscopy to secure the airway. The use of bupivacaine 0.25% with epinephrine 1:200,000 to infiltrate the scalp before the skin incision confers analgesia and decreases the anesthetic requirement and the bleeding. Limiting the total dose to 1 mL/kg of the bupivacaine 0.25% mixture avoids toxicity.

Intraoperative concerns include optimal positioning of the head, maintaining body temperature, and adequately replacing fluid and blood loss. The anesthetic technique (air; oxygen; low concentration of inhaled anesthetic; a nonhistamine-releasing, nondepolarizing muscle relaxant; and a short-acting narcotic) is designed to avoid oversedation and allow early assessment of neurologic function at the completion of surgery. Positioning and hyperventilation may be used to minimize brain swelling. If necessary, mannitol, 0.25 to 1 g given intravenously, and furosemide may be added, although this negates the use of urine output as an indication of intravascular volume status.

A smooth and prompt emergence from anesthesia is desirable. The decision to extubate the trachea of pediatric patients depends not only on the length of the procedure but also on the intraoperative course of events, the extent of the tumor resection, the expected neurologic deficits, the probability of loss of protective airway reflexes and attendant need for airway protection, the possibility of seizures, and the degree of need for postoperative control of ICP. Operation in the posterior fossa may cause either damage to or edema around the brain stem respiratory center or cranial nerves innervating the vocal cords and soft tissues of the upper airway with resultant apnea, stridor, or postextubation airway obstruction. The administration of drugs including phenytoin and the monitoring of ABG, hematocrit, blood chemistry, fluid balance, and neurologic function are continued in the postoperative period.

D. **Surgery for epilepsy.** Patients who require operation for epilepsy have intractable seizures owing to congenital disorders, birth trauma, tumors, or vascular malformations. Continual seizure activity has deleterious effects on the development of the brain and causes psychosocial dysfunction.

Perioperative risks arising from status epilepticus include severe hypoxemia and sudden death. The chronic use of large doses of anticonvulsant (e.g., phenytoin and carbamazepine) for the medical management of seizures may alter pharmacologic response because of enzyme induction, liver dysfunction, and jaundice. This may result in rapid metabolism and clearance of anesthetic drugs including narcotics and muscle relaxants. Anesthetic requirements are therefore increased, and patients require more frequent administration of anesthetic drugs.

1. **Preoperative assessment.** Assessment involves determining the age of onset, type, and frequency of the seizures and any deleterious effects on mental status and development. Recent changes in the level of consciousness and the appearance of new motor deficits must be recognized preoperatively and documented. Liver function tests and a coagulation profile are performed preoperatively.

   When targeting important areas of the brain such as the motor cortex and the speech centers, surgery is performed under local anesthesia if the patient is a cooperative older child or adolescent. Young children and those with evidence of anxiety, developmental delay, and psychiatric illness need general anesthesia. For awake procedures, establishing rapport with the patient and explaining the state of dissociation, lack of pain (neuroleptanalgesia), and need for cooperation are essential for the success of the operation. No sedatives or anticonvulsants are administered for 48 hours if electrophysiologic studies are to be conducted intraoperatively. All patients receive dexamethasone for 48 hours to control brain swelling. Ultrashort-acting barbiturates are readily available to control seizure episodes in the perioperative period. A comfortable position and constant visual contact between the patient and anesthesiologist are essential.

   Blood loss may occur from a large craniotomy, especially in the smaller patient, so blood must be available. The fluid warmer is used to maintain normothermia. The patient well padded because these procedures may be lengthy.

2. **Monitoring.** Routine monitors, including a urinary catheter, are employed, and normocapnia is maintained during the procedure. Intravenous catheters, arterial catheters, and nerve stimulators are placed on the limbs not being used by the surgeons to observe motor function during the localization of the seizure focus. This is discussed with the surgeons in advance and explained to the patient. Neurophysiologic monitoring is used to guide the actual resection of the epileptogenic focus because it may be in close proximity to areas in the cortex controlling memory, speech, and sensory and motor function. General anesthesia can affect the sensitivities of these modalities.

3. **Anesthesia.** All inhalational anesthetics depress cerebral activity and are avoided during EEG studies. The successful use of low concentrations of isoflurane in combination with narcotics has

been reported in several centers. N_2O is avoided for repeat craniotomies, as for removal of electrocorticographic leads or depth electrodes, until the dura is opened because intracranial air may persist for up to 3 weeks after the initial craniotomy. Propofol induces dose-dependent changes in the EEG with an increase in beta activity at low infusion rates and an increase in delta activity, followed by burst suppression, at high infusion rates. Etomidate is not recommended because it produces interictal spiking and might induce clinical seizures in these patients. Ketamine activates epileptogenic foci in epileptic patients and is not recommended. A combination of droperidol and fentanyl or propofol and fentanyl can be used during awake craniotomies. The propofol is discontinued 20 minutes before electrophysiologic monitoring is to begin.

Nondepolarizing relaxants have no effect on electrical activity. The dose requirements are higher due to the interaction with the anticonvulsant drugs. No muscle relaxant is used during the period of direct cortical stimulation so that the surgeons can observe motor activity. This is essential when cortical stimulation of the motor strip is performed under general anesthesia.

4. **Postoperative management.** Careful monitoring of neurologic function is vital during the first 24 hours after the operation. Motor, memory, or speech dysfunction or increased seizure activity may occur in the postoperative period. The hematocrit is monitored because blood loss from a large cranial incision can be considerable. Postoperative pain must be controlled to avoid episodes of hypertension. Short-acting barbiturates or propofol must be available to treat seizure activity.

E. **Head trauma.** Skull fractures occur at all ages as a result of birth injury, traffic and playground accidents, domestic negligence, or abuse. They may be depressed, open, or basal skull fractures and increase morbidity and mortality if unrecognized.

1. Traumatic sequelae include epidural, subdural, and intracerebral hematomas, cerebral contusion, and edema with signs of intracranial hypertension.

a. **Epidural hematomas.** Epidural hematomas account for 25% of all intracranial hematomas and are considered to be true medical emergencies. Most frequently caused by a tear in the middle meningeal artery, epidural hematomas can lead to a decreasing level of consciousness, pupillary dilatation, hemiparesis, posturing, or coma. Patients require urgent surgical evacuation of the hematoma and achievement of intracranial hemostasis.

   b. Subdural hematomas. Subdural hematomas result from parenchymal contusion or blood vessel tears sustained during birth trauma or shaking, as in shaken baby syndrome. They can cause brain edema and progressive neurologic dysfunction.

   c. Skull fractures. Skull fractures are of concern if they involve major blood vessels. Depressed fractures require surgical elevation and might be associated with dural lacerations. Signs and symptoms depend on the extent of cortical injury. Basilar fracture might cause periorbital ecchymoses, hemotympanum, changes in the level of consciousness, and seizures.

2. Preoperative considerations. A CT scan helps in the assessment of the extent of neurologic injury and possible intracranial hypertension. Establishing an airway, maintaining adequate ventilation and circulation, and determining the level of consciousness, associated injuries causing cardiovascular instability, and thermoregulatory problems are of paramount concern. The cervical spine is evaluated and immobilized until the presence of a cervical fracture is ruled out. Renal function must be investigated and the urine checked for hematuria. Blood for transfusion must be available and circulating blood volume restored with blood or crystalloid or both. The need for preoperative evaluation of hematocrit, coagulation profile, and acid–base and electrolyte balance depends on the type and extent of injury. Blunt trauma to the abdomen and long-bone fractures can be major sources of blood loss.

3. Monitoring. Routine monitors, urinary catheter, and arterial catheter for direct blood pressure monitoring are essential. Adequate intravenous access is necessary for volume resuscitation.

4. Anesthesia. The trachea is intubated with the head in "neutral position" to avoid any injury to the cervical spine, and ventilation is controlled to avoid increasing ICP. Volume resuscitation precedes the rapid-sequence induction of anesthesia, which is achieved by the administration of thiopental or propofol, a narcotic, and a nondepolarizing muscle relaxant of rapid onset. The dose of sedative-hypnotic is reduced in hypovolemic patients. Maintenance of anesthesia with air, oxygen, low-dose inhalational anesthetic, and narcotic allows prompt emergence for early neurologic assessment. Poor preoperative condition and adverse intraoperative events mitigate against early awakening and extubation.

5. **Postoperative care.** Control of ICP is vital in the postoperative period. The patient may remain asleep and mechanically ventilated in the intensive care unit if there is concern about either neurologic or organ system dysfunction.

F. **Meningomyelocele and encephalocele.** Embryologic neural tube fusion takes place during the first month of gestation. Failure of fusion causes herniation of the meninges (meningocele) or elements of the neural tube (myelomeningocele) and can occur at any level of the spinal cord. Abnormality occurring at the level of the head is referred to as *encephalocele.* Defects arising at higher levels in the spine can produce bowel, bladder, and lower extremity dysfunction. Most patients also have Arnold-Chiari malformation and hydrocephalus. Surgery is performed at the earliest opportunity (usually in the first week of life) to avoid infection of the CNS. It is important to note that these patients frequently have or may develop latex allergy, either because of repeat exposure (as from frequent catheterization) or because of a genetic propensity, and need to be treated from birth as if the patients do have a latex allergy. The anaphylactic reaction that may result from exposure to latex ranges from airway involvement (tingling of the lips, facial swelling, wheezing) to cardiovascular collapse. Severe anaphylaxis is treated with the administration of fluid, epinephrine, vasopressors, steroids, and diphenhydramine (Benadryl).

1. **Preoperative preparation.** Patients are evaluated for signs and symptoms of hydrocephalus and the presence of any airway problems due to a large encephalocele or thoracic myelomeningocele. There may be considerable evaporative losses with consequent problems in maintaining body temperature and fluid balance. Hematocrit must be checked preoperatively and blood made available for transfusion because blood loss may occur during the repair of large defects. The defect should be well padded in the perioperative period to avoid further complications from compression, CSF leak, bleeding, and infection.

2. **Monitoring.** Routine monitoring is used. Patients who are expected to incur blood loss should have adequate intravenous access for transfusion, an arterial line, and a urinary catheter. Electromyographic monitoring is used to identify functional nerve roots during operation for tethered cord release. The goal is to minimize injury to nerves innervating muscles of the anal sphincter and lower extremities.

3. **Anesthesia.** Intravenous access should be established before induction. Positioning and airway management may be particularly challenging with a large encephalocele. The patient is placed

in the lateral or supine position with the encephalocele or myelomeningocele padded in a "doughnut" support. Intravenous atropine is given and the trachea intubated either awake or after the intravenous administration of a sedative-hypnotic (e.g., thiopental, propofol) and a nondepolarizing muscle relaxant. The eyes are taped closed, the patient turned to the prone position, and the limbs padded. Additional relaxant should not be given if the surgeons plan to use intraoperative nerve stimulation and electromyographic monitoring, and anesthesia is maintained with a low concentration of inhalation agent and a narcotic suited to the length of the procedure. Temperature, blood loss, and fluid balance are monitored closely during the procedure. The trachea is extubated after the patient awakens at the end of the procedure and neurologic integrity has been confirmed. Infants who are at risk of postoperative apnea should have oxygen saturation and apnea monitors in place for overnight observation.

G. **Craniofacial surgery.** Cranial deformities are syndromes associated with premature closure of the cranial sutures. Premature closure may be one manifestation of a number of congenital syndromes and is often associated with anomalies involving the heart or other organs. Patients may be born prematurely and have respiratory dysfunction in addition to a difficult airway from the craniofacial deformity.

1. **Preoperative preparation**
   a. Detailed evaluation of the etiology of the craniofacial abnormality as well as the presence of associated anomalies is vital. Careful note of any anticipated airway management problems must be made. Previous anesthesia records must be reviewed if the patient has had cardiac or other corrective surgeries in the past.
   b. The choice of laboratory investigations depends on the specific craniofacial defect and may include an echocardiogram or consultation with a cardiologist.
   c. Consideration of tracheotomy for airway management in the perioperative period is an important aspect of patient evaluation.
   d. Massive blood loss is always a concern during these procedures. Therefore, adequate amounts of blood and blood products should be available.
   e. The ambient temperature in the operating room is increased to facilitate the maintenance of body temperature and airway humidity during what frequently turns out to be a lengthy procedure.

      f. Fluid warmers are used to warm infusions. Blood replacement is started early and continued in the postoperative period.

2. **Monitoring** involves the use of routine monitors, Doppler if the patient's head is positioned above the heart during surgery; direct arterial blood pressure measurement, which also facilitates the measurement of ABGs, hematocrit, and electrolytes; and a urinary catheter.

3. **Anesthesia**

      a. Establishment of good intravenous access is important because these procedures tend to be long and involve massive blood loss.

      b. Every attempt is made to keep the patient warm during surgery by increasing the ambient temperature and using a forced-air warming blanket, heated humidifier, and fluid warmer.

      c. The successful maintenance of fluid balance is ascertained by hematocrit and urine output.

      d. The coagulation profile is checked after replacement of one blood volume, especially if continued loss and replacement are expected.

      e. Air embolism is a concern when there is extensive bone dissection.

      f. Resuscitation drugs should be available during the procedure.

Anesthesia can be induced with either an inhalational anesthetic (e.g., sevoflurane) if airway problems are anticipated or with intravenous drugs if the patient has an intravenous catheter in place and there is no potential problem with the airway. The endotracheal tube must be well secured, especially if the patient will be operated in the prone position. Eyes are lubricated with hypoallergenic ointment and taped securely closed. All pressure points must be well padded. Surgeons can request the intraoperative reduction of intracranial volume to help with the retraction of the frontal lobes during dissection of the orbital structures. Maintenance of anesthesia is usually with air, oxygen, a long-acting nondepolarizing muscle relaxant, and a narcotic for analgesia.

4. **Postoperative care.** Intubation of the trachea continues into the postoperative period mainly to ensure adequate ventilation. Airway and breathing problems may arise owing to the length of the procedure, expected fluid shifts from massive transfusion, and the use of intraoperative narcotics. Postoperative transfusion might be required because of continued oozing from the surgical site.

H. **Vascular anomalies.** Large arteriovenous malformations (AVMs) are associated with high-output congestive heart failure in infants who may require hemodynamic support.

The initial treatment is by the interventional neuroradiologist who performs selective intravascular embolization. Because the operation for the ligation of an AVM is associated with considerable blood loss, hemodynamic monitoring and good intravenous access are essential. The anesthesiologist also needs to be prepared to treat the sudden hypertension and hyperemic cerebral edema that may develop after ligation of the AVM. This treatment includes hyperventilation and the administration of labetalol and sodium nitroprusside.

MoyaMoya disease is a chronic vasculo-occlusive disorder of the carotid arteries so named because, on angiography, the vessels appear as a "puff of smoke." The syndrome is associated with neurofibromatosis, Down's syndrome, previous intracranial radiation, and hematologic disorders. Patients present with either transient ischemic attacks or recurrent strokes. Anesthetic management involves the enhancement of cerebral perfusion through adequate preoperative hydration, intraoperative maintenance of the preoperative blood pressure, and maintenance of normocapnia to avoid steal from ischemic areas of the brain. The combination of air, oxygen, and narcotic confers a stable level of anesthesia and permits the use of intraoperative EEG monitoring. Cerebral perfusion is maintained in the postoperative period through optimal intravenous hydration and adequate pain management to avoid cerebral vasoconstriction from hypertension and hyperventilation.

VI. **Neuroradiology**

A. **Anesthetic management of neurodiagnostic and neurointerventional procedures.** Most pediatric patients require general anesthesia for neuroradiologic diagnostic procedures such as CT scanning, MRI, angiography, and myelography, as well as interventional procedures and radiation therapy because of age (infants), anxiety, lack of understanding and cooperation, developmental delay, and inability to remain still for lengthy procedures. Sedation is employed in older, cooperative children undergoing short procedures that do not produce pain and discomfort. Anesthesia is frequently administered in locations remote from the operating suite, which means that the same equipment and level of assistance must be available. In addition, the radiologists and their staff must be oriented so that they understand the anesthesiologist's issues and concerns regarding pediatric patients.

1. **MRI** makes use of the intense magnetic field emanating from the large static magnet. Ferromagnetic objects should *never* be brought into the

room housing the magnet. The patient must also be absolutely still and isolated within the tunneled scanning space (which may induce claustrophobia) during the examination. The procedure does not cause any pain to the patient and usually takes approximately 45 minutes to 1 hour. All ferromagnetic objects must be removed from the patient because they may induce motion artifact in the magnetic field. Patients must also be checked for metal objects such as aneurysm clips and cochlear implants. The intravenous infusion of propofol administered by means of an MRI-compatible pump is an effective anesthetic technique for these procedures. Alternatively, inhalation anesthesia may be administered with an MRI-compatible anesthesia machine using a laryngeal mask (LMA) or an endotracheal tube.

2. **CT scanning** also requires understanding and cooperation on the part of the patient who will need to remain still throughout the procedure to secure diagnostic images of high quality. Sedation is used to enhance patient cooperation. Neonates may be scanned without any sedation because they will fall asleep, but infants might need general anesthesia with intravenous or inhalational drugs for the procedure. Sedation is also required in older children who are either uncooperative or mentally handicapped. Healthy children who are older may be scanned without sedation as long as they are assured it will be painless. Patients undergoing stereotactic-guided radiosurgery require general anesthesia.

3. **Angiography** is used mainly as an adjunct to diagnostic CT scanning and MRI. Its main indication is for the detailed demonstration of AVM's and MoyaMoya disease, as well as the extent of tumor vascularity. Cerebral angiography is usually performed through the transfemoral route with an injection of nonionic contrast agents and requires general anesthesia in small children.

B. **Periprocedural management includes the following activities:**
   1. Review the patient's history and any previous diagnostic or surgical procedures and their management.
   2. Check that the consent form has been signed and the patient has been fasting.
   3. Discuss the procedure with the parent and the older patient and develop rapport with the younger patient.
   4. Ensure adequate functioning of the anesthesia machine and suction apparatus and the availability of equipment for difficulty in airway management and resuscitation.

5. Apply all standard monitors routinely used in the operating room: ECG, blood pressure, pulse oximeter, ET_{CO_2}, and temperature.
6. Institute controlled ventilation with normocapnia for patients undergoing cerebral angiography to achieve good-quality images after the injection of the intravenous contrast.
7. Because allergic or anaphylactic reactions are always a possibility with the contrast material used during CT scan, MRI, and angiographic procedures, document history of any allergic reactions and be prepared to treat a reaction if one occurs during the procedure.
8. Monitor patients in a recovery area until they are fully awake and stable before discharging them from the unit. Patients who exhibit an anaphylactic reaction might require intubation, ventilation, and overnight observation because laryngeal edema is a possible sequela of allergic reactions.
9. Monitor patients during transportation from remote locations if they require recovery in the postanesthesia care unit. In addition, procedures that begin in the radiology suite may be continued in the operating room, necessitating that the patients remain anesthetized and monitored during transportation.

SUGGESTED READINGS

Burrows PE, Robertson RL. Neonatal CNS vascular disorders. *Neurosurg Clin N Am* 1998;9:155–180.

Dierdorf SF, McNiece WL, Rao CC, et al. Failure of succinylcholine to alter plasma potassium in children with myelomeningocele. *Anesthesiology* 1986;64:272.

Hamid RKA, Newfield P. Anesthesia for pediatric spine procedures. In: Porter S, ed. *Anesthesia for Surgery of the Spine.* New York, NY: McGraw-Hill, 1995: 225–280.

Hamid RKA, Newfield P. Pediatric neuroanesthesia. Hydrocephalus. *Anesthesiol Clin North America* 2001;19:207–218.

Lam WH, MacKersie A. Paediatric head injury: incidence, aetiology and management. *Paediatr Anaesth* 1999;9:377–385.

Leelanukrom R, Cunliffe M. Intraoperative fluid and glucose management in children. *Paediatr Anaesth* 2000;10:350–353.

Soriano SG, Eldredge EA, Rockoff MA. Neuroanesthesia in children. In: Winn HR, ed. *Youman's Neurological Surgery*, 5th ed. Philadelphia, PA: Saunders, 2004:3187–3197.

Soriano SG, McCann ME, Laussen PC. Neuroanesthesia. Innovative techniques and monitoring. *Anesthesiol Clin North America* 2002;20:137–151.

Sponheim S, Skraastad O, Helseth E, et al. Effects of 0.5 and 1.0 MAC isoflurane, sevoflurane and desflurane on intracranial and cerebral perfusion pressures in children. *Acta Anaesthesiol Scand* 2003;47:932–938.

Tilford JM, Aitken ME, Anand KJ, et al. Hospitalizations for critically ill children with traumatic brain injuries: a longitudinal analysis. *Crit Care Med* 2005;33:2074–2081.

Wahlstrom MR, Olivecrona M, Koskinen LO, et al. Severe traumatic brain injury in pediatric patients: treatment and outcome using an intracranial pressure targeted therapy—the Lund concept. *Intensive Care Med* 2005;31:832–839.

Neurosurgery in the Pregnant Patient

David J. Wlody and Lela D. Weems

Neurologic disorders requiring operation during pregnancy are surprisingly common, and most anesthesiologists eventually encounter a pregnant woman who has such a disorder. The anesthetic management of these patients can be complicated by the significant maternal physiologic changes that occur during pregnancy. These changes may require alterations in anesthetic management that are in opposition to the techniques that would be appropriate for a nonpregnant patient who has the same neurosurgical condition.

Additionally, while maternal considerations must remain paramount, it is important to recognize that interventions that benefit the mother might have the potential for causing fetal harm. Therefore, the major challenge of neuroanesthesia during pregnancy is to provide an appropriate balance between competing, or even contradictory, clinical goals.

The discussion in this chapter is limited to the anesthetic management of pregnant women undergoing craniotomy for resection of arteriovenous malformations (AVMs) and intracranial neoplasms, aneurysm clipping, and evacuation of spontaneous spinal epidural hematomas (SSEHs). Because the anesthetic management of these procedures is discussed elsewhere in this book, this chapter deals primarily with the ways in which pregnancy alters the anesthetic management.

I. **Maternal physiologic alterations during pregnancy**
   A. **Neurologic changes**
      1. **Inhalation anesthetic requirements.** The minimum alveolar concentration (MAC) for inhalation anesthetics decreases by approximately 30% to 40% during pregnancy, a change that occurs as early as the first trimester. This has been postulated to be a result of increased circulating endorphins. Alternatively, an increase in the concentration of progesterone, a hormone with known sedative effects, might account for the diminished anesthetic requirement. As a result of the increased sensitivity to inhalation anesthetics, inspired anesthetic concentrations that would be appropriate in nonpregnant patients can lead to severe cardiopulmonary depression during pregnancy.
      2. **Local anesthetic requirements.** Local anesthetic requirements for spinal and epidural anesthesia are decreased by 30% to 40% during pregnancy. This decrease is in part due to the

decreased volume of cerebrospinal fluid in the lumbar subarachnoid space secondary to engorgement of the epidural veins. However, the decrease in local anesthetic requirements predates the onset of significant epidural venous engorgement. A progesterone-induced increase in the sensitivity of neurons to the sodium-blocking properties of local anesthetics is thought to be the cause.

B. **Respiratory changes**
   1. **Upper airway mucosal edema.** The accumulation of extracellular fluid produces soft-tissue edema during pregnancy, particularly in the upper airway where marked mucosal friability can develop. Nasotracheal intubation and the insertion of nasogastric tubes should be avoided unless absolutely necessary because of the risk of significant epistaxis. Laryngeal edema can also reduce the size of the glottic aperture, leading to difficult intubation, particularly in preeclamptic patients. A 6 mm endotracheal tube is therefore appropriate for most pregnant patients.
   2. **Functional residual capacity (FRC).** FRC decreases by as much as 40% by the end of the third trimester while closing capacity (CC) remains unchanged. The FRC decreases further in the supine position, a situation in which CC commonly exceeds FRC. When CC exceeds FRC, this leads to small airway closure, increased shunt fraction, and an increased potential for arterial desaturation. Additionally, because FRC represents the store of oxygen available during a period of apnea, decreases in FRC can be expected to lead to the more rapid development of hypoxemia when a patient becomes apneic, as occurs during the induction of anesthesia. Because oxygen consumption increases by 20% during pregnancy, significant desaturation can occur even when intubation is performed expeditiously. This mandates at least 4 minutes of preoxygenation and denitrogenation with a tightly fitting face mask before the induction of general anesthesia during pregnancy.
   3. **Ventilation.** Significant increases in minute ventilation occur as early as the end of the first trimester. At term, minute ventilation increases by 50%, owing to increases in both tidal volume (40%) and respiratory rate (15%). It has been postulated that these increases occur because of a progesterone-induced increase in the ventilatory response to carbon dioxide (CO_2). Because the increase in ventilation exceeds the increase in CO_2 production, the normal arterial partial pressure of CO_2 (Pa_{CO_2}) decreases to approximately 32 mm Hg. The increased excretion of

renal bicarbonate partially compensates for the hypocarbia so that pH increases only slightly, to approximately 7.42 to 7.44.

C. **Cardiovascular changes**

1. **Blood volume.** Blood volume increases by 35% during pregnancy. Because plasma volume increases to a greater extent than red cell mass (50% vs. 20%), a dilutional anemia occurs. Normal hematocrit at term ranges from 30% to 35%.

2. **Cardiac output (CO).** Significant increases in CO occur as early as the first trimester. Capeless and Clapp demonstrated a 22% increase in CO by 8 weeks' gestation, which represents 57% of the total change seen at 24 weeks. CO rises steadily throughout the second trimester. After 24 weeks, it remains stable or increases slightly. Earlier studies demonstrating a decrease in CO in the third trimester reflect measurements made in the supine position with consequent aortocaval compression (see subsequent text).

    CO can increase by an additional 60% during labor. Part of this increase is caused by the pain and apprehension associated with contractions, an increase that can be blunted with the provision of adequate analgesia. There is a further increase in CO, unaffected by analgesia, from the autotransfusion of 300 to 500 mL of blood from the uterus into the central circulation with each contraction. Finally, CO increases further in the immediate postpartum period by as much as 80% above prelabor values because of the autotransfusion from the rapidly involuting uterus as well as the augmentation of preload secondary to alleviation of the aortocaval compression.

3. **Aortocaval compression.** When pregnant women beyond 20 weeks gestation assume the supine position, the enlarged uterus can compress the inferior vena cava against the vertebral column. When this occurs, venous return to the heart decreases, sometimes to a marked extent, leading to decreases in CO and blood pressure. This has the potential for decreasing uterine blood flow (UBF) to a level that can impair uteroplacental oxygen delivery. Supine positioning may also produce aortic compression. If this occurs, upper extremity blood pressure might be normal, but distal aortic pressure and therefore uterine artery perfusion pressure decrease significantly. Because both regional and general anesthesthetics reduce venous return, the effects of aortocaval compression are magnified in the anesthetized patient. Therefore, the supine position must be avoided in pregnant patients undergoing anesthesia. Tilting the operating table 30°

to the left prevents significant aortocaval compression. Placing a roll under the patient's right hip can also achieve this goal.

D. Gastrointestinal changes

1. **Gastric acid production.** The placenta produces ectopic gastrin. This leads to increases in both the volume and the acidity of gastric secretions.

2. **Gastric emptying.** Contrary to common belief, gastric emptying is not significantly altered during pregnancy. With the onset of painful contractions, however, gastric emptying is slowed. Systemic opioids administered during labor have a similar effect.

3. **Gastroesophageal sphincter.** The enlarging uterus causes elevation and rotation of the stomach, which interferes with the pinch-cock mechanism of the gastroesophageal sphincter. This increases the likelihood of gastroesophageal reflux.

4. **Pregnancy and aspiration pneumonia.** The changes described make it more likely that a pregnant patient will regurgitate and aspirate and, if this occurs, the pulmonary injury will be greater because of the increased volume and acidity of the gastric contents. These changes occur by the end of the first trimester if not earlier. Therefore, pregnant patients who have an estimated gestational age of approximately 14 weeks or longer are assumed to have a full stomach. They should therefore receive aspiration prophylaxis with either a nonparticulate antacid or a combination of an H_2 blocking drug and metoclopramide. The presence of a full stomach influences anesthetic induction but, as described in the subsequent text, techniques designed to minimize the risk of aspiration might not be ideal for the patient who has an intracranial lesion.

E. Renal and hepatic changes. Aldosterone levels increase during pregnancy with a concomitant increase in total body sodium and water. This increase in total body sodium and water can increase edema in an intracranial neoplasm and lead either to worsening signs and symptoms or the onset of symptoms from a previously unrecognized mass lesion. Renal blood flow and glomerular filtration rate increase by approximately 60% at term, paralleling the increase in CO. Therefore, blood urea nitrogen (BUN) and creatinine are usually one-half to two-thirds the values seen in nonpregnant women. What would be considered a normal or only mildly elevated BUN and creatinine in nonpregnant women should be a cause for concern during pregnancy.

Slight increases in alanine aminotransferase, aspartic transaminase, and lactate dehydrogenase are not uncommon during normal pregnancy. Plasma cholinesterase levels decrease, but prolonged neuromuscular blockade does not occur in normal parturients receiving succinylcholine.

F. Epidural vascular changes

1. **Epidural venous pressure** is increased mainly by global elevation of intra-abdominal pressure secondary to the pregnant uterus and direct compression of the vena cava. These two factors lead to the diversion of a portion of the venous return from the legs and pelvis into the vertebral venous system with resultant engorgement of the epidural venous plexus. It has been postulated that elevated venous pressure in the epidural space in association with the hemodynamic changes of pregnancy may predispose the pregnant patient to the rupture of a preexisting pathologic venous wall. Epidural veins are a primitive venous system containing no valves. Therefore, abrupt pressure changes, such as straining and coughing, could be transmitted directly from the abdominal cavity to the epidural veins, causing rupture.

2. **Epidural arterial vessels** may undergo degenerative structural changes during pregnancy owing to the excess of estrogen and progesterone. The arterial vessels of pregnant women have been shown to demonstrate fragmentation of the reticulin fibers, diminished acid mucopolysaccharides, loss of normal corrugation of elastic fibers, and hypertrophy and hyperplasia of smooth muscle cells. The combination of these structural changes with hemodynamic alterations during pregnancy, particularly in the third trimester, may predispose susceptible patients to the rupture of the epidural arteries.

II. Effects of anesthetic interventions on UBF

A. Determinants of UBF. At term, normal UBF is approximately 700 mL/minute, which is approximately 10% of total maternal blood flow. The magnitude of UBF is determined by this equation:

$$UBF = (UAP - UVP)/UVR$$

where UAP is the uterine arterial pressure, UVP the uterine venous pressure, and UVR the uterine vascular resistance. Alterations in any of these influences UBF and therefore the delivery of oxygen and nutrients to the fetus.

B. Factors decreasing uterine arterial pressure

1. Hypovolemia
2. Sympathetic blockade
3. Aortocaval compression
4. Anesthetic overdose
5. Vasodilator overdose
6. Excessive positive pressure ventilation

C. **Factors increasing uterine venous pressure**
   1. Vena caval compression
   2. Uterine contractions
   3. Uterine hypertonus
      a. Oxytocin overstimulation
      b. Alpha-adrenergic stimulation
D. **Factors increasing uterine vascular resistance**
   1. Endogenous catecholamines
      a. Untreated pain
      b. Noxious stimulation (laryngoscopy, skin incision)
   2. Preeclampsia
   3. Chronic hypertension
   4. Exogenous vasoconstrictors

   Ephedrine is the drug of choice for treating maternal hypotension. Because of its mixed alpha and beta effects, it increases maternal blood pressure (and therefore UAP) without increasing UVR. It therefore maintains UBF. The use of the pure alpha-agonist **phenylephrine** during pregnancy is being revisited. In high doses, it increases maternal blood pressure but decreases UBF because it is a potent uterine artery vasoconstrictor. UBF is well maintained when phenylephrine is given in low doses of 50 to 100 mcg intravenously. Recent studies have revealed less neonatal acidosis after spinal anesthesia for cesarean section with the combination of phenylephrine and ephedrine for maternal blood pressure support than when ephedrine is used alone.

III. **Uteroplacental drug transfer and teratogenesis**
   A. **Drug transfer.** A detailed consideration of the various mechanisms (active transport, facilitated diffusion, pinocytosis) by which substances are transported across the placenta is beyond the scope of this chapter. The discussion here concentrates on **passive diffusion**, the mechanism by which most anesthetic drugs administered to the mother reach the fetus. This process does not require the expenditure of energy. Transfer can occur either directly through the lipid membrane or through protein channels that traverse the lipid bilayer.
      1. **Determinants of passive diffusion**
         a. **Concentration gradient** is the primary determinant of the rate of transfer of drugs across the placenta. As an example, the initial rate of transfer of an inhalation anesthetic is quite rapid. As the partial pressure of the drug increases in the fetus, the rate of transfer decreases.
         b. Substances that have a low **molecular weight** cross the placenta more readily than those that have a higher weight.
         c. Drugs that have high **lipid solubility** readily traverse the placenta.
         d. **Ionization** limits placental transfer.

e. **Membrane thickness** can be increased in certain pathologic states, including chronic hypertension and diabetes. The effects of these conditions on drug transfer are of less concern than the resultant limitation of the transportation of oxygen and nutrients. This can lead to intrauterine growth restriction or, in severe cases, fetal demise.

2. **Specific drugs**

a. The **inhalation agents** cross the placenta freely, owing to their low molecular weight and high lipid solubility. The longer the period of fetal exposure to the drug (induction to delivery interval), the more likely the newborn is to be depressed.

b. The **induction drugs**, thiopental, etomidate, and propofol, are highly lipophilic and unionized at physiologic pH. Placental transfer is quite rapid. Because most of the blood returning to the fetus from the umbilical vein passes through the fetal liver, extensive first-pass metabolism occurs and neonatal depression after an induction dose of these drugs is uncommon.

c. Both depolarizing and nondepolarizing **muscle relaxants** are highly ionized at physiologic pH. Placental transfer is minimal.

d. The **opioids** freely traverse the placenta because of their high lipid solubility and low molecular weight.

e. The **reversal drugs**, neostigmine and edrophonium, are highly ionized and demonstrate minimal placental transfer.

f. The **anticholinergic drugs**, atropine and scopolamine, freely pass the placenta. **Glycopyrrolate** is highly ionized and therefore crosses the placenta to a minimal degree.

g. The commonly used **anticoagulants**, heparin and warfarin, have remarkably different placental transfer. Heparin, a highly ionized polysaccharide molecule, does not reach the fetus. Warfarin, which is uncharged and has a molecular weight of only 330, readily passes across the placenta. Because warfarin can cause birth defects, its use is contraindicated during the period of organogenesis (see subsequent text).

h. **Antihypertensive drugs.** The **beta-blocking drugs** that have been studied all cross the placenta. Labetalol appears to have the least placental transfer of this group of drugs. High-dose infusions of **esmolol** have been reported to cause persistent fetal bradycardia lasting up to 30 minutes after the termination of the infusion. The effect of a single dose is not known, but numerous cases of its safe use as a bolus during anesthetic induction have been reported. **Sodium nitroprusside** (SNP) freely passes the placenta and has implications for fetal toxicity (see subsequent text).

B. **Anesthesia during pregnancy and the risk of birth defects**
   1. **Principles of teratology.** It is an established principle that any substance, if administered in large enough quantities for a prolonged period of time during critical periods of gestation, can produce fetal injury ranging from growth restriction to major structural anomalies to death. Therefore, it should be a goal of the anesthesiologists caring for pregnant women to minimize the exposure of their fetuses to potentially toxic substances. Nevertheless, fears regarding the potential for injury should be tempered by the following considerations:
      - Most anesthetics are administered for such a brief period of time that the potential for toxicity is minimal.
      - There is no convincing **human** evidence that any of the commonly used anesthetics is dangerous to the fetus.
      - Maternal hypotension and hypoxemia pose a much greater risk to the fetus than do any of the anesthetic drugs.
      - Maternal well-being must be our paramount concern. If avoiding a potentially teratogenic drug leads to a poor maternal outcome or maternal death, fetal outcome will be equally compromised.
   2. **Evaluation of teratogenic potential.** Because of the ethical and logistical difficulties inherent in large-scale prospective studies of the teratogenic effects of anesthetics in humans, we must rely on more indirect evidence to evaluate the teratogenic potential of these drugs. The principal investigative tools used are small animal studies, retrospective studies of the offspring of women who underwent anesthesia during pregnancy, and, in the case of inhalation anesthetics, studies of operating room personnel who were exposed to low-level waste anesthetic gases during pregnancy. The discussion of specific drugs that follows refers to the studies supporting or opposing their teratogenic potential.
   3. **Specific drugs**
      a. Animal studies of the potent **inhalation anesthetics** have demonstrated conflicting results. Reproductive effects appear to be dose related. These effects are more likely to

be from the physiologic disturbances (hypothermia, hypoventilation, poor feeding) produced by the anesthetic state rather than the anesthetic drug itself. When animals are exposed to inspired concentrations that do not impair feeding behavior or level of consciousness, reproductive effects are minimal. Neither studies of operating room personnel exposed to trace anesthetics nor of women undergoing surgery during pregnancy support any teratogenic potential for the potent inhaled anesthetics. Fetal loss is increased in women operated upon during pregnancy, but this is primarily because of the underlying condition requiring surgical intervention and the increased incidence of preterm delivery in women undergoing surgery in close proximity to the uterus.

b. **Nitrous oxide** has clearly been shown to increase the incidence of structural abnormalities and fetal loss in rats. This was initially thought to be the result of inhibition of the enzyme **methionine synthetase** and subsequent decreases in the levels of methionine and tetrahydrofolate. This mechanism has been called into question, however, because maximal inhibition of methionine synthetase activity occurs at levels of anesthetic exposure that do not produce teratogenic effects. More recent evidence suggests that the fetal effects of nitrous oxide come from alpha-adrenergic stimulation and subsequent decreases in UBF, which can be reversed by simultaneously administering a potent inhalation drug. Studies of operating room personnel exposed to trace levels of nitrous oxide and of women receiving nitrous oxide anesthesia fail to show any teratogenic effect.

c. **Muscle relaxants** do not have any teratogenic effect at clinically appropriate doses.

d. **Opioids** have not been shown to be teratogenic in either human or animal studies.

e. Several human studies have suggested that chronic **benzodiazepine** therapy during pregnancy increases the incidence of cleft lip and cleft palate. These studies have been faulted for failure to control for concomitant exposure to other potentially teratogenic substances. There is little evidence to suggest that a single dose of a benzodiazepine during pregnancy poses any risk to the fetus.

f. There is no human evidence suggesting that **local anesthetics** are teratogenic. Chronic **cocaine** abuse has been linked to birth defects.

g. **Coumadin** therapy during pregnancy has been correlated with ophthalmologic, skeletal, and central nervous system abnormalities, presumably from microhemorrhages during organogenesis. Because **heparin** does not cross the placenta, it is the drug of choice in women requiring anticoagulation during pregnancy.

IV. **Epidemiology of intracranial disease in pregnancy and the effect of pregnancy on intracranial disease**

A. **Subarachnoid hemorrhage (SAH): aneurysm and AVM.** The causes of SAH during pregnancy are numerous, including hypertensive intracerebral hemorrhage, vasculitis, and bacterial endocarditis, but by far the most common are aneurysmal rupture and bleeding from an AVM. The overall incidence of SAH during pregnancy is approximately 1 in 10,000, which is similar to the incidence in the general population. SAH is responsible for approximately 4% to 5% of maternal deaths and has been reported to be the fourth most common nonobstetric cause of death after trauma, malignancy, and cardiac disease.

In 1990, Dias and Sekhar published a review of 154 published cases of SAH during pregnancy. The ratio of aneurysms to AVMs was approximately 3:1. There was no link between increasing parity and the incidence of hemorrhage. For both AVMs and aneurysms, there was an increasing incidence of hemorrhage with advancing gestational age, which may be from increases in CO or possibly hormonal influences on vascular integrity. Interestingly, few women bled during labor and delivery, which is consistent with the observation that >90% of all hemorrhages in nonpregnant patients occur at rest. Of the patients whose rupture occurred during labor and delivery, 34% had hypertension, proteinuria, or both, suggesting that the differentiation between SAH and preeclampsia may be difficult on clinical grounds alone.

B. **Neoplastic lesions.** The incidence of intracranial neoplasms does not appear to be appreciably different in pregnant compared with nonpregnant women. However, as mentioned previously, some tumors appear to grow more rapidly or become symptomatic during pregnancy. This may be because of an increase in either peritumoral edema secondary to increased sodium and water retention or blood volume in vascular tumors such as meningiomas.

Considerable evidence indicates that hormonal influences affect the growth of brain tumors, particularly meningiomas. The incidence of meningioma is higher in women than in men but decreases significantly after menopause. Progesterone receptors have been identified in both meningiomas and gliomas. Accelerated tumor growth during pregnancy is likely, owing in part to the high levels of circulating progesterone that occur with gestation.

V. **Management of anesthesia for craniotomy during pregnancy**

A. **Timing of surgery in relation to delivery**

1. **General concerns.** When craniotomy during pregnancy is contemplated, the physicians caring for the pregnant woman must decide whether to allow the pregnancy to proceed to term or whether simultaneous operative delivery will occur. The gestational age of the fetus, with 32 weeks commonly used as the cutoff, determines the decision. Before 32 weeks, pregnancy is allowed to continue; after 32 weeks, cesarean delivery is performed and followed by immediate craniotomy. This determination is not only because viability improves at 32 weeks but also the risks of preterm delivery are believed to become less than the risks to the fetus of such maternal therapies as controlled hypotension, osmotic diuresis, and mechanical hyperventilation.

2. **Aneurysm clipping.** Dias and Sekhar demonstrated a significant improvement in survival for both mother and fetus when aneurysm clipping was performed after SAH as compared with nonsurgical management. Therefore, in patients who have good grades after SAH, aneurysm clipping should be performed as soon as possible to prevent rebleeding. Clipping unruptured contralateral aneurysms can be delayed until the postpartum period.

3. **AVM resection.** Resection of unruptured AVMs can be delayed until after delivery with no apparent increase in maternal mortality. Conversely, resection of symptomatic AVMs is usually performed regardless of gestation. The management of women who have a ruptured AVM but are neurologically stable is controversial. Dias and Sekhar showed improved maternal outcome with early operation, but this difference did not reach statistical significance. Therefore, the question of early operation for ruptured AVM during pregnancy remains unanswered at this time.

4. **Neoplasm resection.** Resection of a histologically benign neoplasm such as a meningioma can be delayed until after delivery but only if frequent follow-up and careful monitoring for neurologic deterioration can be ensured. Surgery for presumed malignant tumors and for those masses producing worsening neurologic deficits should be performed regardless of gestational age.

B. **Anesthetic management**

1. Sedative **premedication** may be appropriate in extremely anxious patients, but the risk of

hypoventilation, hypercarbia, and subsequent increases in intracranial pressure (ICP) should be considered and guarded against. It might be more appropriate to defer the administration of sedative medications until the patient arrives in the preoperative holding area where careful observation can be maintained. Because pregnant patients must be considered to be at increased risk for regurgitation and aspiration of gastric contents, medications to decrease the acidity and the volume of the gastric contents should be administered. These include a nonparticulate antacid; metoclopramide, 10 mg; and an H_2 blocking drug such as ranitidine, 150 mg.

2.   Anesthetic **induction** in the pregnant patient who has an intracranial lesion provides the clearest example of the need to reconcile competing clinical goals. A rapid-sequence induction designed to prevent aspiration does little to prevent the hemodynamic response to intubation that can be catastrophic for the patient who has an intracranial aneurysm or increased ICP. At the same time, a slow "neuro induction" with thiopental, a narcotic, a nondepolarizing muscle relaxant, and mask ventilation does little to decrease the risk of aspiration. This technique can also be expected to lead to neonatal depression should a cesarean section be performed as part of a combined procedure.

One acceptable technique for anesthetic induction is described in the Table 15-1; other approaches that accomplish the stated goals are equally acceptable. As described previously, aspiration prophylaxis is mandatory. Cricoid pressure should be maintained from the point at which consciousness is lost until intubation is confirmed by capnography. If cesarean delivery is performed as part of a combined procedure, the physician caring for the newborn should be alerted to the likelihood of neonatal depression and the need to provide ventilatory support.

3.   In addition to the standard maternal monitors, **fetal heart rate (FHR) monitoring** can be extremely useful during craniotomy, not because

Table 15-1.   Anesthetic induction for craniotomy

Thiopental	5–7 mg/kg
Fentanyl	3–5 mcg/kg
Lidocaine	75 mg
Rocuronium	0.9–1.2 mg/kg
Mask ventilation with cricoid pressure, 100% O_2	

Table 15-2.   Anesthetic maintenance for craniotomy

Fentanyl	1–2 mcg/kg/hr
Isoflurane	0.5–1%
Nondepolarizing muscle relaxant	
	Thiopental 5–6 mg/kg/hr for "tight brain"

an ominous FHR indicates when cesarean delivery should be performed but because it should lead to a rapid search for potentially reversible causes of decreased uteroplacental perfusion, such as hypotension or hypoxemia. FHR monitoring usually becomes technically feasible at approximately 20 weeks of gestation. Note that decreases in short- and long-term variability, as well as a decreased baseline FHR, are commonly seen even in the healthy, uncompromised fetus whose mother is receiving general anesthesia.

4. **Anesthetic maintenance** is not appreciably different between the pregnant and nonpregnant patient undergoing craniotomy (Table 15-2). As is the case during induction of anesthesia, every effort should be made to maintain hemodynamic stability as well as to avoid increases in cerebral blood volume that could interfere with surgical exposure. As stated previously, potentially teratogenic drugs should be avoided, but the commonly used anesthetics do not appear to fall into this category.

5. **Adjuvants to surgery**
   a. Osmotic diuresis with **mannitol** is commonly used to decrease brain bulk and facilitate exposure during craniotomy. Because mannitol has been demonstrated in both animal and human studies to produce fetal dehydration, some have advised against its use during pregnancy. However, the doses given in these early studies were considerably higher than those currently in clinical use. There is no evidence that mannitol, 0.5 to 1 g/kg, has any significant adverse effect on fetal fluid balance.
   b. **Maternal hyperventilation** can facilitate surgical exposure by decreasing cerebral blood volume. Severe hypocarbia may impair fetal oxygen delivery, however, by shifting the maternal oxygen-hemoglobin dissociation curve to the left. Hyperventilation can also decrease maternal CO by increasing intrathoracic pressure. Modest hyperventilation to a Pa_{CO_2} of 28 to 30 mm Hg should

provide adequate surgical conditions without compromising the fetus.

c. **Controlled hypotension** is becoming less common during aneurysm surgery because of the growing use of temporary clip occlusion of proximal vessels. Some situations, however, make this technique necessary. Because UBF varies directly with perfusion pressure, severe hypotension can lead to fetal asphyxia. Blood pressure should therefore be lowered only to that level deemed necessary for maternal well-being and for as brief a period as possible. FHR monitoring might alert the anesthesiologist to the development of fetal hypoxia and lead to the restoration of blood pressure if the need for hypotension is not critical at that time.

There is an additional concern when **SNP** is used as the hypotensive agent. Because of the limited ability of the fetal liver to metabolize cyanide, it is possible for fetal intoxication to occur in the absence of any signs of maternal toxicity. Although there are several case reports of the safe use of SNP during pregnancy, the duration of administration should be limited to that period deemed essential to maternal well-being. The total dose of SNP can also be limited through the administration of adjuvants such as beta-blocking drugs and inhalation anesthetics.

d. It has been suggested that mild **hypothermia** (33°C to 35°C) has cerebral protective effects. This level of hypothermia has no significant fetal effects. More profound hypothermia, however, can cause fetal arrhythmias and should be avoided.

6. **Emergence.** Before the removal of the endotracheal tube, the pregnant patient should be fully awake and airway reflexes intact to minimize the risk of aspiration. An alert patient also facilitates early neurologic evaluation and eliminates the need for emergent radiologic evaluation of the persistently obtunded patient. At the same time, however, every effort should be made to prevent coughing and straining on the endotracheal tube because this may cause a catastrophic intracranial hemorrhage. Prevention of coughing and straining on the endotracheal tube may be accomplished through the administration of lidocaine, 75 to 100 mg, and fentanyl, 25 to 50 mcg, at the end of the operation. Because the placement of the head dressing is associated with movement that produces airway stimulation, maintaining neuromuscular blockade until the dressing has been secured is

appropriate. These guidelines do not apply to the patient who was obtunded preoperatively or who had a significantly complicated intraoperative course with bleeding, brain swelling, or ischemia. The trachea of such patients should remain intubated until their neurologic status can be evaluated.

VI. **Epidemiology of SSEH during pregnancy**

A. **SSEH.** SSEH is a rare cause of spinal cord compression. Only a handful of case reports having a clear etiology for the pregnant and nonpregnant population have been published since 1869. Bidzinski described the earliest case of SSEH in pregnancy in 1966. Spontaneous, or atraumatic, spinal epidural hematomas are usually associated with congenital or acquired bleeding disorders, hemorrhagic tumors, spinal AVMs, or instances of increased intrathoracic pressure. Considering the physiologic changes of pregnancy and the inherent hypercoagulable state, very few cases have been reported. To date, the English-language literature has reported only six cases. Jea reviewed the cases that involved healthy women in their twenties who were in their second trimester or later. All of the women had profound neurologic deficits, were managed operatively, and exhibited significant neurologic improvement after surgery. Pregnancy was carried to term in three cases, and an emergency cesarean section was performed before evacuation of the spinal epidural hematoma in three cases.

VII. **Management of anesthesia for evacuation of spinal epidural hematoma**

A. **Timing of surgery in relation to neurologic symptoms**

1. **Surgical management.** When the hematoma occurs in the thoracic or lumbar region, initial neurologic symptoms and signs consist of lower extremity radicular pain as well as bladder and bowel dysfunction. Motor and sensory deficits are usually progressive within hours of presentation. The definitive diagnosis is made radiologically, and magnetic resonance imaging appears to be the safest imaging modality during pregnancy. For patients who have profound and progressive neurologic deficits, the treatment of choice is surgical evacuation of the hematoma within 4 to 32 hours of the onset of symptoms as recommended in the literature reviewing the cases of pregnant patients. Lawton concluded that neurologic outcome appeared to depend on the length of time that elapsed between the onset of the neurologic deficits and the surgical intervention.

2. **Conservative management. There are no case reports of the conservative management of pregnant patients with SSEH.** However, Duffill reported the successful nonoperative management of SSEH in nonpregnant patients. There is some consensus that patients who demonstrate rapid improvement of neurologic symptoms after SSEH may be managed without surgery although these patients must be closely monitored for any renewed deterioration of neurologic status. The decision to manage SSEH conservatively may be influenced by the gestational age of the fetus: being near term may alter the risk considerably. **Labor**, vaginal delivery, and the related hemodynamic changes can precipitate the expansion of the hematoma and potentially worsen the patient's neurologic status when neurosurgical intervention may be rendered difficult or impossible. Also, cesarean section may be inappropriate during conservative management because there is no way to assess the patient's potentially unstable neurologic status during delivery secondary to the general or regional anesthetic needed for the procedure. If the neurologic status improves **dramatically** in the pregnant patient who has SSEH and an immature, nonviable fetus (<24 weeks' gestation), conservative management may be appropriate with close neurologic monitoring for potential deterioration. To date, no case of successful conservative management of SSEH in a pregnant patient has been reported. Therefore, caution is indicated in applying the experiences observed in the nonpregnant population to the pregnant patient.

B. **Timing of delivery in relation to surgery** depends on gestational age. If the fetus is deemed viable (>25 weeks' gestation) when SSEH is diagnosed, the cesarean section may be performed before neurosurgical evacuation of the hematoma to facilitate optimal neurologic outcome for the patient. If the fetus is determined to be nonviable (at or below 24 weeks' gestation), neurosurgical intervention should be undertaken as soon as possible to improve neurologic outcome with implementation of specific considerations for surgery in the pregnant patient.

C. **Anesthetic management of evacuation of SSEH.** The concerns and techniques outlined for anesthetic management of intracranial lesions should be followed for cesarean section and evacuation of hematoma with or without cesarean section, including the recommendations for **sedative premedication, anesthetic induction, FHR monitoring, and emergence.**

1. **Anesthetic maintenance** is not appreciably different from for that in patients undergoing operation for intracranial lesions except for the need to maintain the mean arterial blood pressure in the high normal range (70 to 85 mm Hg in normotensive patients) to ensure optimal UBF until decompression is completed. To avoid uterine atony, the end-tidal concentration of the volatile anesthetic is maintained at a low concentration (0.3%), relying on an opioid-based technique and a nondepolarizing muscle relaxant for maintenance.

2. **Positioning considerations** are extremely important in the pregnant patient before thoracic or lumbar laminectomy for hematoma evacuation. Aortocaval compression must be avoided to prevent significant reductions in maternal CO, systemic blood pressure, and UBF in patients for whom prior cesarean section is not performed. Physiologic studies reveal improved relief of uterine compression of the large maternal vessels in the prone position as compared to the sitting or lateral position. The lateral position actually demonstrates an increased incidence of aortocaval compression.

   Jea described the use of the four-post Wilson frame with two posts placed just below the clavicles on the chest and the other posts centered on the anterosuperior iliac spines to support the pelvis. With this configuration, the protuberant abdomen hung free of compression between the four posts, encouraging the gravid uterus to migrate off the large vessels. Positioning the patient on the Jackson table would similarly reduce aortocaval compression.

3. **Emergence** is managed as for pregnant patients undergoing surgery for intracranial lesions. Additional precautions must be taken to assess the patient's readiness for extubation after remaining in the prone positioning for surgery because of possible edema of the airway. A leak test should be performed when the patient is fully awake before removing the endotracheal tube.

SUGGESTED READINGS

Bidzinski J. Spontaneous spinal epidural hematoma during pregnancy. *J Neurosurg* 1966;24:1017–1018.

Capeless EL, Clapp JF. Cardiovascular changes in early phase of pregnancy. *Am J Obstet Gynecol* 1989;161:1449.

Carroll SG, Malhotra R, Eustace D, et al. Spontaneous spinal extradural hematoma during pregnancy. *J Matern Fetal Med* 1997;6(4):218–219.

Cohen SE. Physiologic alterations of pregnancy: anesthetic implications. *Am Soc Anesthesiol Refresher Course Lectures* 1993;21:51.

Cohen SE. Nonobstetric surgery during pregnancy. In: Chestnut DPI, ed. *Obstetric Anesthesia*. St. Louis, MO: Mosby, 1994:273–293.

Cywinski JB, Parker BM, Lozada LJ. Spontaneous spinal epidural hematoma in a pregnant patient. *J Clin Anesth* 2004;16:371–375.

Dias MS, Sekhar LN. Intracranial hemorrhage from aneurysms and arteriovenous malformations during pregnancy and the puerperium. *Neurosurgery* 1990;27:855.

Donaldson JO. *Neurology of Pregnancy*, 2nd ed. London: WB Saunders, 1989.

Duffill J, Sparrow OC, Millar J, et al. Can spontaneous spinal epidural hematoma be managed safely without operation: a report of four cases. *J Neurol Neurosurg Psychiatr* 2000;69:816–819.

Herman NL. The placenta: anatomy, physiology, and transfer of drugs. In: Chestnut DH, ed. *Obstetric Anesthesia*, 3rd ed. St. Louis, MO: Mosby, 2004:49–76.

Jea A, Moza K, Levi AD, et al. Spontaneous spinal epidural hematoma during pregnancy: case report and literature review. *Neurosurgery* 2005;56:1156.

Lawton MT, Porter RW, Heiserman JE, et al. Surgical management of spinal epidural hematoma: relationship between surgical timing and neurological outcome. *J Neurosurg* 1996;84:308.

16A

Anesthetic Management of Therapeutic Interventional Neuroradiologic Procedures

Shailendra Joshi, Sundeep Mangla, and William L. Young

The endovascular approach has opened new options in the treatment of vascular and nonvascular intracranial and spinal diseases. Interventional neuroradiologic (INR) procedures may seem technically straightforward, yet they carry a significant morbidity. Approximately 0.2% to 1% of the patients develop transient or permanent neurologic signs and symptoms after diagnostic cerebral angiography. When compared with diagnostic angiography, therapeutic interventions are associated with significantly more risks of neurologic complications. The primary goals of anesthesia for INR procedures are to control the level of sedation in a manner that permits prompt neurologic examination, to render the patient immobile, and to manipulate cerebral hemodynamics.

Many INR procedures such as diagnostic angiography, carotid angioplasty and stenting (CAS), and embolization of cerebral arteriovenous malformations (AVMs) can be undertaken with intravenous sedation. General anesthesia is required, however, for a growing number of INR procedures including intracranial angioplasty and embolization of aneurysms and some high-flow AVMs, diagnostic procedures in children and uncooperative adults, and prolonged procedures such as those on the spinal cord. Often the choice of anesthetic technique is a collaborative decision by the radiologist and the anesthesiologist on the basis of their assessment of each individual patient.

I. **Neurovascular access and methods**
   A. **Vascular access.** INR procedures typically involve the insertion of catheters into the arterial circulation of the head or the neck, usually through the transfemoral route. As illustrated in Figure 16A-1, transfemoral arterial access is accomplished by the placement of a large introducer sheath into the femoral artery, usually 5 to 7.5 Fr in size. A 5 to 7.5 Fr coaxial catheter is positioned through the introducer sheath into either the carotid or vertebral artery by fluoroscopic control. Finally, a 1.5 to 2.8 Fr superselective microcatheter is introduced into the cerebral circulation to deliver drugs, embolic agents, or balloons to distal regions of the brain. The transfemoral placement site is usually infiltrated with a local anesthetic,

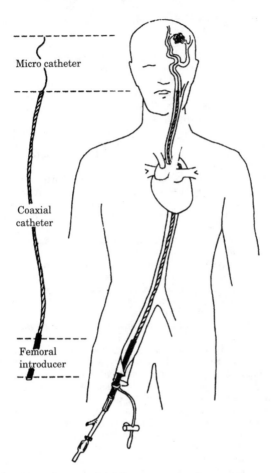

Figure 16A-1. Representation of a typical arrangement of a transfemoral coaxial catheter system showing the femoral introducer sheath, the coaxial catheter, and the microcatheter. (From Young WL. *Clinical Neuroscience Lectures.* Munster, IL: Cathenart Publishing, 1999, with permission.)

which can cause femoral nerve block and a temporary weakness of the quadriceps muscle. Transfemoral venous access can also be used to reach the dural sinuses and, in some cases, the arterial side of an AVM. Direct percutaneous puncture is used to access superficial lesions of the head and neck, such as tumors and arteriovenous and venous malformations.

B. Imaging technology. Radiologic imaging techniques needed for INR procedures include high-resolution fluoroscopy and high-speed digital subtraction angiography (DSA) with road-mapping functions. DSA enables the visualization of only those vessels that are opacified by contrast injection. The road-mapping function enables the radiologist to observe the advance of the catheter against the background map of the patient's cerebral vessels "in real time." DSA involves subtraction of the images obtained before and after the injection of the radiocontrast drug. Any displacement of the cerebral vessels because of the movement of the head profoundly degrades the DSA images. Hence, it is critical that the patient remain immobile during the procedure.

    C. Materials for embolization and infusion. Factors that affect the choice of the embolic agent include the nature of the disease, the purpose of embolization, the size and penetration of emboli and vessels, and the permanency of occlusion. The ideal choice and the combination of agents remain controversial. Embolic agents include balloons, coils, polyvinyl alcohol (PVA) particles, gelatinous embolization spheres, and glue. As used for embolization, N-butyl cyanoacrylate (NBCA) glue is available as a liquid monomer that rapidly polymerizes in contact with ionic solutions such as blood and saline.

II. Anesthetic considerations. Briefly, the primary functions of the anesthesiologist in the intervention suite are (a) to provide to the patient the level of sedation that permits prompt neurologic assessment when needed, (b) to render the patient physiologically stable and immobile, (c) to manipulate systemic blood pressure optimally as dictated by the needs of the procedure, and (d) to provide emergent management of catastrophic complications.

III. Conduct of anesthesia for INR procedures

    A. Preoperative assessment. A careful assessment of the airway must be made. A history of snoring may suggest that partial airway obstruction might occur with sedation. Snoring results in movement artifacts that may degrade the quality of images during cerebral angiography. Patients who have a history of adverse reaction to radiocontrast drugs require pretreatment with steroids and antihistaminic drugs. The population of patients who have occlusive cerebrovascular disease might also require adequate treatment of hypertension, heart failure, or angina. Preoperative communication should exist with the INR team to develop a clear strategy for sedation and hemodynamic interventions that might be needed during the procedure.

    B. Preoperative investigations. The routine guidelines for indicated laboratory investigations before surgery are applicable to INR procedures. Of particular interest is the baseline coagulation screen because anticoagulation is required for the procedure.

C. **Premedication.** Anxiolytics may be administered depending on the condition of the patient. Minimal premedication is required for INR procedures. Either oral nimodipine or transdermal nitroglycerin is sometimes used to decrease intraoperative vasospasm.

D. **Room preparation.** The INR suite should have the same anesthesia equipment as is available in a standard operating room. Suction, gas evacuation, oxygen, and nitrous oxide (N_2O) should be available from the wall outlets. Ideally, the anesthesia machine should have the capacity to provide carbon dioxide (CO_2) for deliberate hypercapnia. An extended anesthetic breathing system is necessary to reach the remotely located patient's airway. Rapid access to all critical equipment should be possible at all times during the procedure. Induction and emergency drugs must be prepared and ready for immediate use.

E. **Patient positioning.** Because INR procedures may last for several hours, it is essential that the patient be made as comfortable as possible before the start of sedation.

F. **Intravenous access.** During INR procedures, patients are often moved cephalad toward the image intensifier and away from the anesthesiologist to check the position of the catheters. This limits access to venipuncture sites and injection ports during the procedure. Therefore, adequate vascular access and a sufficient length of intravenous tubing should be in place before the start of the procedure. In adults, two intravenous cannulae are usually inserted for this purpose; one cannula is at least 18 gauge in size. The anesthetic and vasoactive drugs should be in line before the patient is draped.

G. **Monitoring**
  1. **Arterial pressure.** Because of the need to manipulate systemic hemodynamics and the emergent need, at times, for hemodynamic interventions, it is usually desirable to obtain direct measurement of systemic arterial pressure during INR procedures. This is most conveniently achieved by transducing the side arm of the femoral introducer sheath. If a relatively large coaxial catheter passes through the introducer, however, the arterial pressure trace is "damped." Despite damping, the mean pressure is still reliable in this situation. To avoid excessive damping of the femoral arterial trace, the introducer sheath should be at least 0.5 Fr larger than the coaxial catheter. Radial artery cannulation may be desirable when systemic arterial pressure needs to be monitored before inserting the femoral introducer sheath. Radial arterial line may be required during the induction of general anesthesia for the coil occlusion of an intracranial aneurysm or when monitoring blood pressure in the postoperative period is indicated.

During a typical intracranial INR procedure, two other pressures may be measured in real time in addition to the systemic arterial pressure: either the internal carotid or vertebral artery pressure through the coaxial catheter or the distal cerebral arterial pressure through either the microcatheter or a balloon-tipped catheter. The coaxial catheter pressure is monitored to detect either thrombus formation or vasospasm at the catheter tip as evidenced by a damped arterial trace. A high volume of heparinized flush solution is infused continuously through the coaxial tip to discourage thrombus formation; hence, the pressure reading characteristically increases by 10 to 20 mm Hg when recorded through the coaxial catheter. The setup for measuring arterial pressures is shown in Figure 16A-2. The pressure transducers and access stopcocks for zeroing and withdrawal of blood are mounted, depending on the institutional preferences, either on the sterile field or toward the anesthesiologist. Measurements of the distal cerebral arterial pressure made through the microcatheter are useful during embolization of

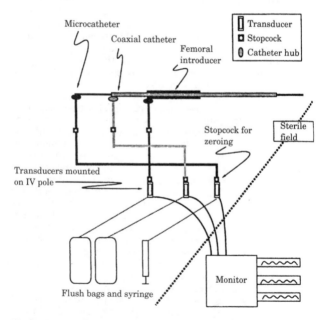

Figure 16A-2. Schematic representation of pressure monitoring and the continuous flush systems. (From Young WL. *Clinical Neuroscience Lectures.* Munster, IL: Cathenart Publishing, 1999, with permission.)

AVMs (see **VI.B**). When a balloon-tipped catheter is used for internal carotid artery (ICA) occlusion, pressure measurements at the tip of the catheter provide the stump pressure (see **VI.D**).

2. **Other systemic monitoring.** Other monitors include five-lead electrocardiogram, preferably with ST segment trending and respiratory trace, automated blood pressure, end-tidal CO_2, and peripheral temperature probe. Pulse oximeter probes are placed on each of the great toes and are useful for qualitatively comparing distal pulses in the lower limbs. Loss of the oximeter pulse trace on the side of the femoral introducer sheath might provide an early warning of the occurrence of thromboembolism, vasospasm, or mechanical obstruction.

3. **Central nervous system (CNS) monitoring.** During many procedures, neurologic examination provides adequate monitoring of the integrity of the CNS. Adjuncts especially useful during general anesthesia or planned proximal occlusions include electroencephalogram, somatosensory and motor evoked potentials, transcranial Doppler (TCD) ultrasound, and ^{133}Xe cerebral blood flow (CBF) monitoring.

4. **Urinary output.** Most patients undergoing INR procedures require catheterization of the bladder to assist in fluid management and to increase their level of comfort. Diuresis may also occur during the procedure from the increase in intravascular volume attendant upon continuous flushing of the intravascular lines and from the osmotic load conferred by the injection of either mannitol or the radiocontrast drug. The timing and volume of the injected radiocontrast need to be monitored, especially during prolonged procedures.

5. **Laboratory tests.** A baseline arterial blood gas at the time of initial arterial puncture is useful to assess the gradient between the arterial oxygen tension (Pao_2) and the hemoglobin saturation (Sao_2) and between the arterial CO_2 tension ($Paco_2$) and the end-tidal CO_2 ($ETco_2$). The activated clotting time (ACT) is used to monitor coagulation. The patients receive large volumes of fluid and radiocontrast and can diurese considerably, so that determination of a baseline hematocrit is helpful as well.

H. **Dynamic sedation.** The primary goals guiding the choice of anesthetic for conscious sedation are anxiolysis, the alleviation of pain and discomfort, and the assurance of patient immobility. At the same time, the anesthesiologist must provide for a rapid decrease in the level of sedation when neurologic testing is required. The procedures are not generally painful with the exception of sclerotherapy and chemotherapy. However, an element of pain is associated with distention of and traction on the vessels; the injection of contrast into the carotid artery is frequently described as "burning." Discomfort might also be caused by prolonged periods of immobilization, bladder catheterization, and, to a lesser extent, the femoral puncture site. The patient might find the procedure psychologically stressful because of the potential risk of stroke during the procedure. However, **immobilization of the patient, whether by conscious effort or deep sedation, is essential.** Movement not only degrades the quality of the images but can also result in vascular injury.

Anesthetic drugs are selected to achieve controlled sedation, adequate analgesia and desired immobility. The primary approach to conscious sedation is to establish a base of **neuroleptic anesthesia** by the titration of fentanyl, 2 to 4 mcg/kg; droperidol, 2.5 to 5 mg; and midazolam, 3 to 5 mg, after intravenous access and monitoring have been established and oxygen administration has begun. In men, a small bolus of propofol is useful just as the urinary catheter is passed. The bolus dose of propofol also helps the anesthesiologist to assess the patency of the airway under deep sedation and determine whether a nasopharyngeal airway is required. The insertion of the nasopharyngeal airway after anticoagulation can result in troublesome bleeding and is best avoided.

When the patient is in final position, draping is begun and an infusion of **propofol** is started at a very low dose of 10 to 20 mcg/kg/minute and then increased slowly to render the patient immobile yet breathing spontaneously. The recent availability of the alpha$_2$ agonist, **dexmedetomidine,** offers an alternative to propofol and has the advantage of improved maintenance of the airway during sedation. Dexmedetomidine, administered as a loading dose of 0.5 to 1 mcg/kg over 20 minutes followed by an infusion of 0.01 to 1 mcg/kg/hour also permits neurologic examination during awake craniotomy. Some evidence, however, indicates that the recovery of cognitive functions might be delayed in patients after receiving dexmedetomidine during INR procedures. Further, patients who have received this drug tend to have lower blood pressures in the recovery period. This may not be desirable in patients who are critically dependent on the maintenance of adequate perfusion pressure to the collateral circulation. Therefore, the choice of anesthetics is on the basis of the experience of the anesthesiologist, the needs of the patient, and the requirements of the procedure.

I. **General anesthesia with endotracheal intubation.** General anesthesia with endotracheal intubation in the INR suite is similar to that in the operating room for both adult and pediatric patients. The primary reason for employing general anesthesia is to reduce motion artifact and improve the quality of the images. This is especially pertinent to the INR treatment of spinal pathology during which extensive multilevel angiography is sometimes performed. In view of the fact that chest excursion during positive-pressure ventilation can interfere with road mapping, radiologists frequently request periods of apnea during DSA for certain procedures; this can best be accomplished with endotracheal anesthesia. A theoretic' argument can be made in the context of INR for eschewing the use of N_2O because of the possibility of expanding the volume of air emboli introduced into the cerebral circulation.

J. **Anticoagulation.** Careful management of coagulation is required to prevent thromboembolic complications from the presence of catheters, which act as foreign bodies, and from endothelial injury associated with the passage of microcatheters. After insertion of the femoral introducer sheath, a baseline ACT is obtained. **Heparin,** 2,000 to 5,000 U/70 kg, is given intravenously and another ACT is measured approximately 3 to 5 minutes later. The target ACT depends on the clinical needs and could be two to three times the baseline value. Additional heparin may be required throughout the procedure to maintain adequate anticoagulation. On occasions, at the completion of the INR procedure, heparin's anticoagulant effect is reversed with protamine, and the femoral artery catheter is removed in the angiography suite. The proliferation of percutaneous closure devices has improved hemostasis at the arteriotomy site, particularly in patients receiving thrombolytic and antiplatelet drugs.

K. **Deliberate hypotension.** Two primary indications for deliberate hypotension are to decrease blood flow through an arteriovenous fistula during the injection of glue and to test the cerebrovascular reserve of the patient undergoing carotid occlusion. In most instances, the level of sedation is decreased to permit neurologic examination during the period of deliberate hypotension. The induction of hypotension in awake or minimally sedated patients can be fairly challenging because large doses of hypotensive drugs may be required to reduce the blood pressure in these patients. Adrenergic-blocking drugs that do not directly affect CBF might be preferable to drugs that are potential cerebral vasodilators. Typically, large doses of **esmolol** as a 1 mg/kg bolus followed by an infusion of approximately 0.5 mg/kg/minute are required in these patients. Supplemental **labetalol** might also be needed during the infusion of esmolol. Drugs such as **sodium nitroprusside** and **nitroglycerin** may also be used. Because hypotension may cause nausea and vomiting, supplemental doses of antiemetic drugs such as droperidol, 1.25 mg; ondansetron, 4 mg;

or dolasetron, 12.5 mg, may be given before decreasing the blood pressure.

L. Flow arrest. Transient flow arrest has been used successfully for treating high-flow cerebral AVMs in relatively healthy (American Society of Anesthesiologists [ASA] status I and II) patients with the embolization of NBCA glue. When flow arrest is planned, the patient is prepared for a general anesthetic. In addition to the usual preparation, a central venous catheter is inserted to inject drugs. Intravenous **adenosine** as a 10 to 90 mg bolus has been used for this purpose. Either external pacing pads or a transvenous pacing line is inserted for treating any persistent arrhythmias. The procedure is generally conducted in two parts. In the first part, the target feeding artery is identified and the safety of embolizing the vessel is assessed by performing a superselective Wada test under minimum alveolar concentration sedation. In the second part with the catheter positioned in the desired location, general anesthesia is induced. Conducting a dose-response study to determine the optimal dose of adenosine is recommended. The dose of intravenous adenosine is geared to produce 5 to 15 seconds of asystole and ranges from 10 to 90 mg. Small amounts of either esmolol or nitroprusside might be necessary to treat rebound hypertension or tachycardia.

M. Deliberate hypertension. During the occlusion of a cerebral artery, planned or inadvertent, systemic blood pressure might need to be increased to augment CBF through collateral vessels. The extent to which the blood pressure needs to be increased depends on the condition of the patient and the nature of the disease. During deliberate hypertension, the systemic blood pressure typically is raised either to 30% to 40% above the patient's baseline or until the ischemic symptoms resolve. The electrocardiogram and ST segments should be inspected for myocardial ischemia. **Phenylephrine** is the first-line drug for deliberate hypertension. **Dopamine** might be useful in patients who have a low heart rate.

N. Deliberate hypercapnia. Deliberate hypercapnia to a Pa_{CO_2} of 50 to 60 mm Hg may be induced during the treatment of venous malformations of the head and neck. The rationale for employing hypercapnia is to increase cerebral venous outflow relative to extracranial venous drainage and to create a pressure gradient that would divert sclerosing agents away from the intracranial veins. This is usually achieved by decreasing minute ventilation. Alternatively, CO_2 may be added to the inspired gases.

O. Radiation safety. The INR suite has three sources of radiation: direct radiation (from the x-ray tub), leakage (through the collimator's protective shielding), and scattered (or reflected from the patient and the area surrounding the body part being imaged). It is important to realize that the amount of exposure drops proportionally to the square of the distance from the source of radiation (inverse square law). It should also be realized that DSA delivers considerably more radiation than fluoroscopy. Everyone working in the INR suite must wear a lead apron, a thyroid shield, and a radiation exposure badge. Although they are heavy, using leaded glasses is a consideration for anyone who must be near the source of the radiation.

IV. **Management of procedural catastrophes.** Complications arising from cerebrovascular instrumentation can be rapid and dramatic and require a multidisciplinary approach to management. A **catastrophe plan** such as that shown in Table 16A-1 should be clearly defined by the anesthesia team for every INR procedure. Drugs and equipment required to secure the airway must be available without any delay. Protamine should be available for immediate injection if the decision is made to reverse the heparinization. There must be effective communication between the INR team and the anesthesiologist. The appropriate neurologic and neurosurgical consultants should be contacted as soon as possible. The anesthesia team has the primary responsibility to secure the airway and ensure adequate ventilation. While securing the airway, the anesthesiologist must communicate with the INR team to determine whether the problem is occlusive or hemorrhagic.

Table 16A-1. Management of neurologic catastrophes[a]

Initial resuscitation: Communicate with radiologists. Call for assistance. Secure the airway and hyperventilate with 100% O_2. Determine if problem is hemorrhagic or occlusive.

Hemorrhagic: Immediate heparin reversal (1 mg protamine for each 100 U heparin given) and low-normal pressure.

Occlusive: Deliberate hypertension, titrated to neurologic examination, angiography, or physiologic imaging studies (e.g., TCD, CBF).

Further resuscitation: Head-up 15° in neutral position.
Titrate ventilation to a $Paco_2$ of 26 to 28 mm Hg.
Give 0.5 g/kg mannitol, rapid intravenous infusion.
Anticonvulsants: phenytoin (give slowly, 50 mg/min) and phenobarbital. Titrate thiopental infusion to electroencephalogram burst suppression. Allow body temperature to fall as quickly as possible to 33°C to 34°C. Consider dexamethasone 10 mg.[b]

[a]These are only general recommendations, and drug doses must be adapted to specific clinical situations and in accordance with a patient's preexisting medical condition. In some cases of asymptomatic or minor vessel puncture or occlusion, less aggressive management might be appropriate.
[b]Steroids are of dubious value in the treatment of focal cerebral ischemia but might have a place in reducing mass effect from a hemorrhage, if clinically appropriate.
TCD, transcranial Doppler; CBF, cerebral blood flow.

A. **Occlusive catastrophes.** In the case of vascular occlusion, the primary strategy is to increase distal cerebral perfusion either by augmentation of the blood pressure or by thrombolysis. Both therapies may be combined.

B. **Bleeding catastrophes** may be heralded by headache, nausea, vomiting, and vascular pain related to the area of the vascular perforation. The radiologist might see extravasation of the contrast only seconds before the patient becomes symptomatic. In the case of the puncture of a vessel, reversal of the heparin before withdrawing either the offending wire or the catheter back into the lumen of the vessel keeps the perforation partially occluded until hemostatic function has been restored. Immediate reversal of heparin is indicated as soon as an intracranial hemorrhage has been diagnosed. Protamine, 1 mg for every 100 U of heparin given, is administered without undue regard for systemic blood pressure. An ACT may be obtained later to adjust the final dose. When active bleeding occurs, the blood pressure must be kept as low as possible. Once the bleeding has been controlled, the target blood pressure should be discussed with the INR team. If vascular occlusion has been used to control the hemorrhage, the INR team may request deliberate hypertension. Allergic reactions to protamine are rare but can occur.

V. **Postprocedural considerations.** Patients are usually observed in the intensive care unit for the first 24 hours after intracranial and spinal procedures. The groin is monitored for bleeding from the femoral puncture site. In general, INR procedures have their own inherent potential complications and require frequent neurologic, metabolic, and hemodynamic monitoring. For example, after embolization of an AVM, the tissue edema might be minimal but still sufficient to cause deterioration in the patient's neurologic status during the course of the first evening after the procedure.

VI. **Specific procedures**

A. **Superselective anesthesia and functional examination (SAFE) or superselective Wada** is routinely performed before therapeutic embolization to minimize the risk of occluding a nutritive vessel to eloquent regions of either the brain or the spinal cord. This could happen if the microcatheter tip is proximal to the origin of the nutritive vessel. Not all interventionalists, however, recognize the need for SAFE before embolization. The level of sedation is decreased before testing by discontinuing the infusion of propofol. In rare instances, it might be necessary to use naloxone or flumazenil to antagonize other intravenous drugs. The INR team performs a baseline focused neurologic examination under residual light sedation.

Sodium amobarbital, 30 mg/mL, or lidocaine, 30 mg/mL, mixed with contrast is injected through the superselective catheter to obtain an angiogram with the drug/contrast mixture. Sodium amobarbital is used to investigate the gray matter. Lidocaine can be used to evaluate the integrity of the white matter tracts, especially in the spinal cord. The injection of lidocaine into cortical areas, particularly those close to the motor strip, can precipitate seizures, however. Such seizure activity can cause transient neurologic deficits. Postictal paralysis may also confuse the interpretation of the test. For this reason, the barbiturate is usually given first, followed by lidocaine. If the amobarbital test is negative, the amobarbital can protect against seizures but will not interfere with the assessment of lidocaine's effect on white matter tracts.

B. **Superselective angiography and therapeutic embolization of AVMs.** Typically, patients who present for embolization have large, complex, parenchymatous AVMs, which are composed of several discrete fistulae with multiple feeding arteries. The goal of the therapeutic embolization is to obliterate as many of the fistulae as possible. The procedure can last up to 4 to 5 hours, depending on the complexity of the lesion. Various embolic materials have been used to obliterate AVM fistulae including polyvinyl chloride particles. More durable results have been achieved with NBCA glue.

In rare cases, INR treatment is aimed at total obliteration. More commonly, however, embolization is employed as an **adjunct in preparation for either surgery or radiotherapy** and can be beneficial in several ways. First, embolization may facilitate operation by obliterating deep feeding arteries that are difficult to approach surgically and thereby reduce the surgical risk. Second, staging the obliteration of the arteriovenous shunts also theoretically allows the surrounding brain to accommodate to the alterations in hemodynamics and may **prevent normal perfusion-pressure breakthrough.** Third, the obliteration of high-flow feeders can benefit patients who have either progressive neurologic deficits or intractable seizures. Neurologic improvement after high-flow AVM embolization has been attributed to the decease in cerebral steal and a decrease in the mass of the lesion. Finally, approximately 10% of patients with AVM harbor intracranial aneurysms. Such aneurysms appear to increase the risk of spontaneous hemorrhage from AVMs. The **obliteration of intranidal aneurysms** during the initial embolization may decrease the rate of recurrent hemorrhage during the course of treatment.

Once the catheter has been positioned for potential glue injection, SAFE is performed. If SAFE is positive (i.e., if focal neurologic deficits develop), either the catheter is repositioned or embolization of that pedicle is aborted. If the test is negative, either glue or another embolic material may be injected. Controlled deposition of the glue is necessary to decrease complications from pulmonary embolism or obstruction of the AVM's venous drainage. The achievement of flow arrest through the fistula is necessary during injection of the glue to facilitate polymerization and solidification of NBCA glue. Techniques for **flow arrest** include deliberate hypotension, balloon occlusion of the proximal vessel, and circulatory pause with either adenosine or controlled ventricular fibrillation. In most instances, deliberate hypotension suffices for flow arrest, which can be achieved when the mean systemic blood pressure is reduced to approximately 50 mm Hg. Flow arrest is usually not needed for embolization with PVA particles.

The measurement of the **immediate postembolization pressure** has been suggested as a way to follow the course of hemodynamic changes and predict postprocedure complications. A large increase in the pressure of the feeding artery after embolization may be associated with intracranial hemorrhage. Because the AVM's feeding arteries supply normal vascular territories to a variable degree, the abrupt restoration of normal perfusion pressure to a chronically hypotensive vascular bed might overwhelm its autoregulatory capacity and result in either hemorrhage or swelling, the phenomenon known as *normal perfusion-pressure breakthrough.* For this reason, the target range for maintenance of posttreatment blood pressure is at or slightly below the normal blood pressure of the patient.

C. **Embolization of spinal cord lesions.** Embolization can be used to treat intramedullary spinal AVMs, dural fistulae, and tumors invading the spinal canal. For cases performed under general anesthesia with endotracheal intubation, an **intraoperative "wake-up test"** may be requested. The wake-up test must be explained to the patient the night before and on the day of surgery. A N_2O/narcotic anesthetic technique with concurrent administration of propofol may be employed for the procedure. Neuromuscular blockade, if required, should be readily reversible for the wake-up test. For selected lesions, somatosensory and motor evoked potentials may be helpful in both anesthetized and sedated patients. When motor evoked potentials are monitored, the degree of neuromuscular blockade should be titrated to the monitoring needs.

D. **Carotid test occlusion and therapeutic carotid occlusion.** Test occlusion of the carotid artery is undertaken either before the anticipated sacrifice of the vessel or when temporary carotid occlusion may be required during surgery. During the test occlusion, a catheter with a distal balloon and a lumen is placed in the ICA. A baseline neurologic examination is performed. Flow velocity is measured over the middle cerebral artery by TCD ultrasound, if available, and the CBF can be measured by the intracarotid ^{133}Xe injection technique. Baseline femoral and carotid artery pressures are also noted. The balloon is then inflated and the pressure in the carotid artery distal to the balloon is recorded. The inflation of the balloon can cause headache and at times an increase in the systemic blood pressure. Aggressive treatment of the hypertension is probably not warranted because it may decrease collateral perfusion pressure. The anesthesiologist should be prepared to treat bradycardia with atropine. The neurologic examination is repeated a few minutes after occlusion, and TCD and ^{133}Xe CBF measurements are taken again. After ^{133}Xe washout data have been obtained, a radioactive tracer for single-photon emission computerized tomography (SPECT) studies may be injected. This provides a snapshot measurement of regional CBF during ICA occlusion. Because SPECT tracers usually have a long half-life and bind avidly to cerebral tissues, the imaging part of a SPECT study may be undertaken in the nuclear medicine department after the patient leaves the INR suite.

To assess the patient's cerebrovascular reserve, the systemic blood pressure can be decreased if the patient has not demonstrated any neurologic impairment during the initial ICA occlusion. The neurologic examination is repeated at frequent intervals while the blood pressure is reduced. The distal ICA or stump pressure at which neurologic deterioration occurs and whether the patient starts yawning—often a sign of impending cerebral ischemia—are noted and correlated with the corresponding TCD flow velocity. Depending on the clinical condition of the patient, another ^{133}Xe measurement is obtained. If overt neurologic symptoms develop, the balloon is immediately deflated, hypotensive drugs are discontinued, and vasopressors might be required to increase the blood pressure to normal levels, depending on the clinical situation.

Although uniform guidelines for **interpreting the results of test occlusion** are yet to be formulated, a new neurologic deficit, significant asymmetry on SPECT imaging, and a 25% to 30% reduction in CBF as measured after occlusion by either ^{133}Xe CBF or TCD may be considered as relative indications for an extracranial to intracranial bypass procedure before sacrifice of the carotid artery.

E. **Aneurysm ablation.** Many intracranial aneurysms are amenable to endovascular treatment. As the techniques of interventional therapy have continued to evolve, endovascular ablation is increasingly considered to be the primary treatment modality for ruptured and unruptured intracranial aneurysms. The indications for open surgical versus endovascular therapy are currently a topic of vigorous discussion. There are two basic approaches for endovascular obliteration of intracranial aneurysms: (a) the occlusion of the proximal parent artery, such as the carotid artery, which was discussed earlier and (b) obliteration of the aneurysmal sac itself. **Endovascular obliteration of the aneurysmal sac** is usually accomplished through the use of detachable coils manufactured by a wide variety of vendors. Complicated aneurysms that have wide necks and large sacs may require advanced techniques involving either temporary balloon remodeling or placing an intracranial stent. These procedures may be prolonged and require general anesthesia with endotracheal intubation. The anesthesiologist should be prepared for the occurrence of aneurysmal subarachnoid hemorrhage (SAH) either spontaneously or as a result of the intravascular manipulations. **Occlusive complications** may also develop and require additional maneuvers to enhance CBF and initiate revascularization. Occlusion and thrombosis of the aneurysm may be ongoing immediately after intervention. Therefore, careful attention to the control of blood pressure in the postprocedure period remains critical, especially in patients who have presented with SAH.

F. **Angioplasty.** Either mechanical angioplasty or pharmacologic dilatation may be indicated for vasospasm after SAH and for atherosclerotic cerebrovascular disease.

1. **Angioplasty for cerebral vasospasm** is usually undertaken in patients who, despite maximum medical management, continue to demonstrate neurologic signs and symptoms of cerebral ischemia. These patients are often in extremis: their tracheas are frequently intubated, they are receiving vasopressor drugs, and they have either an external ventricular drain or other device in place to monitor intracranial pressure. Angiography is first undertaken to demonstrate that a significant degree of spasm in large proximal vessels (anterior, middle, and posterior cerebral arteries) exists. A balloon catheter is guided under fluoroscopy into the spastic segment and inflated to distend the constricted area mechanically. If deliberate hypertension is being used to ameliorate a focal neurologic deficit before angioplasty, the blood pressure should be reduced to the patient's normal range after angiographic demonstration of significant widening of the spastic segment.

2. **Pharmacologic dilatation** is also used for the treatment of cerebral vasospasm by direct intra-arterial injection of vasodilators under fluoroscopic guidance. Although the technique was originally described for **papaverine,** the selection of vasodilators has now expanded to include the more frequent use of calcium-channel–blocking

drugs such as **verapamil** and **nicardipine.** During recirculation, the anesthesiologist needs to monitor for systemic side effects of these drugs, which include hypotension and bradycardia, especially with the calcium-channel–blocking drugs.

3. **Angioplasty for atherosclerosis.** At present, patients who have high-risk factors for carotid endarterectomy are considered favorable candidates for **cervical carotid angioplasty and stenting** (CAS, Stenting and Angioplasty with Protection in Patients at High Risk for Endarterectomy [SAPPHIRE] Trial). Studies evaluating the safety and efficacy of carotid stenting in traditional "low-risk" patients are ongoing (Carotid Revascularization Endarterectomy versus Stent Trial [CREST]), with encouraging preliminary results. These patients generally require **balloon dilatation and placement of a vascular stent.** In many cases, the insertion of a cerebroprotective device may be used to decrease the risk of distal thromboembolism. Angioplasty of the ICA is usually undertaken with minimal sedation. General anesthesia is required for treating segments of the intracranial arteries. **Intracranial angioplasty and stenting** procedures for atherosclerosis have a higher level of risk secondary to the inherently more delicate nature of intracranial vessels. Intracranial arteries have a thinner media and therefore are more prone to dissection and perforation. The selection of **anesthetic technique** also depends on the patient's medical condition and ability to cooperate during the procedure as well as the presence of anticipated technical difficulty in negotiating the stenosed segment. Deliberate hypertension may be required to augment collateral blood flow. The considerations for general anesthesia are similar to those for carotid endarterectomy.

G. **Thrombolysis for acute stroke.** It is possible to recanalize the occluded vessel after an acute thromboembolic stroke by either **mechanical means or superselective intra-arterial delivery of thrombolytic agents,** such as recombinant tissue plasminogen activator, streptokinase, or urokinase. Significant improvement in neurologic outcome has been demonstrated when either pharmacologic thrombolysis is completed within 6 hours of the onset of ischemic symptoms (Prolyse in Acute Cerebral Thromboembolism II [PROACT II]) or mechanical thrombolysis is performed within 8 hours (Mechanical Embolus Removal in Cerebral Ischemia [MERCI] Trial). Techniques for mechanical means of clot retrieval, balloon angioplasty, and laser ablation are also being developed. These methods can restore arterial flow more rapidly than intra-arterial thrombolysis, which may require up to 2 hours. In the vertebro-basilar circulation, treatment may be effective even when administered as long as 24 hours after the onset of symptoms. The main risk of intra-arterial thrombolysis is hemorrhagic conversion of the ischemic infarct, which has a high mortality when it occurs.

Anesthetic considerations in these patients include those for elderly people and for patients who have widespread arterial disease. Hypertension occurs spontaneously after acute thromboembolic stroke and, in the face of nonhemorrhagic focal neurologic deficits, should not be treated aggressively. Once clot lysis has been accomplished, the blood pressure is maintained in the patient's normal range and ideally titrated to some index of CBF to prevent hyperperfusion injury.

H. Treatment of other CNS vascular malformations

1. **Dural AVMs.** Dural AVMs induce venous hypertension, and, when cortical venous drainage is involved, may cause intracranial hemorrhage. Multiple intracranial and extracranial arteries may feed these dural AVMs so that multistage embolization is usually performed. SAFE are required, as in the case of intracranial AVMs. Transarterial embolization with NBCA glue is a commonly utilized technique, as is the transvenous coil occlusion of pathologic venous pouches.

2. **Carotid cavernous fistulae.** Skull-base trauma is the most common etiology of carotid cavernous fistula. Traumatic fistulae can also occur between the vertebral artery and the paravertebral veins. Such arteriovenous fistulae can lead to chronic hypotension of the surrounding normal vascular territories. The treatment may include either transarterial occlusion with detachable balloons or transvenous occlusion of the involved cavernous sinus. The obliteration of these fistulae might result in normal perfusion-pressure breakthrough. Therefore, after obliterating these lesions, the blood pressure should be maintained in the range of 10% to 20% below the normal pressure of the patient.

3. **Vein of Galen malformations.** These relatively uncommon but complicated lesions usually present in infancy and childhood. The patients may have congestive heart failure, intractable seizures, hydrocephalus, and mental retardation. Several approaches have been attempted including transarterial and transvenous methods. Concerns during general anesthesia for INR therapy are the same as for surgical treatment. In the setting of congestive heart failure, preexisting right-to-left shunts, and pulmonary hypertension, a relatively small glue embolus can be fatal.

I. Intra-arterial chemotherapy and embolization of tumors. Preoperative embolization as a means of decreasing blood loss during surgery can be performed for many hypervascular intracranial or spinal tumors. Paragangliomas can cause catecholamine release from the tumor during embolization, and means of treating the ensuing hypertensive crisis should be at hand. Superselective administration of chemotherapeutic agents can also be used for treating neoplasms refractory to conventional therapy.

J. Spinal compression fracture therapy. Vertebroplasty and kyphoplasty procedures involve the intravertebral body administration of acrylic bone cement compounds via a percutaneous, often transpedicular, approach. Many patients report significant pain relief after these procedures. The demographics of this population (elderly, frail, osteoporotic) and prone positioning require extra care during the preparation process. Most of these procedures fortunately can be performed and well tolerated with mild sedation.

VII. Conclusions. Interventional neuroradiology offers a new approach to several intracranial and spinal disorders. To some extent, the risk/benefit ratio of INR procedures remains to be elucidated when compared with traditional surgical approaches. The anesthetic management of these procedures, while similar to traditional operative approaches, is beset with hazards and requires certain accommodations.

SUGGESTED READINGS

Duong H, Hacein-Bey L, Vang MC, et al. Management of cerebral arterial occlusion during endovascular treatment of cerebrovascular disease. *Probl Anesth: Controv Neuroanesth* 1997;9:99–111.

Gobin YP, Starkman S, Duckwiler GR, et al. MERCI 1: a phase 1 study of mechanical embolus removal in cerebral ischemia. *Stroke* 2004;35(12):2848–2854.

ISAT investigators. International Subarachnoid Aneurysm Trial (ISAT) of neurosurgical clipping versus endovascular coiling in 2143 patients with ruptured intracranial aneurysms: a randomized trial. *The Lancet* 2002;360:1267–1274.

Pile-Spellman J, Young WL, Hacein-Bey L. Perspectives on interventional neuroradiology. In: Maciunas RJ, ed. *Endovascular Neurological Intervention*. Park Ridge, IL: AANS, 1995:279–284.

Schell RM, Cole DJ. Cerebral protection and neuroanesthesia. *Anesthesiol Clin North Am* 1992;10:453–469.

Yadav JS, Wholey MH, Kuntz RE, et al. Stenting and Angioplasty with Protection in Patients at High Risk for Endarterectomy Investigators. Protected carotid-artery stenting versus endarterectomy in high-risk patients. *N Engl J Med* 2004;351(15):1493–1501.

Young WL, Pile-Spellman J. Anesthetic considerations for interventional neuroradiology (review). *Anesthesiology* 1994;80:427–456.

Young WL, Pile-Spellman J, Hacein-Bey L, et al. Invasive neuroradiologic procedures for cerebrovascular abnormalities: anesthetic considerations. *Anesthesiol Clin North Am* 1997;15:631–653.

Anesthetic Management of Diagnostic Neuroradiology

Deborah M. Whelan, Melissa A. Laxton,
and Patricia H. Petrozza

The introduction of the first computed tomographic (CT) scanners in 1975 revolutionized the imaging of neurosurgical lesions. Since that time, the diagnostic armamentarium of the neuroradiologist in terms of neuroimaging has expanded progressively. Diagnostic procedures usually involve limited pain so that the neuroradiologist frequently administers sedation. The anesthesiologist is involved, however, in cases for which difficulty with sedation is anticipated for a myriad of reasons. These include extreme ages, claustrophobia, serious neurologic or systemic illness, and the inability of patients to remain motionless to be able to achieve high-quality images.

Many radiology departments have recently adopted the guidelines for the sedation of children formulated by the American Academy of Pediatrics Committee on Drugs. These guidelines address patient selection, dietary precautions, equipment, monitoring, and discharge criteria. Furthermore, strict selection criteria minimize sedation-related side effects. The screening of patients before the procedure often reveals those who have either anticipated airway difficulties or serious medical conditions for whom the presence of an anesthesiologist becomes advisable. In one study, 13.1% of patients were inadequately sedated for their procedure, resulting in failure of 3.7% of procedures. Older children and those undergoing magnetic resonance imaging (MRI) and CT scans experienced higher failure rates. In addition, Malviya found that 5.5% of children sedated by nonanesthesiologists experienced an untoward respiratory event. These events occurred more commonly in American Society of Anesthesiologists (ASA) status III and IV patients.

I. **General considerations.** Once involved in the neuroradiologic procedure, the anesthesiologist faces the usual problems of providing anesthesia in an environment foreign to and far from the operating room. Nonferromagnetic equipment and monitoring modalities are required in the MRI suite, and most neuroradiographic procedures require that the anesthesiologist be positioned at a distance from the patient. Additionally, the issue of contrast media with their attendant osmolar effects and potential for toxic and allergic reactions must be considered. Finally, the design of modern medical facilities often requires that patients be either recovered by qualified personnel in an area adjacent to the radiology suite or transported over relatively large distances through the medical center to the regular postanesthesia care unit.

A. **Evaluation.** A thorough preoperative evaluation should be performed for each patient scheduled for a neurodiagnostic procedure. In addition to elucidation of the patient's medical and surgical history, experience with sedatives and anesthetics, allergies, and medications, particular attention must be directed to the neurologic examination. Patients must be carefully evaluated for signs of increased intracranial pressure (ICP), preexisting neurologic deficits, and, in the case of the emergency patient, concomitant injury to the spine and other major organ systems.

B. **Equipment.** Equipment available in the radiology suite should include compatible anesthesia delivery systems, adequate supplies of medical gases, suction apparatus, age-appropriate drugs and airway equipment, and monitors for oxygen saturation, end-tidal carbon dioxide (CO_2), electrocardiogram (ECG), and blood pressure compatible with the imaging modality.

II. **Computed tomographic scan**

A. **Basic considerations.** Ionizing radiation is delivered to the patient during CT scanning. Radiation detectors are permanently fixed all of the way around the CT gantry. For each image, an x-ray tube rotates in a circle within the detector ring emitting a beam of ionizing radiation that passes through the body. The multiple detectors record the quantity of the x-ray beam that is attenuated or absorbed as it passes through the patient's tissues. This information from various angles is electronically integrated and the average attenuation value of each point in space is expressed in Hounsfield units.

Attenuation by a substance is directly related to its electronic density. Therefore, structures are hypodense (of lower attenuation), isodense (of similar attenuation), or hyperdense (of higher attenuation) relative to the brain parenchyma. The attenuation of vascular structures is increased by the use of iodinated contrast drugs. While CT axial images are displayed initially, high-resolution thin images can be transformed into coronal or sagittal sections through computer reformatting.

CT scanning is relatively insensitive for viewing structures within the posterior fossa because of image degradation by the artifact produced by the interface of bone and brain parenchyma. This modality remains the choice, however, for the detection of skull fractures and acute subarachnoid hemorrhage in the emergent setting. **Spiral acquisition CT scan** is also popular because larger anatomic regions can be imaged quickly, which is particularly useful in the trauma situation. For example, visualization from the aortic arch to the circle of Willis can be accomplished in <1 minute of scan time. With spiral acquisition scanning, unlike conventional CT scan, the patient is moved at a constant speed through the scanning field while the x-ray tube rotates continuously. CT angiography utilizes spiral acquisition scanning during the administration of iodinated contrast as an intravenous bolus. Complex intracranial aneurysms of <2 mm in diameter can also be visualized with CT angiography.

B. Management

   1. **Sedation.** With the current rapid CT scanners, very few adults or school-aged children require sedation for CT scanning. Occasionally, either intravenous midazolam in titrated doses of 0.5 mg may be effective, or an infusion of propofol at a dose of 25 to 100 mcg/kg/minute will sedate an anxious adult patient for the brief procedure. If an adult or older child manifests symptoms of increased ICP or serious airway compromise, it could be better to proceed with general anesthesia rather than attempt sedation. Several suggested techniques for the sedation of small children are listed in Table 16B-1. In addition to concerns about equipment, monitoring, and airway management, it must be remembered that the temperature of children within the cold radiology suite environment must be carefully maintained.

   2. **General anesthesia.** In the clinical situation where increased ICP is a critical factor, the intravenous induction of general anesthesia can be accomplished in children through an indwelling catheter, the insertion of which has been facilitated by the prior application of EMLA (lidocaine 2.5% and prilocaine 2.5%) cream to the dorsum of the patient's hands. In adults, an intravenous induction utilizing thiopental, 3 to 4 mg/kg, or propofol, 1 to 2 mg/kg, followed by

Table 16B-1. Sedation techniques for small children

Drug	Dose	Route	Onset (min)	Peak effect (min)
Chloral hydrate	20–75 mg/kg (2 g maximum)	p.o., p.r.	20–30	30–90
Pentobarbital sodium	2–4 mg/kg 5–7 mg/kg (120 mg maximum)	i.v., i.m.	5–10	60–90
Midazolam	0.02–0.15 mg/kg 0.3–0.75 mg/kg	i.v. p.o., p.r.	1–5 (i.v.)	20–30
Methohexital[a]	1–2 mg/kg 20–30 mg/kg	i.v. p.r.	5 10–15	45

[a] Might exacerbate temporal lobe seizures.
p.o., by mouth; p.r., rectally; i.v., intravenously; i.m., intramuscularly.

succinylcholine, 1 mg/kg, with the addition of a small dose of narcotic such as fentanyl, 50 to 100 mcg, and lidocaine, 1 mg/kg, to deepen the anesthetic is appropriate for endotracheal intubation. In small children, the issue of an undiagnosed muscular dystrophy mitigates against the use of succinylcholine. An induction utilizing either rocuronium, 0.6 to 1 mg/kg, or mivacurium, 0.2 to 0.25 mg/kg, for relaxation is often indicated. Anesthesia in children is maintained with an intravenous infusion of propofol, 25 to 100 mcg/kg/minute, or low concentrations of inhaled anesthetics. Rapid awakening at the end of the procedure is desirable. An infusion of remifentanil, 0.1 to 0.2 mcg/kg/minute, is an alternative in adults.

III. **MRI.** MRIs are acquired when protons on water molecules within the patient's body are excited through a combination of a strong magnetic field and intermittent radiofrequency (RF) pulses. Additional magnetic fields are applied to create gradients and excite the protons to different orientations within the basic magnetic field. In the excited state, these protons gain energy and shift from a low energy state to a high-energy state. This process is termed *resonance*. When the RF pulse is turned off, the protons lose energy in two ways: T1, the longitudinal relaxation time, and T2, the transverse relaxation time. Fortunately, no ionizing radiation is employed with MRI, but a large, powerful, external magnetic field is necessary.

Standard MRI sequences include T1-weighted images, proton density, and T2-weighted images, as well as T1 images with the intravenous administration of gadolinium contrast material. Conventional double-echo T2-weighted imaging has largely been supplanted by fast-scan echo or hybrid rapid acquisition relaxation enhancement (RARE) sequencing. Additional imaging sequences include gradient echo, blind-attenuated inversion recovery, magnetic resonance angiography (MRA), perfusion imaging, and diffusion weighting. Through constant technologic improvement, MRI has achieved increased accuracy with difficult clinical scenarios. Currently, the areas optimally imaged by MRI include the limbic system, pineal gland region, sella and parasellar structures, cranial nerves, internal auditory canal, cerebellopontine angle, leptomeninges, and posterior fossa. Flair imaging can detect processes in the area of the periventricular and cortical surfaces.

While MRA provides images of arterial and dural sinus blood flow, functional MRI is being utilized with increasing frequency in patient evaluation. Precise three-dimensional anatomic localization and a contrast effect dependent on the level of blood oxygenation facilitate functional studies of sight and hearing. These permit the lateral identification of the areas responsible for language before epilepsy surgery. Diffusion-weighted imaging is useful in the detection of acute cerebral infarctions and is able to identify regions of ischemia within minutes. Perfusion-weighted imaging that utilizes intravenous gadolinium contrast can be added to a diffusion-weighted study to demonstrate the presence of cerebral tissue at risk for further ischemia.

The frequency of adverse reactions to gadolinium-based contrast of all types is much lower than the frequency of adverse reactions to iodinated contrast material. The reactions to gadolinium can, however, range from mild erythema of the skin to severe life-threatening reactions including periorbital edema, respiratory distress, and cardiovascular collapse. In patients who report a previous reaction to gadolinium-based contrast, pretreatment with corticosteroids, famotidine (Pepcid), and diphenhydramine (Benadryl) and substituting a different gadolinium-based contrast agent can be helpful.

A. **Monitoring.** The MRI suite presents a hostile environment to the anesthesiologist. The following summarizes several of the safety considerations:

1. Metallic objects within the patient can be affected, depending on their metallic properties. Implants (including vascular surgical clips, stents, cochlear implants, and intrauterine devices) are subject to magnetic flux, which can induce electrical currents and cause local heating and movement. The function of pacemakers, cardiac catheters, and insulin pumps can be altered with exposure to the magnetic field. The radiologist most commonly assesses the hazards of metallic implants.

2. External metal wires, such as the ECG leads and temperature probe, can burn the skin. It is therefore necessary to use nonferromagnetic monitoring modalities especially designed for and compatible with the magnetic resonance (MR) scanner. Pulse oximeters, even nonferrous and fiberoptically cabled ones, should be placed on a distal extremity as far from the scanner as possible. The occurrence of scan artifacts and local skin irritation and swelling has been reported in patients who have either permanent eye makeup or tattoos that contain ferromagnetic pigments.

3. Small loose metal objects can be pulled toward the magnet and are obviously dangerous. Large objects such as oxygen cylinders can also be pulled into the magnet with considerable force and can be a serious threat to both patients and health care personnel. In general, no metallic objects are allowed in the scanning room.

4. Noise is a problem in the MR scanner. The torque on the loops of wire in which gradient currents are induced during the RF pulses causes vibration and audible noise that can average 95 decibels in a 1.5-Tesla scanner. Newer 3T machines generate twice the noise, hampering communication and necessitating ear protection for patients regardless of whether they are awake, sedated, or asleep.

5. RF heating from induced currents is a potential problem, particularly in small infants. Periodic assessment of body temperature must be conducted. Infants can also become cold within the magnet because of the low ambient temperature in the scanning room.

6. Newer, more powerful 3T MR scanners can induce electric currents in patients that can stimulate the peripheral nervous system. Paresthesias, cephalgia, and muscle contractions have all been reported. The RF impulse–induced electric currents can also cause burns.

7. The anesthesiologist must find the point of least distortion by orienting monitors in various positions relative to the magnetic field. Most ECG artifacts cannot be eliminated and monitors should be MR-compatible and have good artifact suppression characteristics. It is important to twist the ECG cables, keeping the electrodes close together, and position the electrodes near the center of the imager with the cables padded to avoid direct contact with the skin, to get the best images and to reduce the possibility of burns.

   Specialized equipment compatible with MRI is currently available for monitoring blood pressure, $ETCO_2$, Doppler, oxygen saturation, and ECG. Compatible anesthesia machines and ventilators are available as well. Plastic laryngoscopes are also available although the batteries in the handle could still be pulled into the magnetic field. Problems remain in terms of patient accessibility, hypothermia, and the physical limitations of positioning obese patients within the magnet's bore.

B. **Anesthetic management.** Many sedative techniques have proven quite reasonable for MR scanning, including the scanning of infants shortly after a meal to take advantage of postprandial drowsiness. The anesthesiologist is called to assist with MRI, however, when a patient is complicated neurologically, manifests serious illness, or has significant airway difficulties. In general, securing the airway with an endotracheal tube and then supplying ventilatory assistance through hand ventilation, an MRI-compatible ventilator, or a long circuit ensure an optimum combination of monitoring, airway protection, and anesthetic delivery. Certain centers have utilized an intravenous infusion of propofol, either with or without a laryngeal mask airway, to achieve the same goals. Whatever the technique, the ability to maintain adequate control of the airway in the face of limited accessibility remains of paramount importance.

IV. **Positron emission tomography (PET) and single-photon emission computed tomography (SPECT).** These nuclear imaging modalities are used to measure glucose consumption (PET) and regional cerebral blood flow (SPECT), thereby providing an indirect measurement of tissue metabolism and oxygen utilization. PET scans use positron-labeled molecules of which the most common is 2-[^{18}F] fluoro-2-deoxy-D-glucose (FDG). The FDG is injected intravenously and taken up into cerebral tissue. Because FDG cannot diffuse out of the brain after phosphorylation, it is well suited for imaging cerebral metabolism. PET scans are used in the investigation of malignancy because tumor cells have a much higher glucose metabolism. A PET scan of the brain takes 15 to 30 minutes.

SPECT scans use radiotracers that emit single photons. Three radiopharmaceutical agents have been approved by the United States Food and Drug Administration (FDA) for brain perfusion and SPECT scanning. Of the three, Tc-99m hexamethylpropyleneamine oxime ([^{99m}Tc]HMPAO) is used most commonly. It reaches maximum uptake 10 minutes after injection but has a constant distribution for hours afterward, which makes scheduling a scan very flexible. SPECT scans are used to investigate malignancy, cerebral ischemia, neurodegenerative disorders, epilepsy, cortical visual loss, and migraine headaches. A SPECT scan of the brain takes 20 to 45 minutes. Almost all of the radiopharmaceuticals are cleared through the urinary tract. For both PET and SPECT scans, the radiation exposure for the patient is usually equivalent to a CT scan but may be as high as ten effective dose equivalents.

A. **Anesthetic considerations.** Many anesthetic drugs have been shown to alter cerebral blood flow and metabolism, but, because of the stability of the tracers after injection, anesthetizing a patient for a scan should not interfere with the results. Anesthetic considerations include the necessity to provide all appropriate monitoring modalities, medical gases, drugs, suction, and airway equipment in a remote location. Unlike MRI, PET scanners do not require nonferromagnetic monitors, and the visualization of and access to the patient are more easily accomplished.

V. **Cerebral angiography.** Cerebral angiography continues to be important in the evaluation of subarachnoid hemorrhage and carotid artery disease. The safest and most widely used arterial access is the common femoral artery so that the use of a transfemoral catheter has replaced direct puncture of the carotid artery. Digital subtraction angiography reduces the volume of intra-arterial contrast required and the overall duration of the procedure. Unfortunately, neurologic problems related to the angiography itself still occur. In a prospective study of 1,002 angiograms, the overall rate of ischemic events within 0 to 24 hours of the procedure was 1.3% and 2.5% in patients studied for cerebrovascular disease. Complications from the catheters include transient global amnesia, cortical blindness, multiple cholesterol emboli syndrome, and vascular complications such as hematoma and pseudoaneurysm at the puncture site.

A. **Anesthetic management.** Although anesthesiologists are asked to participate in diagnostic angiography on rare occasions, they must bear in mind that contrast media cause vasodilatation and a burning discomfort. Often the degree of sedation needs to be increased in anticipation of an intra-arterial injection of contrast. As always, there is the possibility that a reaction to the contrast material can occur.

VI. **Myelography.** Myelography is utilized to define the contents of the thecal sac and any intrinsic or extrinsic impressions. Contrast agents are introduced directly into the subarachnoid space, thereby bypassing the blood-brain barrier. The newest myelographic contrast agents are nonionic, of low osmolarity, and mix well with cerebrospinal fluid. The main complications related to myelography include headache, contrast-related complications, either subdural or epidural contrast injection, hematoma of the spinal canal, meningitis, seizures, and various forms of neurologic injury. The incidence of adverse events is higher in women and increases with cervical versus lumbar puncture and with the use of 22-gauge bevel-tipped versus 24-gauge Sprotte needles. Among the anesthetic considerations is the need to carefully position infants and children while the myelogram table is rotated to achieve good flow of the contrast material.

VII. **Contrast material.** In addition to CT scan, iodinated contrast is used for catheter angiography and myelography. High-osmolar contrast agents are ionic monomers at concentrations ranging from 60% to 76% by weight. This material possesses five to eight times the osmolality of human serum (280 mOsm/kg H_2O). Nonionic monomers and dimers as well as ionic dimers are considered low-osmolar contrast agents (LOCAs) when they have from two to three times the osmolality of human serum. The LOCAs demonstrate more hydrophilia and less tendency to bind to tissue and are therefore more biologically inert. Despite their higher cost, LOCAs are used for most neurodiagnostic procedures.

Iodinated contrast agents are nephrotoxic. After an initial mild vasodilatation, the renal vascular tree undergoes prolonged vasoconstriction. Patients who have preexisting renal insufficiency, diabetes mellitus, and low cardiac output syndromes are at risk for developing contrast agent-induced nephrotoxicity. Renal insufficiency can be ameliorated or prevented with adequate hydration and the withholding of any other nephrotoxic medications before the procedure. The use of fenoldopam, N-acetylcysteine, and dopamine has consistently failed to preserve renal function more effectively than hydration alone. Patients at risk should receive limited amounts of iodinated contrast media. Diabetic patients who have nephropathy and who receive metformin should be carefully monitored for the development of metformin-induced lactic acidosis after receiving iodinated contrast.

The hypertonicity of iodinated contrast media is responsible for the side effects that occur after injection. These include pain, flushing, nausea, and vomiting. Patients' responses to iodinated contrast material can range from a warm flushing and a metallic taste during contrast injection to an anaphylactoid reaction. Large multi-institutional studies have demonstrated that patients given nonionic contrast material have a 1 in 10,000 chance of having a severe reaction. Patients likely to have a problem with contrast include those who have had previous idiosyncratic contrast reactions, patients who have either asthma or multiple food and medication allergies, and patients who have other illnesses including preexisting azotemia and cardiac disease. The use of corticosteroids such as oral methylprednisolone, 32 mg, both 6 to 24 hours before and 2 hours before the injection of the contrast material, markedly reduces the chance of a severe reaction to contrast. Additionally, some centers add antihistamines and H_2 blocking drugs to the steroid regimen.

Not infrequently, a few hives about the face, neck, and chest are the sole reaction that a patient manifests to contrast. Often the only therapy necessary in such cases is reassurance with perhaps a dose of diphenhydramine, 25 mg to 50 mg intravenously (i.v.). A severe reaction to contrast, manifested by generalized skin irritation, respiratory difficulties, and hypotension, requires treatment with epinephrine, 100 mcg i.v., and glucagon for refractory hypotension. Equipment must be available in the radiology suite for immediate airway control and the administration of additional adjuncts such as beta$_2$-agonists including albuterol for treating bronchospasm. Occasionally, large volumes of fluid as well as vasoactive drugs are necessary to support the blood pressure. A prolonged stay in the intensive care unit could be necessary to stabilize the patient.

Delayed reactions can be seen in 1% to 3% of patients receiving x-ray contrast material. These are usually mild and consist of rashes and hives.

SUGGESTED READINGS

Blake P, Johnson B, VanMeter JW. Positron emission tomography (PET) and single photon emission computed tomography (SPECT): clinical applications. *J Neuroophthalmol* 2003;23:34–41.

Frush DP, Bisset GS, Hall SC III. Pediatric sedation in radiology: the practice of safe sleep. *Am J Roentgenol* 1996;167:1381–1387.

Gandhi D. Computed tomography and magnetic resonance angiography in cervicocranial vascular disease. *J Neuroophthalmol* 2004;24:306–314.

Goldenberg I, Matetzky S. Nephropathy induced by contrast media: pathogenesis, risk factors and preventive strategies. *Can Med Assoc J* 2005;172:1461–1471.

Gooden CK, Dilos B. Anesthesia for magnetic resonance imaging. *Int Anesthesiol Clin* 2003;41:29–37.

Guidelines for Nonoperating Room Anesthetizing Locations. American Society of Anesthesiologists. Approved by House of Delegates on October 19, 1994, and last amended on October 15, 2003. Available at: http://www.asahq.org/publicationsAndServices/standards/14.pdf. Accessed July 8, 2005.

Jager HR, Grieve JP. Advances in non-invasive imaging of intracranial vascular disease. *Ann R Coll Surg Engl* 2000;82:1–5.

Krauss B, Green SM. Sedation and analgesia for procedures in children. *N Engl J Med* 2000;342:938–945.

Malviya S, Voepel-Lewis T, Eldevik OP. et al. Sedation and general anaesthesia in children undergoing MRI and CT: adverse events and outcomes. *Br J Anaesth* 2000;84:743–748.

Morcos SK, Thomsen HS. Adverse reactions to iodinated contrast media. *Eur Radiol* 2001;11:1267–1275.

Murphy KJ, Brunberg JA, Cohan RH. Adverse reactions to gadolinium contrast media: a review of 36 cases. *Am J Roentgenol* 1996;167:847–849.

Schlüzen L, Vafaee MS, Cold GE, et al. Effects of subanaesthetic and anaesthetic doses of sevoflurane on regional cerebral blood flow in healthy volunteers. A positron emission tomographic study. *Acta Anaesthesiol Scand* 2004;48:1268–1276.

Veselis RA, Feshchenko VA, Reinsel RA, et al. Propofol and thiopental do not interfere with regional cerebral blood flow response at sedative concentrations. *Anesthesiol* 2005;102:26–34.

Postanesthesia Care Unit & Intensive Care

Complications in the Postanesthesia Care Unit

Jean G. Charchaflieh and Samrat H. Worah

I. **Complications after operation for supratentorial tumor**
   A. **Increased intracranial pressure (ICP).** The cranial cavity has a limited capacity to accommodate increased intracranial volume without a significant increase in pressure. Increased volume of any of the three components of the intracranial cavity—brain cells, blood, and cerebrospinal fluid (CSF)—may increase ICP. Increased ICP causes injury to the brain by compression, herniation, and ischemia. Brain ischemia in turn enhances brain edema, propagating a cycle of vascular insufficiency and swelling.

   Intracranial hemorrhage, hydrocephalus, and cerebral edema are the most common postoperative causes of increased ICP. Intracranial hypertension leads to headache, nausea, vomiting, decreased level of consciousness, and neurologic dysfunction. These signs are not specific for increased ICP and are not uncommon postoperatively. Detection of increased ICP relies on clinical signs and symptoms, direct measurement of ICP, and imaging studies such as computed tomographic (CT) scanning. Prevention and treatment seek to avoid and alleviate factors that can aggravate intracranial hypertension such as arterial hypertension, impaired cerebral venous drainage, blocked or malfunctioning surgical drains, postoperative pain, respiratory depression, nausea and vomiting, shivering, and seizures.
   1. Cerebral edema is minimized by intraoperative and postoperative use of dexamethasone, loading dose 10 to 20 mg intravenously (i.v.); then 4 mg i.v. every 6 hours and mannitol, loading dose 0.25 to 2 g/kg i.v. over 30 minutes; then every 6 hours as needed, with careful monitoring of fluid intake and output and control of blood pressure and central venous pressure.
   2. Cerebral venous drainage is facilitated by head elevation to 30°, blood pressure permitting.
   3. Postoperative ventilation and oxygenation should be monitored and supplemental oxygen and ventilatory support should be provided as needed.
   4. Pain is treated with small doses of fentanyl, 0.5 to 1 mcg/kg i.v. every 1 to 2 hours; morphine, 0.025 to 0.05 mg/kg i.v. every 1 to 2 hours; or hydromorphone, 0.2 to 1 mg i.v. every 2 to 3 hours.

5. Postoperative nausea and vomiting are minimized by intraoperative use of dexamethasone (see **I.A.1**) and 5HT3 receptor antagonists such as dolasetron, 12.5 mg i.v. in adults and 0.35 mg/kg i.v. in children; or ondansetron, 4 mg i.v. over 4 minutes for adults and children weighing >40 kg and 0.1 mg/kg i.v. over 4 minutes for children weighing <40 kg.

6. Postoperative shivering is treated by gradually rewarming the patient and administering small doses of meperidine, 12.5 mg i.v.

7. Postoperative seizures are treated with phenytoin, loading dose 10 to 20 mg/kg i.v. no faster than 50 mg/minutes (1,000 mg over 20 minutes in typical adults) and then 5 to 7 mg/kg/day; or fosphenytoin, loading dose phenytoin equivalent (PE) 15 to 20 mg/kg i.v. no faster than 100 to 150 mg/minute (1,000 mg PE over 10 minutes in typical adults) and then 4 to 6 PE mg/kg/day.

II. **Complications after operation for infratentorial tumor**

A. **Increased ICP.** The elastance of the infratentorial compartment is greater than that of the supratentorial compartment, which means that it takes smaller increases in volume to produce significant increases in pressure. Furthermore, increased pressure in the posterior fossa is more life threatening because it can compress or herniate the brain stem, which contains the respiratory and vascular centers. Brain stem herniation can occur downward through the foramen magnum or upward through the tentorium, which is most common after resection of tumors of the cervical medullary junction. Brain stem compression is manifested by a decreased level of consciousness and respiratory and cardiovascular abnormalities including collapse. Measures to control ICP should be continued in the postoperative period: head elevation; prevention and treatment of hypertension; treatment of pain, nausea, and vomiting; prevention and treatment of shivering; and maintenance of adequate ventilation and oxygenation (see **I.A.1–7**). Decreased level of consciousness or the development of respiratory or cardiovascular abnormalities should prompt surgical consultation.

B. **Brain stem injury** can occur intraoperatively. This presents postoperatively as failure to regain consciousness or resume spontaneous respiration with cardiovascular abnormalities such as bradycardia and hypertension/hypotension. Pharmacologic causes of such manifestations should be ruled out by ensuring adequate reversal of anesthetic agents and muscle relaxants. Supportive care in the form of mechanical ventilation and hemodynamic therapy is provided as needed.

C. **Injury to cranial nerves IX, X, and XII** may compromise the patient's ability to maintain a patent and protected airway due to difficulty in swallowing and clearing secretions. Tracheal extubation should be performed only after the integrity of protective upper airway reflexes is evident. After extubation, respiratory monitoring should continue with readiness to reintubate the trachea and reinstitute mechanical ventilation if the patient fails to maintain adequate ventilation and a patent and protected airway. Injury to the ophthalmic division of the trigeminal nerve (cranial nerve V) may impair protective reflexes of the cornea and require external protection with an eye patch.

D. **Edema of the mucosa** of the upper airway may occur after prolonged surgery, especially in the sitting position. It is more significant in children due to the small diameter of their airways. Tracheal extubation should be performed only after absence of airway edema is ascertained by deflating the cuff of the endotracheal tube and confirming the ability of the patient to breathe around the tube. If airway edema is suspected, the trachea should remain intubated and the patient sedated, if needed, until the edema resolves. Inhaled racemic epinephrine, 0.5 mL of 2% solution in 3 mL saline, decreases localized mucosal edema and might relieve upper airway obstruction. Macroglossia may accompany upper airway edema, causing complete airway obstruction. If this occurs, cricothyroidotomy, tracheotomy, or insertion of laryngeal mask airway may be the fastest way to reestablish the airway.

E. **Pneumocephalus** occurs after craniectomy, especially in the sitting position, and is usually of little clinical consequence. Tension pneumocephalus, which may decrease the level of consciousness due to brain compression, is more common in patients after ventricular shunting and aggressive drainage of CSF, which allows air trapping in the space that surrounds the brain that has been drained of CSF. Pneumocephalus is diagnosed by a CT scan or x-ray of the head and is effectively treated with a burr hole, which can be done under local anesthesia and usually produces rapid recovery of consciousness once the trapped air has been released.

F. Patients who develop intraoperative venous air embolism may subsequently develop postoperative **pulmonary edema** requiring mechanical ventilation and diuresis. Extubation is performed after resolution of pulmonary edema as documented by clinical examination, chest x-ray, and arterial blood gases. Patients with functionally patent foramen ovale may develop paradoxical air embolism, which is manifest postoperatively by neurologic deficits, decreased level of consciousness, and cardiac abnormalities.

III.   Complications after operation for pituitary tumor

A. **Endocrine complications** include adrenocortical insufficiency, hypothyroidism, and diabetes insipidus (DI).

1. All patients receive corticosteroid coverage until testing indicates an intact pituitary-adrenal axis.

2. Thyroid hormone replacement is reserved for patients who were hypothyroid preoperatively.

3. DI occurs in 10% to 20% of patients, usually develops within 12 to 24 hours of surgery, and lasts for a few days. Decreased release of antidiuretic hormone results in the excretion of excessive amounts (4 to 14 L/day) of dilute urine and leads to dehydration, hypernatremia, increased serum osmolality (>300 mOsm/kg), decreased urine osmolality (<200 mOsm/kg), and decreased urine specific gravity (<1.005). Symptoms of hypernatremia are nonspecific and include decreased level of consciousness, tremulousness, muscle weakness, irritability, ataxia, spasticity, confusion, seizures, coma, and possibly intracranial bleeding due to increased serum osmolality. Treatment of DI consists of hydration and hormonal supplementation. The amount and content of intravenous fluids are guided by urine volume, serum electrolytes, and serum osmolality. Free water (H_2O) deficit can be estimated using the following formula:

Free H_2O deficit =

$$\frac{(\text{Serum Na}^+ - 140) \text{ body weight (kg)} \times 0.6}{140}$$

If fluid is replaced early, it is not necessary to administer free water (D_5W). Rather, a hypotonic solution such as 0.45% sodium chloride (NaCl) or lactated Ringer's may be given. Insulin and potassium supplementation might be required when dextrose-containing fluids are used, especially if corticosteroids are used concomitantly. When hormonal replacement is required, 1-deamino-8-D-arginine vasopressin (DDAVP), a synthetic analog of the natural hormone arginine vasopressin, can be given intravenously, subcutaneously, orally, or intranasally. The latter might not be feasible after transnasal transsphenoidal pituitary surgery. The usual intravenous or subcutaneous dose is 0.3 mcg/kg/day, divided and given twice daily. The dose by mouth is 0.05 to 1.2 mg/day, divided and given two to three times a day. The intranasal dose is 10 to 40 mcg one to three times a day. The dose is adjusted according to the patient's sleep pattern and water turnover. Once intravascular volume has been restored, persistent hypernatremia may be treated with thiazide diuretics, such as hydrochlorothiazide, 50 to 100 mg/day i.v.

B. **Rhinorrhea** of CSF may develop after transnasal transsphenoidal operations. Spontaneous resolution occurs commonly, and clinical observation is sufficient in most cases. If signs of infection develop, antibiotic therapy and surgical repair are indicated.

C. **Airway obstruction** from bleeding and accumulation of blood and secretions in the pharynx sometimes occurs after transnasal transsphenoidal surgery. Frequent assessment of the patency of the airway and adequacy of ventilation is mandatory. Excessive bleeding might require reintubation and surgical consultation.

D. **Postoperative nausea and vomiting** might develop due to intraoperative swallowing of blood during transsphenoidal resection of pituitary tumors. To minimize the risk of postoperative nausea and vomiting, the pharynx and stomach are suctioned at the conclusion of surgery, and 5HT3 receptor antagonists are administered prophylactically: dolasetron, 12.5 mg i.v. in adults and 0.35 mg/kg i.v. in children; ondansetron, 4 mg i.v. over 4 minutes for adults and children weighing >40 kg and 0.1 mg/kg i.v. over 4 minutes for children weighing <40 kg, or granisetron, 0.1 to 1 mg i.v.

IV. **Complications after operation for head trauma.** Systemic sequelae of head trauma frequently become apparent in the postoperative period. These include adult respiratory distress syndrome, neurogenic pulmonary edema (NPE), cardiac arrhythmias, electrocardiographic (ECG) changes, disseminated intravascular coagulation, DI, syndrome of inappropriate antidiuretic hormone secretion (SIADH), hyperglycemia, nonketotic hyperosmolar hyperglycemic coma, and gastrointestinal ulcers and hemorrhage.

A. **NPE** is a fulminant form of pulmonary edema that progresses rapidly (within hours to days) toward either resolution or death. The pathologic characteristics of NPE are marked pulmonary vascular congestion, pulmonary arteriolar wall rupture, protein-rich edema fluid, and intra-alveolar hemorrhage. NPE results from a massive transient central sympathetic discharge due to an increase in ICP and is particularly associated with hypothalamic lesions. The pathophysiology includes systemic vasoconstriction and left ventricular failure, redistribution of blood from the systemic to the pulmonary vessels, pulmonary venous constriction, and increased pulmonary capillary permeability. Treatment is aimed at reducing ICP, reducing sympathetic hyperactivity, mainly by using alpha-adrenergic blockers such as diazoxide, 1 to 3 mg/kg i.v. every 5 minutes until blood pressure is controlled, up to 150 mg, or phentolamine, 5 mg i.v. increments, and providing respiratory supportive care and inotropic therapy as needed.

B. **The syndrome of inappropriate antidiuretic hormone (SIADH)** causes water retention with continued urinary excretion of sodium. This leads to dilutional hyponatremia, decreased serum osmolality, increased urine osmolality, and decreased urinary output. Water retention and serum hypo-osmolality might progress to water intoxication, which leads to nonspecific symptoms such as nausea, vomiting, headache, irritability, disorientation, seizures, and coma. Treatment consists of water restriction, loop diuretics, and hypertonic saline. In mild cases, fluid restriction (1 to 1.5 L/day) is sufficient to correct hyponatremia. Furosemide may be added because it impairs renal ability to concentrate urine. Hypertonic saline is usually reserved for serum sodium of <120 to 125 mEq/L. It is given in small amounts for a short time (1 to 2 mL/kg/hour for 2 to 3 hours), after which serum sodium and osmolality are measured. During the acute phase of SIADH, urine output is measured hourly and urine osmolality and specific gravity and serum sodium and osmolality are measured every 6 to 8 hours. Serum sodium should be increased at a rate of no more than 0.5 mEq/L/hour or 12 mEq/L/day. Faster rates of correction may cause osmotic demyelination, which develops over several days. It is associated with nonspecific signs such as behavioral changes, movement disorders, seizures, pseudobulbar palsy, quadriparesis, and coma.

C. **Spinal cord injury** occurring in conjunction with head injury might become apparent only in the postoperative period. Up to 15% of patients with head injury sustain cervical spine injury as well. Precautions to avoid exacerbation of spinal cord injury are continued in the postoperative period until cervical spine injury is ruled out or repaired. Pharmacologic therapy to ameliorate spinal cord injury may be given within 8 hours from injury in the form of methylprednisolone, loading dose 30 mg/kg i.v.; then 5.4 mg/kg/hour i.v. for 23 hours. Acute phase spinal shock (usually during the first week) is treated with fluids, inotropes, and pressors. During the chronic phase of spinal injury (after the first week), adequate analgesia is provided before somatic or splanchnic stimulation in patients with injury above T6 to avoid the risk of autonomic hyperreflexia.

D. **Cardiovascular and respiratory monitoring,** aided with the appropriate imaging and laboratory studies, is aimed at detecting extracranial injuries and complications such as pneumothorax, hemothorax, intra-abdominal or retroperitoneal hemorrhage, and fat embolism.

E. **Prevention of secondary brain injury** is continued in the postoperative period. Hypotension, hypoxia, hyperthermia, hyperglycemia, hypoglycemia, increased ICP, and any aggravating factors such as pain, nausea, vomiting, seizures, hypertension, hypercarbia, and impaired cerebral venous drainage should all be prevented and treated. Conscious, mechanically ventilated patients are sedated with short-acting agents, such as propofol, 10 to 30 mcg/kg/minute i.v., or dexmedetomidine, load 1 mcg/kg i.v. over 10 minutes; then 0.2 to 0.7 mcg/kg/hour for <24 hours, to allow intermittent neurologic assessment. Pain due to the operative procedure or the primary or associated injury is relieved with opioids such as morphine, 0.05 mg/kg i.v., or fentanyl, 0.5 to 1 mcg/kg i.v. Nausea and vomiting are treated with stomach suctioning (after ruling out skull base fracture) and pharmacologic means such as ondansetron, 4 mg i.v.; dolasetron, 12.5 to 25 mg i.v., or granisetron, 0.1 to 1 mg i.v. Seizure prophylaxis after head trauma is somewhat controversial. Phenytoin, loading dose 15 mg/kg i.v. over 20 minutes followed by 5 to 7 mg/kg/day, or fosphenytoin, loading dose PE 15 to 20 mg/kg i.v. and then 4 to 6 PE mg/kg/day, may be given for 2 weeks after head injury if there have been no seizures or longer if there have.

   F. **Clotting** may be impaired because of the release of tissue thromboplastin and a trauma-induced decrease in platelets, prothrombin (factor II), proaccelerin (factor V), and plasminogen and increase in fibrin degradation products.

V. Complications after operation for aneurysm

   A. **Vasospasm.** Angiographic narrowing of blood vessels occurs in approximately 30% of patients between days 4 and 14 after subarachnoid hemorrhage (SAH). Neurologic dysfunction (disorientation, decreased level of consciousness, focal deficit) occurs in approximately 50% of patients who have angiographic narrowing. The risk for developing vasospasm correlates with the amount of blood around the circle of Willis, the preoperative use of antifibrinolytic therapy, and the postoperative development of the cerebral salt wasting (CSW) syndrome. Pharmacologic prophylactic therapy of vasospasm is initiated within 96 hours of SAH and consists of nimodipine, 60 mg by mouth every 4 hours for 21 days or longer. Triple-H therapy (hypervolemia, hypertension, and hemodilution) may be used to treat vasospasm following SAH. It consists of the administration of crystalloid and colloid solutions to achieve a pulmonary capillary wedge pressure of 15 mm Hg and hemoglobin level of 11 g/dL and the use of inotropes and vasopressors to achieve a mean arterial pressure of 120 mm Hg or more. Antidiuretic therapy with vasopressin is sometimes necessary to prevent the diuresis induced by volume loading. Hypotension, heart failure, myocardial ischemia, and pulmonary edema are occasional complications of triple-H therapy.

B. **Obstructive hydrocephalus** due to subarachnoid blood-induced disturbances in CSF circulation may occur after SAH. The resulting increase in ICP may manifest itself as a decreased level of consciousness. CT scan is diagnostic, and ventriculostomy with CSF drainage is the effective therapy.

C. **Hyponatremia** after SAH can be due to CSW syndrome or, less commonly, to SIADH. CSW syndrome is caused by increased secretion of atrial natriuretic peptide, brain natriuretic peptide, and C-type natriuretic peptide. These peptides suppress aldosterone synthesis and lead to natriuresis, diuresis, and vasodilatation. Hyponatremia in the CSW syndrome results from increased renal excretion of sodium (150 to 200 mEq/L), which is followed by water with resultant hypovolemia. Hyponatremia of SIADH is mainly due to water retention in conjunction with renal excretion of sodium in a range of 20 to 30 mEq/L. Treatment of the two forms of hyponatremia is completely different. Patients with CSW require sodium replacement and fluid administration, whereas patients with SIADH require fluid restriction and diuresis. Fluid restriction and diuresis in a patient with CSW can be fatal due to the possibility of severe hypovolemia and cerebral infarction; fluid and salt administered to a patient with SIADH may lead to osmotic demyelination. Hypertonic saline may be used with close monitoring of serum sodium in both CSW syndrome and SIADH.

D. **DI** occurs less frequently than CSW syndrome or SIADH after SAH (see **III.A**). Treatment includes hypotonic fluids in the form of enteral free water or parenteral D_5W, D_5 0.2% NaCl, or 0.45% NaCl plus the administration of DDAVP, 0.3 mcg/kg/day i.v. or subcutaneously, divided and given twice a day; 0.05 to 1.2 mg/day by mouth; or 10 to 40 mcg one to three times a day by nasal spray.

E. **Intracranial hematomas** might develop at the operative site or at the bridging dural veins due to overzealous CSF drainage. Manifestations are those of increased ICP, which may be associated with focal deficit. CT scan is diagnostic, and treatment with surgical evacuation may be required.

F. **Seizure prophylaxis** is continued in the postoperative period due to the high risk of seizures after SAH, especially in hypertensive patients. Phenytoin is usually given for 3 to 6 months after SAH.

G. **NPE** occurs in some patients after SAH due to the sudden increase in ICP, which produces intense sympathetic activation, catecholamine release from the hypothalamus and the medulla, and increased pulmonary vascular pressure and permeability (see **IV.A**). Diagnosis depends on the exclusion of other causes of pulmonary edema such as triple-H therapy and aspiration pneumonia. Treatment includes supplemental oxygen, mechanical ventilation plus positive end-expiratory pressure, and reduction of ICP.

H. After SAH, patients are at moderate risk for developing **deep venous thrombosis (DVT)** and **pulmonary embolus (PE).** Mechanical DVT prophylaxis, in the form of graduated stockings or intermittent pneumatic compression of the lower extremities, is instituted in all patients after SAH. Anticoagulation is contraindicated in the acute postoperative phase. Insertion of an inferior vena cava filter may be necessary for the prevention of recurrent pulmonary embolization.

I. **Cardiac complications** are common after SAH. ECG changes of arrhythmia, ischemia, or infarction, which are detected in >50% of patients, occur within 48 hours of SAH but may be first noted in the early postoperative period. Echocardiography, thallium scintigraphy, and autopsy detect evidence of myocardial injury. These ECG changes may be due to hypothalamic injury and high catecholamine levels. Treatment depends on the severity of the complications, the hemodynamic stability of the patient, and concomitant vasospasm. Infarcted, stunned, or hibernating myocardium might exclude these patients from triple-H therapy.

VI. **Complications after ablation of arteriovenous malformation (AVM).** After surgery for AVM, patients are at risk of developing complications similar to those found after aneurysm surgery (vasospasm, hydrocephalus, and seizures). In addition, these patients are at high risk of developing hyperemic complications.

A. **The syndrome of normal perfusion-pressure breakthrough or cerebral hyperperfusion** is a hyperemic state characterized by cerebral edema, swelling, and/or hemorrhage that develops after resection of AVM. This condition results from the restoration of cerebral blood flow (CBF) to chronically hypoperfused areas or from venous outflow obstruction after AVM ablation. The ensuing cerebral swelling and hemorrhage cause neurologic dysfunction and are a major cause of postoperative morbidity and mortality. Patients who have ischemic rather than hemorrhagic symptoms preoperatively or certain angiographic features such as high or inverse flow in a large, deep, border zone AVM are particularly at risk. Staged repair and strict control of blood flow through the AVM may decrease the risk of hyperemic complications. Treatment of the manifestations of cerebral hyperemia includes mechanical hyperventilation, osmotic diuresis, and barbiturate coma.

VII. **Complications after neuroradiologic procedures.** Cerebral vascular embolization procedures may lead to complications such as SAH, intracerebral hemorrhage, cerebral ischemia, cerebral infarction, reperfusion syndrome, seizures, pulmonary embolism, and contrast reactions. The priority of treatment in all of these complications is to secure a patent and protected airway and maintain adequate cerebral perfusion pressure through the management of blood pressure and ICP.

A. Cerebral hemorrhage may occur either immediately due to vessel perforation by the catheter or guidewire or aneurysmal rupture or later due to hyperemic complications. Most small perforations can be managed conservatively by observation and follow-up. Alternatively, the catheter itself can be used to tamponade the source of bleeding and occlude the perforation. Other treatment measures include reversal of systemic anticoagulants, seizure prophylaxis, analgesic and antiemetic therapy, and insertion of large bore intravenous catheters for fluid resuscitation and possible blood transfusion. These measures should be instituted in consultation with the attending neuroradiologist or neurosurgeon. Large perforations with massive bleeding require emergent surgical intervention. However, the prognosis of extensive bleeding is grave because most of these patients exsanguinate prior to surgery owing to the inability to perform craniotomy and vascular repair in a timely manner, particularly because most of these vessels are situated deep in the cerebral parenchyma.

B. Cerebral ischemia may occur due to the obstruction of venous drainage, unintentional occlusion of surrounding arteries, or local injection of papaverine for treatment of vasospasm. Cerebral ischemia/infarction may manifest themselves as hemiplegia, hemiparesis, cranial nerve palsies, aphasia, nausea, vomiting, and seizures. Treatment of cerebral ischemia/infarction in this setting consists of maintaining adequate cerebral perfusion pressure by blood pressure and ICP management, airway protection, and other supportive care as needed. Intravenous thrombolytic therapy is contraindicated in this setting. Interventional neuroradiologic measures to reestablish perfusion can be attempted.

C. Seizures may occur in patients with preexisting seizure disorders or in patients with no such history. They may occur due to cerebral ischemia or infarction, which could be due to vessel obstruction or trauma, as mentioned earlier (see **VII.B**), or localized cerebral edema, which could follow even successful embolization procedures; or they may be precipitated by the **cerebral hyperperfusion syndrome** (see **VII.F**). Management of seizures should include, in addition to pharmacologic therapy, identification and, when possible, treatment of precipitating factor(s), airway management, and stabilization of hemodynamic parameters. Anticonvulsant therapy includes midazolam, 0.1 to 0.2 mg/kg i.v.; lorazepam, 4 to 8 mg i.v.; thiopental, 3 to 5 mg/kg i.v.; phenytoin, loading dose 10 to 20 mg/kg i.v. no faster than 50 mg/minute (1,000 mg over 20 minutes in typical adult) and then 5 to 7 mg/kg/day; or fosphenytoin, loading dose PE 15 to 20 mg/kg i.v. no faster than 100 to 150 mg/minute (1,000 mg PE over 10 minutes in typical adult) and then 4 to 6 PE mg/kg/day.

D. **Pulmonary embolism** may occur due to either the release of embolization materials into the venous circulation, particularly in AVMs that contain large fistulae or those of the vein of Galen, or from vessels accessed en route to the AVM. Depending on the extent and source of embolism, treatment consists of securing a patent and protected airway, maintaining adequate oxygenation and ventilation, and, in case of cardiopulmonary collapse, performing surgical embolectomy.

E. **Contrast media reactions** may be allergic or nonallergic in nature. Allergic reactions manifest as generalized flushing, hives, hypotension, and bronchospasm. Treatment consists of supportive measures of airway, breathing, and circulation and pharmacologic therapy in the form of epinephrine, 0.5 to 1 mg i.v. or 3 to 5 mL intratracheally of 1:10,000 solution; hydrocortisone, 100 mg i.v. every 6 hours; and diphenhydramine, 25 to 50 mg i.v. every 4 to 6 hours. Nonallergic reactions occur due to the sheer volume of the contrast dye, which may lead to congestive heart failure in susceptible patients or to osmotic diuresis, which may lead to fluid and electrolyte imbalances in patients who are already hypovolemic due to diuretic therapy and/or restricted salt and water intake.

F. **Cerebral hyperperfusion syndrome** may occur in areas surrounding large AVMs due to diversion of blood flow to the AVM. These hypoperfused areas lose their ability to autoregulate blood flow and are usually maximally vasodilated. Following embolization, the large amount of blood flow flowing through the erstwhile AVM is now shunted back to these maximally dilated vessels leading to cerebral hyperemia, edema, and/or hemorrhage. Methods to prevent this sudden increase in blood flow include deliberate hypotension, pretreatment with barbiturates, clamping of the cervical carotid artery, and staged embolization of the feeding vessels to allow the surrounding tissues to regain their autoregulatory function. Pharmacologic treatment of cerebral edema includes administration of furosemide, 0.1 to 1 mg/kg i.v., and mannitol, 0.25 to 1 g/kg i.v. over 20 minutes.

G. **Complications due to materials used for embolization.** Glues such as normobutyl cyanoacrylate (NBCA) and isobutyl 2-cyanoacrylate may cause pulmonary complications manifesting as hemoptysis and pleural pain. Particulate materials such as polyvinyl alcohol (PVA), silicon beads, silk, steel and platinum microcoils, Gelfoam, and collagen may cause pulmonary or systemic embolism. Also, PVA is known to increase the risk of recanalization of the embolized AVM.

VIII. **Complications after carotid endarterectomy (CEA)**

A. **Cardiac ischemia and infarction** are the leading cause of mortality after CEA. Coronary artery disease is common among patients undergoing CEA. Perioperative tachycardia, hypertension, and hypotension increase the risk of perioperative myocardial ischemia and infarction. The alpha-agonists, such as phenylephrine, are preferable in the treatment of hypotension in this setting because they raise blood pressure without significantly increasing heart rate. However, the ensuing hypertension may be detrimental. Combined alpha- and beta-agonists such as ephedrine increase heart rate and have been associated with myocardial ischemia and infarction in this setting.

B. **Occlusion of the operated carotid artery** should be suspected whenever new neurologic symptoms develop postoperatively. This is one cause of postoperative cerebral ischemia that is amenable to surgical intervention. Early diagnosis and treatment significantly alter outcome. A Doppler flow study can detect cessation of flow in the involved vessel, and angiography can confirm vascular occlusion. Surgical reexploration need not await angiographic confirmation but may be undertaken on the basis of the clinical picture and the ultrasound examination.

C. **The cerebral hyperperfusion syndrome** may develop after CEA due to the sudden increase in CBF in a maximally dilated vascular bed that has lost its ability to autoregulate because of longstanding hypoperfusion. This hyperperfusion may lead to cerebral edema or hemorrhage with headache, seizures, decreased level of consciousness, and focal neurologic deficit. Severe carotid stenosis and hypertension contribute to the development of this syndrome. Careful control of blood pressure is essential in preventing hyperperfusion. Mild elevation of blood pressure need not be treated in the postoperative period, whereas moderate to severe hypertension should be reduced to avoid the cerebral hyperperfusion syndrome. Titratable, short-acting agents such as sodium nitroprusside (SNP), 0.25 to 8 mcg/kg/minute i.v., and esmolol, loading dose 500 mcg/kg over 1 minute followed by 50 to 300 mcg/kg/minute i.v., are preferable in this setting. The beta-blocking effects of esmolol offset the sympathetic hyperactivity from SNP.

D. **Hypotension** is poorly tolerated by hypertensive patients who have a rightward shift in their autoregulatory curve. Hypotension can lead to cerebral and cardiac hypoperfusion and can increase the risk of thrombus formation in the operated vessel. Blood pressure is usually kept at 20% above baseline. Hypotension is treated with volume expansion and infusion of a short-acting alpha-agonist such as phenylephrine, 40 to 180 mcg/minute i.v., mixed as 20 mg in 250 mL D_5W at 30 to 160 mL/hour.

E. **Treatment of stroke after CEA** consists of blood pressure management, supportive care, and treatment of complications. Intravenous thrombolytic therapy is contraindicated in the postoperative period. Intra-arterial thrombolytic therapy may be considered in institutions that have the expertise. Neuroprotective therapy, still the subject of clinical trials, has not been approved for clinical use.

F. **Airway obstruction** can result from hematoma formation and can be aggravated by laryngeal edema and cranial nerve injury. Reestablishing airway patency might require suture removal and drainage of the hematoma. This is best accomplished by a surgeon in conjunction with tracheal intubation and racemic epinephrine. If the patient is in extremis, the first person to reach the bedside opens the wound to secure the airway.

IX. **Complications after vertebral column procedures**

A. **Complications after anterior cervical discectomy.** The patient's trachea is usually extubated in the operating room after an uncomplicated discectomy. However, tracheal intubation may be maintained postoperatively if upper airway edema is anticipated after a prolonged operation or one associated with infusion of large volumes of fluid. It is important to prevent the patient from coughing and straining while the trachea is intubated. This may cause the newly placed bone graft to dislodge, which might compress the trachea or the esophagus and require reoperation. After extubation, the patient's voice is evaluated to detect recurrent laryngeal nerve injury, a benign complication that usually resolves over days to weeks.

B. **Complications after cervical corpectomy and stabilization.** These procedures are usually more invasive, more prolonged, associated with more fluid administration, and therefore more likely to cause airway edema at the conclusion of surgery. The patient's trachea usually remains intubated until the airway edema resolves, as evidenced by the ability of the patient to breathe around the endotracheal tube after the cuff has been deflated. Sedation is provided as needed while the trachea is intubated.

C. **Complications after transoral resection of the odontoid and occipitocervical fusion.** This operation is usually performed in two steps: anterior transoral resection of the odontoid and posterior occipitocervical fusion. Airway management involves either tracheotomy or an oral endotracheal tube draped out of the surgical field as for tonsillectomy. The procedure is associated with significant posterior pharyngeal swelling, which requires postoperative intubation for several days. The patient is usually awakened at the conclusion of surgery to undergo a neurologic examination and then sedated again. The degree of resolution of the airway edema is evaluated by deflating the cuff of the endotracheal tube and establishing the ability of the patient to breathe around the endotracheal tube.

D. **Complications after posterior cervical spine procedures.** Complications are related to the patient's intraoperative position and the degree of airway edema and respiratory dysfunction at the conclusion of surgery.

1. The operative positions include prone, sitting, and three-quarters prone. Complications of the prone position include injury at pressure points: eyes, cheeks, lips, breasts, and genitalia. Injury to these structures requires appropriate surgical consultation.

2. Airway edema depends on the duration of surgery, the amount of blood loss, and fluid administration.

3. Respiratory dysfunction may exist preoperatively due to involvement of C3–C5 nerve roots or may result from resection of intramedullary spinal cord tumors. These patients are evaluated before extubation to demonstrate the patency of the airway (lack of airway edema) and adequacy of respiratory function (tidal volume, vital capacity, negative inspiratory force). Postoperative intubation and mechanical ventilation might be required until airway edema resolves and respiratory function recovers.

E. **Complications after scoliosis surgery.** These procedures are performed with the patient in the prone or lateral position or a combination of a lateral-position operation followed immediately or 1 to 2 weeks later by a prone-position operation.

1. Complications related to the prone position are those of pressure point injury, particularly the eyes. Ischemic optic neuropathy (ION) is correlated with intraoperative hypotension and ischemia, regardless of position. Central retinal artery occlusion can occur during prone-position procedures due to improper protection of the eyes. Scoliosis surgery patients are therefore particularly vulnerable to ION, which is manifest

postoperatively by varying degrees of unilateral or bilateral decreases in visual acuity or defects in the visual field. The decrease in visual acuity may resolve over time, but the defects in the visual field usually persist. Postoperative visual examination is performed routinely in these patients; ophthalmologic consultation is requested if any abnormality is detected.

2. Patients with scoliosis may have respiratory dysfunction preoperatively due to skeletal deformities, muscular weakness, central nervous system (CNS) dysfunction, or a combination of factors. This respiratory dysfunction might be aggravated postoperatively by the residual effect of anesthetics, inadequate reversal of muscle relaxants due to hypothermia, restrictive effect of pain, and pneumothorax. Airway edema from positioning, prolonged surgery, and administration of a large volume of fluids contributes to the respiratory compromise. Extubation of the trachea is undertaken only after airway patency and adequacy of respiratory function have been established. Pain control is essential for patient comfort and the maintenance of adequate respiratory function.

3. Postoperative hemorrhage can continue either externally from surgical drains or internally into the operative site. Monitoring of systemic blood pressure, urinary output, central venous pressure (if available), hemoglobin, and hematocrit is necessary. Excessive blood loss is treated with volume expansion, blood transfusion, hemodynamic support, and surgical consultation.

4. Central and peripheral neurologic function is monitored postoperatively. Patients might develop spinal cord injury due to instrumentation or hematoma formation and CNS dysfunction due to pharmacologic or hemodynamic factors. Neurologic dysfunction should prompt a thorough examination of the patient, review of medication, hemodynamic and laboratory workup, surgical consultation, and supportive therapy as needed.

F. **Complications after lateral extracavitary and percutaneous endoscopic procedures.** A factor common to these two operations is the intraoperative use of double-lumen endotracheal tubes or other forms of one-lung ventilation. Pulmonary edema may develop with reexpansion of the lung after one-lung ventilation for >3 hours, most likely within 1 hour of reexpansion. If mechanical ventilation is to be maintained in the postoperative period, the double-lumen tube is exchanged for a single-lumen one. Alternatively, a univent tube, which is a single-lumen tube with a movable endobronchial blocker, may be used intraoperatively and postoperatively during weaning and until extubation.

X. Complications after spinal cord procedures

A. Complications after syringomyelia repair.
Respiratory complications are the main concern. Preoperative respiratory dysfunction is due to skeletal deformities, autonomic dysfunction, and chronic aspiration (from depressed gag reflex and vocal cord paralysis). This respiratory dysfunction may be exacerbated in the postoperative period by airway edema, residual anesthetic effects, and incomplete reversal of muscle relaxants, which could be aggravated by the hypothermia of autonomic dysfunction. Extubation is performed only after the adequacy of respiratory function and airway patency have been established. Respiratory monitoring and support are maintained in the postoperative period as needed.

B. Complications after resection of spinal cord tumors.
Significant cord edema may develop up to 24 hours after resection. The edema-induced respiratory dysfunction associated with the resection of upper cervical cord tumors might not become apparent in the immediate postoperative period. Respiratory monitoring of these patients in an intensive care setting for at least 24 hours postoperatively is therefore necessary.

C. Complications after spinal cord injury.
Patients with spinal cord injury develop complications related to sympathectomy, skeletal muscle denervation, immobilization, chronic instrumentation, decreased respiratory force, and coexisting injuries involving other organs. Approximately 50% of patients with cervical spine injury have concurrent head trauma and approximately 25% have injuries to the chest, abdomen, or extremities.

1. The severity and mechanism of the initial spinal shock, which lasts for 2 to 3 weeks after injury, are related to the level of the injury. With mid-thoracic lesions (T6-7), hypotension may not be severe and is mainly due to vasodilatation. With higher lesions (T4 or above), hypotension may be profound when vasodilatation is added to a decrease in heart rate, contractility, and compliance from loss of cardiac accelerator fibers (T1-4).

2. Succinylcholine may cause hyperkalemia in patients who have denervated muscle because of the increased number and sensitivity of their neuromuscular cholinergic receptors. These receptor changes start 3 days after the injury and persist for 6 to 8 months. Succinylcholine is therefore avoided in spinal cord injury patients from 48 hours to 8 months after the injury.

3. Autonomic hyperreflexia is caused by noxious stimulation below the level of the lesion in a patient with a sympathectomy at or above T6.

   a. The risk of autonomic hyperreflexia is highest during the fourth week after injury but continues thereafter. At this time, while the patient is recovering from the spinal shock phase, which lasts for 2 to 3 weeks after the initial injury, the flaccid paralysis changes to spastic paralysis because of the absence of the effect of central inhibitory pathways. The efferent sympathetic fibers recover from the initial injury but remain unaffected by central inhibitory input from the brain stem and hypothalamus.

   b. The severity and manifestations of autonomic hyperreflexia are affected by the level of the sympathectomy. With mid-thoracic lesions below the level of cardiac accelerator fibers, hypertension is accompanied by reflex bradycardia transmitted via cardiac accelerator fibers and the vagus. In patients whose sympathectomy is above the level of the thoracic cardiac accelerator fibers, tachycardia may occur because cardiac accelerator fibers become part of the efferent sympathetic activity rather than part of the central inhibitory input from the brain stem and hypothalamus. Arrhythmias and occasionally heart block may accompany changes in heart rate. Clinical manifestations of autonomic hyperreflexia include vasodilatation, decreased sympathetic activity, and increased vagal activity above the level of the lesion such as nasal congestion, flushing, headache, dyspnea, nausea, and visceral muscle contraction. Vasoconstriction and increased sympathetic activity below the level of the lesion cause vasoconstrictive pallor, sweating, piloerection, and somatic muscle fasciculation. Patients also develop hypertension with headache, blurred vision, myocardial infarction, and retinal, subarachnoid, and cerebral hemorrhages that may lead to syncope, convulsions, and death.

   c. Autonomic hyperreflexia may be prevented or attenuated by regional or deep general anesthesia, but this is usually impractical in the postanesthesia care unit. Pharmacologic means of preventing and treating autonomic hyperreflexia include alpha-blockers such as diazoxide, 1 to 3 mg/kg i.v. every 5 minutes up to 150 mg, or phentolamine, 5 mg i.v. increments, vasodilators such as

SNP, 0.25 to 8 mcg/kg/minute i.v., and selective beta-blockers such as esmolol, loading dose 500 mcg/kg followed by 50 to 300 mcg/kg/minute i.v., for supraventricular tachycardia.

SUGGESTED READINGS

Dodson BA. Interventional neuroradiology and the anesthetic management of patients with arteriovenous malformations. In: Cottrell JE, Smith DS, eds. *Anesthesia and Neurosurgery*. St. Louis, MO: Mosby, 2001:399–424.

Newfield P, Weir BDA, Hamid RKA. Intracranial aneurysms and A-V malformations. In: Albin MS, ed. *Textbook of Neuroanesthesia with Neurosurgical and Neuroscience Perspectives*, Chapter 26. New York, NY: McGraw-Hill, 1997:845–900.

Petrozza PH, Prough DS. Postoperative and intensive care. In: Cottrell JE, Smith DS, eds. *Anesthesia and Neurosurgery*. St. Louis, MO: Mosby, 2001:623–662.

Respiratory Care of the Neurosurgical Patient

Irene Rozet and Karen B. Domino

This chapter discusses specific considerations of respiratory pathology and care in the neurosurgical intensive care unit (NICU). The development of pulmonary complications contributes significantly to mortality in critically ill neurosurgical patients and worsens neurologic outcome. Prompt recognition and treatment of pulmonary disorders are therefore important in the management of neurosurgical patients.

I. **Respiratory disorders**
   A. **Clinical physiology of oxygen transfer.** Arterial hypoxemia commonly occurs in patients after central nervous system (CNS) injury, adversely affecting neurologic outcome, especially in patients who have sustained head trauma. Arterial hypoxemia (PaO_2 <50 mm Hg) causes cerebral vasodilatation and increases in cerebral blood flow and cerebral blood volume, which could have a detrimental impact on intracranial pressure (ICP). The major causes of arterial hypoxemia are (a) a decrease in alveolar oxygen tension (PAO_2) owing either to hypoventilation or to decreased inspired oxygen tension (PIO_2) or (b) an increase in alveolar-arterial oxygen tension difference ($P[A\text{-}a]O_2$). Inspired gas is mixed with gas in the functional residual capacity (FRC) to make up alveolar gas. Mixed venous blood equilibrates with alveolar gas and is distributed to the systemic circulation as mixed arterial blood.
   B. **Causes of decreased PAO_2.** PAO_2, the major driving factor for arterial oxygenation, may be reduced because of either a decrease in PIO_2 or diminished alveolar ventilation from respiratory depression, increased dead space, or mechanical impairment. PAO_2 is determined by the barometric pressure (PB), the fraction of inspired oxygen (FIO_2), and the ratio of oxygen consumption ($\dot{V}O_2$) to alveolar ventilation ($\dot{V}A$):

$$PAO_2 = PB \times (FIO_2 - \dot{V}O_2/\dot{V}A). \qquad (18.1)$$

As far as $\dot{V}A$ is directly proportional to carbon dioxide production

$(\dot{V}_{CO_2})$, $\dot{V}A = \dot{V}_{CO_2}/PA_{CO_2} \times (k)$, and $PA_{CO_2} \sim Pa_{CO_2,}$

Equation 18.1 can be transformed into the alveolar gas equation 18.2:

$$PAO_2 = FIO_2(PB - 47) - (Pa_{CO_2}/R_Q), \qquad (18.2)$$

where R_Q = respiratory quotient, $R_Q = \dot{V}_{CO_2} / \dot{V}_{O_2}$ (0.8 in resting state), and 47 = saturated water vapor pressure at the PB in mm Hg.

1. **Respiratory depression (hypoventilation).** Respiratory depression can be either central (from CNS disease, narcotics, or sedatives) or peripheral (from neuromuscular disease, muscle relaxants).

    a. **Traumatic brain injury (TBI).** Variations in both the depth and rate of spontaneous respirations occur in 60% of patients who have CNS injury. Five respiratory patterns are observed in patients who have head injuries and brain tumors (Fig. 18-1). Pathologic

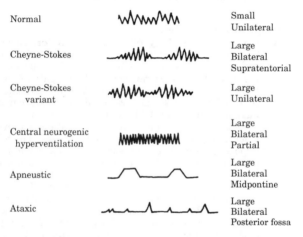

Normal	Small Unilateral
Cheyne-Stokes	Large Bilateral Supratentorial
Cheyne-Stokes variant	Large Unilateral
Central neurogenic hyperventilation	Large Bilateral Partial
Apneustic	Large Bilateral Midpontine
Ataxic	Large Bilateral Posterior fossa

Figure 18-1. Respiratory patterns associated with closed head injury.
Normal breathing in an awake patient with a small, unilateral lesion. *Cheyne-Stokes* ventilation is a periodic breathing pattern in which hyperpnea alternates with apnea. The hyperpneic phase lasts longer than the apneic phase. The *Cheyne-Stokes variant* has a shorter apneic phase and is associated with large unilateral injuries. *Central neurogenic hyperventilation* is a sustained, regular, rapid, fairly deep hyperpnea. It occurs with a large pontine lesion, systemic hypoxia, or metabolic acidosis. It is often associated with brain stem tumors, including lymphomas and astrocytomas, and metastatic disease. *Apneustic breathing* occurs with large bilateral midpontine lesions. There is a brief 2- to 3-second pause at the end of inspiration, alternating irregularly with expiratory pauses. It has a very poor prognosis. *Ataxic respiration* is a pattern of irregular breathing in which shallow and deep breaths alternate randomly with irregular pauses. It is associated with medullary compression and has a very poor prognosis. The irregularity distinguishes it from Cheyne-Stokes ventilation. (Reprinted with permission from Plum F, Posner JB. *The Diagnosis of Stupor and Coma*, 2nd ed. Philadelphia, PA: FA Davis Co., 1972.)

hypoventilation and hyperventilation lead to hypoxemia, pH disturbances, and electrolyte imbalance.

b. **Spinal cord injury (SCI).** High cervical spinal cord lesions impair ventilation because of either partial or complete loss of innervation of the diaphragm (C3-5), with loss of the ability to cough. The diaphragm is spared when injury is below C6-7. However, injury at the thoracic level results in the loss of intercostal and abdominal muscle function, which reduces FRC and creates paradoxical ventilation (chest retraction on inspiration and expansion during expiration), loss of cough, and reduced ability to handle secretions. All lung volumes, except residual volume, are markedly decreased. With a C5-6 lesion, ventilation may be inadequate and forced vital capacity (FVC) decreased to 30% of predicted capacity. Improvement of FVC occurs with time because of the strengthening of the accessory muscles (clavicular portion of the pectoralis major and sternocleidomastoid), development of spasticity (which stops the paradoxical chest wall motion), improvement of diaphragmatic function, and decreased usage of narcotics and sedatives. At 5 months after injury, FVC reaches 60% of predicted values.

c. **Associated airway injuries** in multiple trauma patients including tracheobronchial fistula, tracheobronchial disruption, and rupture of diaphragm cause acute hypoventilation and profound hypoxemia.

2. **Increased airway dead space.** Dead space increases with drug administration (such as atropine and nitroprusside for deliberate hypotension), mechanical ventilation with positive end-expiratory pressure (PEEP), hypovolemia, hypotension, hypocapnia, and cardiopulmonary disease.

3. **Mechanical impairment.** Airway obstruction from oropharyngeal soft tissue, uncleared secretions, hemoptysis, foreign bodies, bleeding, or bronchospasm can cause mechanical impairment of effective alveolar ventilation. The restriction of free chest movement from surgical positioning, surgical retraction of the chest and abdomen, traumatic rupture of the diaphragm, pneumothorax, hemothorax, flail chest and restrictive lung disease can reduce alveolar ventilation significantly. Proper recognition and treatment of traumatic chest injuries are crucial to the successful management of patients after traumatic injury.

C. **Causes of increased P(A-a)o$_2$.** The P(A-a)o$_2$ may be increased as the result of both pulmonary and extrapulmonary factors. Pulmonary disorders can increase

$P(A-a)O_2$ because of a (a) shunt, (b) $\dot{V}A/\dot{Q}$ mismatch, and (c) limitation of diffusion. Most pulmonary disorders increase the $\dot{V}A/\dot{Q}$ mismatch and shunt but seldom affect diffusion capacity. Decreases in cardiac output and either a respiratory or metabolic alkalosis are important extrapulmonary factors that increase $P(A-a)O_2$ in the presence of lung disease.

1. **Extrapulmonary factors.** Two extrapulmonary factors that commonly contribute to hypoxemia in neurosurgical patients who have preexisting lung disease are (a) hyperventilation to reduce ICP and (b) excessive depletion of intravascular volume from fluid restriction and the administration of diuretics.

   a. **Respiratory alkalosis.** Hyperventilation to induce hypocapnia results in a decrease in venous return and cardiac output. Hypocapnia increases pulmonary shunt, especially in the presence of lung disease. The mechanism is unclear but might be related to hypocapnic bronchoconstriction and inhibition of hypoxic pulmonary vasoconstriction. In addition, the oxyhemoglobin dissociation curve shifts to the left, resulting in a lower PaO_2 for any given oxygen saturation (Fig. 18-2). This is

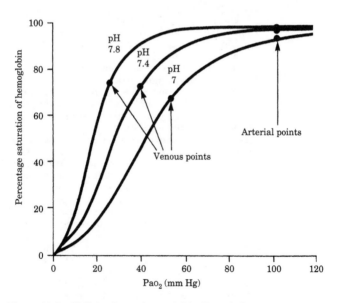

Figure 18-2. Shift in the oxyhemoglobin dissociation curve with change in blood pH.

especially noticeable when the Pao_2 is equal
to or <70 mm Hg.

b. **Hypovolemia and decrease in $P\bar{v}o_2$.** Pao_2
is lower when the mixed venous oxygen ten-
sion ($P\bar{v}o_2$) is decreased, as can occur with
decreased cardiac output, increased oxygen
consumption, or severe anemia with increased
oxygen extraction. The effect of $P\bar{v}O_2$ can be
quite significant, especially when there are areas of low $\dot{V}A/\dot{Q}$ and shunt (Fig. 18-3). For instance, in the presence of $\dot{V}A/\dot{Q}$ mismatch,
$Pao_2 = 80$ mm Hg when $P\bar{v}o_2$ is 50 mm Hg.
If $P\bar{v}o_2$ is decreased to 20 mm Hg from a decrease in cardiac output, then Pao_2 decreases
to 40 mm Hg without any change in the degree
of $\dot{V}A/\dot{Q}$ inequality or shunt. Therefore, low
cardiac output from hypovolemia or myocar-
dial depression increases $P(A-a)o_2$ and might
result in hypoxemia, especially in the presence
of pulmonary disease.

2. **Pulmonary factors that increase $P(A-a)o_2$ in
critically ill neurosurgical patients** consist of

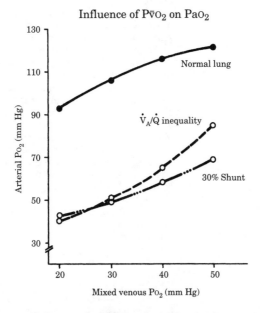

Figure 18-3. Influence of mixed venous oxygen tension on arterial
oxygen tension. (Reprinted with permission from Dantzker DR.
Ventilation-perfusion inequality in lung disease. Chest 1987;
91:749–754.)

neurogenic pulmonary edema (NPE), $\dot{V}_A/\dot{Q}$ mismatch, and abnormalities of lung parenchyma.

a. **Neurogenic etiologies of increased $P(A\text{-}a)O_2$**

   (1) **Reduced FRC.** The FRC is often reduced after TBI and SCI at the cervical and thoracic levels. Head trauma patients might exhibit a reduction in FRC and pulmonary compliance and an increase in pulmonary shunting without evidence of pulmonary disease on the chest radiograph.

   (2) **NPE.** Classic NPE develops in severe CNS injury, such as TBI, SCI, and subarachnoid hemorrhage (SAH). Of immediate onset, NPE becomes clinically recognizable 2 to 12 hours after injury. NPE is generally of short duration and resolves within hours to days. The pathogenesis of NPE is complex and related to circulatory hyperactivity owing to catecholamine release, particularly norepinephrine, which causes an increase in the permeability of the alveolar capillary barrier.

   (3) **Neurogenic alterations in $\dot{V}_A/\dot{Q}$ matching.** Hypoxemia and increased pulmonary shunting have been observed in animals and patients who have CNS disorders in the absence of pulmonary disease. The etiology of these changes in $\dot{V}_A/\dot{Q}$ regulatory mechanisms is multifactorial. Release of inflammatory and anti-inflammatory mediators in patients after TBI may cause acute lung injury (ALI). Brain thromboplastin is released into the blood with TBI, causing deposition of fibrin microemboli and platelet aggregates in the pulmonary capillaries. Neutrophil accumulation and the release of vasoactive substances might also cause local $\dot{V}_A/\dot{Q}$ abnormalities. Patients who have an increase in fibrin spit products are also more likely to develop respiratory failure.

b. **Pulmonary etiologies of increased $P(A\text{-}a)O_2$**

   (1) **Gastric aspiration.** Aspiration of gastric contents occurs frequently in comatose neurosurgical patients and in trauma patients because of intoxication from alcohol and street drugs and abdominal injury. Aspiration of large

volumes of fluid with a low pH or particulate matter results in aspiration pneumonitis and ALI. The aspiration of large foreign bodies, such as gravel, gum, or teeth, might also cause bronchial obstruction, atelectasis, and hypoxemia, and potentially may lead to necrotizing pneumonia. Treatment of aspiration is primarily supportive. Antibiotics are not indicated.

(2) **Atelectasis** and lung consolidation are common in the neurosurgical patient. Central respiratory depression, cervical and thoracic spine injury, hypoventilation from pain, altered levels of consciousness, bronchial obstruction from mucous plugs or aspiration of particulate matter, and compression of adjacent lung by traumatic pneumothorax, hemothorax, or pleural effusion all contribute to the formation of atelectasis. Prevention and treatment of lung collapse through hyperventilation, recruitment maneuvers (PEEP, inverse-ratio ventilation where inspiration is longer than expiration, "sigh" breaths), and aggressive physiotherapy can prevent the development of lung infection. Because SCI patients are not able to clear secretions adequately, therapeutic bronchoscopy, bed rotation, and turning the patient into the prone position can help clear secretions.

(3) **Nosocomial pneumonia (NP)/ ventilator-associated pneumonia (VAP).** VAP is an NP that develops in patients 48 hours or more after endotracheal intubation. NP is the second most common (after urinary tract infection) and the most serious infection in hospitalized patients. VAP occurs in 5% to 30% of intensive care unit (ICU) patients and is responsible for 30% to 40% of all ICU-acquired infections. NP/VAP develops in about half of critically ill neurosurgical patients who have isolated TBI and SCI and in nearly two-thirds of patients after cervical SCI. Pulmonary complications, particularly pneumonia, represent an independent risk factor for death in SCI.

(a) **Risk factors for NP/VAP** are presented in Table 18-1.

(b) **Early onset NP/VAP and late-onset VAP** are distinguished by their respective times of onset and

Table 18-1. Diagnostic criteria for nosocomial pneumonia/ventilator-associated pneumonia

Clinical Criteria	Bacteriological Criteria

I. *"Classic" clinical criteria* (sensitivity and specificity 50%–60%)
A. Change in chest x-ray: new and persistent pulmonary infiltrates, or new pleural effusion, *and*
B. Two or more findings from the following:
  1. Fever >38°C or hypothermia <36°C
  2. White blood cell count (mm³) ≥12,000 or ≤5,000
  3. Purulent tracheobronchial secretions
  4. Impaired oxygenation
II. *Clinical Pulmonary Infection Score* ≥6 (includes scoring system with points for temperature, white blood cell count, tracheal secretions, oxygenation, pulmonary radiography, tracheal aspirate)
	I. *Noninvasive techniques*
	A. Endotracheal tube aspirates
	  1. *Qualitative cultures* (sensitivity 90%, specificity <50%)
	  2. *Quantitative culture* ≥10^5–10^6 cfu/mL
	B. Mini-BAL with aspirates from lower respiratory tract with blind protected telescopic catheters (*quantitative cultures*)
	
	I. *Invasive bronchoscopic techniques with quantitative cultures* (sensitivity and specificity 70%–90%)
	A. BAL: ≥10^4 cfu/mL
	B. Protected specimen brushing: ≥10^3 cfu/mL
	C. Gram stain: ≥5% infected leukocytes (containing intracellular microorganisms) is optional

BAL, bronchoalveolar lavage; cfu/mL, colony-forming units per milliliter.

pathogens. In the general ICU population, early onset NP/VAP develops within the first 5 days of hospitalization while late-onset VAP develops after 5 days. Early onset NP/VAP is characterized by community-acquired microorganisms including gram-positive cocci (*Staphylococcus aureus, Haemophilus influenzae, Streptococcus pneumoniae*), Enterobacteriaceae, and anaerobes. In late-onset VAP, the causative pathogens are hospital-acquired (nosocomial), highly virulent, antibiotic-resistant microorganisms (e.g., *Pseudomonas aeruginosa, Acinetobacter baumannii, Klebsiella, methicillin-resistant Staphylococcus aureus* [*MRSA*], *vancomycin-resistant Enterococcus*). The extreme virulence and the antibiotic resistance of the flora are responsible for the high mortality rate of 40% to 60%, which can go as high as 80% in late-onset VAPs. Community-acquired organisms predominate as the causative agents of pneumonia in critically ill TBI patients in the first 10 days after admission. With comatose patients, VAP develops most frequently between hospital days 4 and 7.

(c) **Pathogenesis** of late-onset NP/VAP in terms of sources of infection includes major aspirations, nasal colonization by *S. aureus*, and microaspiration of colonized oral, upper airway, and gastric secretions, all of which can lead to the development of microabscesses in the lung. Hypoventilation with resultant insufficient alveolar aeration and consequent alveolar collapse and consolidation hastens the onset of infection.

(d) **Diagnosis** (Table 18-2). Unfortunately, there is no "gold standard" for diagnosis of VAP. Along with clinical criteria, early bacteriological detection of causative microorganisms is important for appropriate antibiotic treatment. If not supported by bacteriological

Table 18-2.   Risk factors for nosocomial pneumonia/ventilator-associated pneumonia

Patient Related	Intervention Related
Aspiration	Endotracheal intubation
Bacterial colonization of nasopharynx	Mechanical ventilation for >48 hours
Coma, decreased level of consciousness	
Atelectasis	Barbiturate use
Older age	Traumatic brain injury
>30 in early onset pneumonia	Histamine type 2 blocking drugs, antacids
>60 in late onset pneumonia	Muscle relaxants
Serum albumin <2.2	Excess sedation
Adult respiratory distress syndrome	Supine position
Chronic obstructive pulmonary disease	Frequent ventilator circuit changes
Multiorgan dysfunction syndrome	Reintubation/unplanned extubation
High gastric pH	Intracranial pressure monitoring
Sinusitis	Nasogastric tube/enteral nutrition
Uremia	Parenteral nutrition
	Patient transport
	Length of stay in intensive care unit[a]

[a]Controversial in long-term intensive care unit survivors.

results, empiric antibiotic treatment is often inadequate. The use of invasive bronchoscopic techniques (bronchoalveolar lavage and protective specimen brushing) with quantitative cultures of the specimen allows precise adjustment of antibiotic therapy. However, finalizing quantitative cultures takes 2 to 3 days, which inevitably leads to delay in instituting appropriate treatment.

(e)   Choice of antibiotic **treatment** depends on onset of NP/VAP, risk factors, and the severity of the illness. In general, in early onset NP/VAP, monotherapy with amoxyclavulanate, a second-generation or non-pseudomonal third-generation cephalosporin, or carbapenem for

5 to 7 days is effective in early onset NP/VAP. Late VAP requires broad coverage of resistant pathogens, and empiric combination therapy with two or three antibiotics should be initiated with an antipseudomonal cephalosporin or carbapenem with amikacin or quinolone. For MRSA coverage, linezolid or vancomycin should be added, although linezolid is more effective than vancomycin. After quantitative cultures have been finalized, empiric antibiotic coverage should be adjusted to the particular pathogen and continued for at least 7 to 21 days, depending on the microorganism and the severity of illness.

(f) **Preventive strategies** for VAP are directed at preventing aerodigestive tract colonization, aspiration, and lung consolidation. Routine hand washing with either water and soap or alcohol gel is the most effective strategy for reducing colonization of nosocomial infections. Other modalities include restriction of antibiotic usage, attention to oral hygiene, isolation of patients who have antibiotic-resistant pathogens, and selective digestive decontamination. Semirecumbent positioning, subglottic drainage, prevention of unexpected extubation, and avoidance of nasal intubation, gastric overdistention, and oversedation can reduce the chance of aspiration.

(4) **Acute lung injury (ALI)/Adult respiratory distress syndrome (ARDS)**

(a) **Definition.** ALI/ARDS is a clinical syndrome of diffuse lung injury that results in noncardiogenic, high-permeability pulmonary edema. ALI/ARDS consists of the following: (a) acute onset, (b) bilateral pulmonary infiltrates on the chest radiograph, (c) noncardiogenic origin of edema: pulmonary capillary occlusion pressure of <18 mm Hg, (d) hypoxemia, as defined by a ratio of the partial pressure of arterial oxygen to the fraction of inspired oxygen (Pa_{O_2}/F_{IO_2}) that is ≤ 300 in ALI, and ≤ 200 in ARDS. The incidence of ALI/ARDS in North America and Europe varies from 1.5 to 75 cases/100,000 population. ALI/ARDS is a severe disease with a significant mortality rate of 22% to 32% for ALI and approximately 40% to 70% for ARDS. One-third of ALI cases progress to ARDS in the first week, particularly in trauma patients. One-third of patients who have isolated TBI develop ALI/ARDS; this significantly increases mortality and worsens neurologic outcome. The major cause of death in patients with ALI/ARDS is sepsis and multiorgan failure. Only approximately 10% to 20% of patients dying from ARDS die from hypoxemia per se.

   (b)   Risk factors (Table 18-3). Primary ARDS is caused by direct lung injury and primarily pneumonia and has a higher mortality rate than that of secondary ARDS, which is caused by indirect lung injury.

   (c)   Pathogenesis   and   clinical course. ALI/ARDS usually develops within the first 72 hours of the initiating event with 60% to 70% of cases occurring within the first 24 hours. The initial step in the pathogenesis of ALI/ARDS is endothelial cell activation in the pulmonary microvasculature by various insulting agents such as microbial products, different cytokines, and histamine, which leads to microcirculatory distress, microcoagulation, neutrophil activation and imbalance

Table 18-3.   Risk factors for adult respiratory distress syndrome

Primary ARDS: Direct Lung Injury	Secondary ARDS: Indirect Lung Injury
Pneumonia	Sepsis
Aspiration	Trauma with shock
Pulmonary contusion	Blood transfusions
Fat emboli	Subarachnoid hemorrhage
Near drowning	Traumatic brain injury
	Acute pancreatitis

ARDS, adult respiratory distress syndrome.

between proinflammatory and anti-inflammatory mediators, impairment of the alveolar-capillary barrier, and influx of protein-rich fluid into the alveoli. The alveolar epithelium is damaged, resulting in the disruption of the epithelial ion and fluid transport system, impairment of surfactant production, and loss of the epithelial barrier. Disorganized epithelial repair leads to fibrosis. The degree of epithelial injury correlates with the severity of illness and outcome. Significant abnormalities of pulmonary vascular permeability usually persist for 1 week after the onset of ARDS. The acute phase may either resolve in the first week or progress to fibrosis with persistent hypoxemia. Patients who do not improve in the first week have a poor prognosis. In late phases, pulmonary hypertension can develop from elevated pulmonary vascular resistance, primarily from arteriocapillary obstruction, rather than pulmonary vasoconstriction. Pulmonary compliance decreases. The chest computed tomographic (CT) scan often shows diffuse interstitial thickening and honeycombing. In survivors of ARDS, muscle wasting and weakness are the most prominent extrapulmonary conditions that persist for a year after recovery.

3. **Ventilator-induced lung injury (VILI)/ ventilator-associated lung injury** is an inflammatory syndrome of diffuse alveolar damage that worsens the outcome in patients who have ALI/ ARDS. Several mechanisms are suggested for the pathophysiology of VILI: oxygen toxicity, alveolar overdistension from either high tidal volumes (volutrauma) or high airway pressures (barotrauma), and repeated alveolar opening and collapse during the ventilatory cycle. Because ALI/ARDS is a heterogenous lung disease, positive-pressure ventilation causes uneven distribution of volume and alveolar pressure to the extent that even moderate tidal volumes can overstretch healthy alveoli, leading to inflammatory responses and exacerbation of inflammatory processes. PEEP diminishes VILI by recruiting alveoli and preventing alveolar collapse.

4. **Treatment.** Lung protective strategies for mechanical ventilation have contributed to the decline in mortality along with the prevention and treatment of nosocomial infection such as pneumonia and sepsis, prophylaxis against upper gastrointestinal bleeding, and prevention of thromboembolism.

   a. **Lung-protective ventilation** is the cornerstone of ALI/ARDS management. Positive-pressure ventilation with a tidal volume of 6 mL/kg of ideal body weight and plateau pressure <30 cm H_2O significantly decreased mortality compared to conventional ventilation. PEEP should be adjusted to allow for an F_{IO_2} of <0.6 to prevent oxygen toxicity. The oxygenation goal is either a Pa_{O_2} of >60 mm Hg or an oxygen saturation of 90% or better.

   b. **Permissive hypercarbia.** Lung-protective ventilation can inevitably lead to hypoventilation. Hypercarbia with a Pa_{CO_2} of 60 mm Hg to 100 mm Hg and a pH of 7.25 can be safely tolerated. However, because CO_2 is a potent cerebral vasodilator, permissive hypercarbia is contraindicated in neurosurgical patients who have intracranial hypertension.

   c. **Prone position.** Turning the patient from the supine to the prone position improves oxygenation through favorable redistribution of ventilation-perfusion matching by recruitment of collapsed alveoli. In patients who have SAH and normal ICP, the prone position enhances brain tissue oxygenation but can increase ICP slightly. Risks of the prone position include accidental extubation, loss of intravenous access, hemodynamic instability, coughing, and late complications such as edema and pressure sores.

   d. **Nitric oxide (NO).** Although not proven to affect survival, inhaled NO improves oxygenation and can be used in life-threatening hypoxemia unresponsive to other maneuvers. NO can be used safely in patients who have increased ICP and in situations where it is not possible to turn the patient to the prone position.

   e. **Diuresis and fluid restriction.** Regardless of origin, diuresis and fluid restriction are beneficial in ALI/ARDS but may be impossible to achieve in patients who have vasospasm after SAH and require hypertensive hypervolemic hemodilution (triple-H) therapy.

   f. **Glucocorticosteroids.** Moderate doses of glucocorticosteroids in the late phase of hypoxemic ARDS may suppress fibroproliferation in the lung and could be beneficial in patients who do not have signs of infection.

5. **Cardiogenic pulmonary edema.** Pulmonary edema of cardiogenic etiology can occur in the neurosurgical patient. Left ventricular dysfunction may be from myocardial ischemia or infarction, adverse drug reactions, tachyarrhythmias, severe hypertension, or fluid overload. Older patients are at greater risk; however, myocardial ischemia from severe anemia, hypotension, fluid overload, excessive mannitol administration, and triple-H therapy can precipitate pulmonary edema in the younger patient. Treatment involves diuresis, fluid restriction, and supportive care.

6. **Pulmonary embolism.** Pulmonary emboli are common in critically ill neurosurgical patients. In SCI, the incidence of deep vein thrombosis reaches 100% without prophylaxis and 10% to 25% with prophylaxis. Pulmonary emboli occur in >10% of SCI patients and usually originate from venous thrombosis in lower extremities and, less commonly, from either the pelvic or prostatic venous plexi or the right ventricle. Pulmonary embolism causes acute pulmonary hypertension, right ventricular failure, and a reduction in cardiac output. The diagnosis of smaller pulmonary emboli should be considered in patients who have unexplained tachypnea and chest pain. The Pao_2 is usually normal, and the $Paco_2$ is decreased in the tachypneic patient who has small pulmonary emboli. Massive pulmonary embolism causes acute cardiorespiratory failure. In the past decade, the multidetector row spiral CT scan has become the first-line diagnostic tool for the diagnosis of pulmonary embolism. If the multidetector row spiral CT scan is not available, CT scan and pulmonary angiography are indicated. Definitive treatment is predominantly supportive and involves anticoagulation. If anticoagulation is contraindicated, an inferior vena cava filter should be placed.

II. **Respiratory care**
   A. **Administration of oxygen and airway management.** All TBI patients should be considered hypoxic until proven otherwise, and supplemental oxygen (O_2) should be administered. A Pao_2 of >60 mm Hg is necessary to maintain adequate cerebral oxygenation in patients after TBI and SCI.
   1. **Endotracheal intubation** is indicated in the neurosurgical patient for the following conditions:
      Inability to protect the airway or clear secretions
      Need to reduce ICP by control of ventilation
      Pao_2 <60 mm Hg in spite of supplemental O_2 by mask
      $Paco_2$ >50 mm Hg
      pH <7.2

Respiratory rate >40/minute or <10/minute
Tidal volume <3.5 mL/kg
Vital capacity <10 to 15 mL/kg
Muscle fatigue
Airway compromise
Hemodynamic instability

a. **Orotracheal intubation.** Orotracheal intubation is preferable for urgent intubation in the presence of increased ICP, hypoxemia, and/or hemodynamic instability. In the hemodynamically stable patient, either thiopental, 3 to 5 mg/kg, or propofol, 2.5 mg/kg, and succinylcholine, 1.5 mg/kg, can be used to prevent coughing and an increase in ICP. Alternatively, rocuronium, 1 to 1.5 mg/kg, can be used for muscle paralysis. Etomidate, 0.1 to 0.3 mg/kg and lidocaine, 1 to 1.5 mg/kg, can be used in the less stable patient. With patients who have a full stomach, a modified rapid sequence induction with cricoid pressure and ventilation by mask might be used to avoid marked increases in ICP from hypoxemia and hypercarbia. The head and neck should be stabilized by an assistant (manual in-line stabilization) to prevent head movement in the presence of potential cervical spine injury. Manual in-line stabilization may make a difficult intubation more difficult and result in more movement of unstable structures lower in the neck.

b. **Nasotracheal intubation.** Nasotracheal intubation is of minimal use in NICU patients because of the possibility of resultant obstruction of sinus drainage, which increases the risk of sinusitis, pneumonia, and subsequent sepsis and ALI/ARDS. Nasotracheal intubation is absolutely contraindicated in the presence of a basilar skull fracture. Awake nasotracheal intubation might increase ICP in the head-injured patient.

2. **Tracheotomy** is absolutely indicated in the presence of high SCI (higher than C5). Emergency tracheotomy or cricothyrotomy could be required in patients who have TBI and multiple facial fractures rendering bag-and-mask ventilation difficult. Compared with endotracheal intubation, tracheotomy decreases anatomical dead space and the work of breathing slightly, improves access for suctioning, provides more comfort to the patient, and reduces sedation requirements, all of which may be beneficial to patients who have difficulties in weaning from the ventilator. Early tracheotomy is considered in the first week of admission. Although there is no consensus as to the beneficial effects of early surgical tracheotomy, performing

a bedside percutaneous dilatational tracheotomy (PDT) on the second or third day after injury significantly reduces the incidence of pneumonia, the ICU length of stay, and the mortality in patients who were expected to need mechanical ventilation for >14 days. Therefore, early bedside PDT should be considered in patients who have significant neurologic injury, absent gag reflex, or inability to protect their airway and clear secretions and for patients who are in a persistent vegetative state. Because of the advantages of bedside PDT, including negation of the need to involve the operating room and to transport a critically ill patient, this technique has gained popularity in recent decades. The procedure requires the participation of two physicians (surgeon, otolaryngologist, intensivist) and consists of cricothyroidotomy and tracheal dilatation using the Seldinger technique with bronchoscopic guidance through the endotracheal tube by an experienced bronchoscopist. Although complications are rare with an experienced team, the major complication is bleeding (1% to 2%).

3. **Invasive mechanical ventilation** is used to improve gas exchange after nasal or oral endotracheal intubation. Vital signs should be monitored and arterial blood gases measured 30 minutes after changing ventilator settings.

   a. Controlled mechanical ventilation is used in the operating room and occasionally in the NICU in selected patients who have no ventilatory efforts owing to neuromuscular blockade, high cervical SCI, absent ventilatory drive, drug overdose, or brain death.

   b. For patients in whom spontaneous ventilation is preserved, the preferred assisted modes of ventilation are those in which the ventilator delivers a breath triggered by the patient's inspiratory effort (Fig. 18-4). Along with classic volume-controlled and pressure-controlled modes of mechanical ventilation (assist-controlled, synchronized and nonsynchronized intermittent mandatory ventilation, and pressure support ventilation), modern ventilators provide a variety of new ventilation modes. These modes include "dual-controlled" mechanical ventilation with preset tidal volume and inspiratory pressure ("volume-assured pressure support" or "pressure augmentation" mode), airway-pressure release ventilation (the mode of pressure-controlled inverse-ratio ventilation, allowing spontaneous breathing), and proportional assist ventilation.

   c. PEEP is used to increase arterial oxygenation by alveolar recruitment and increasing

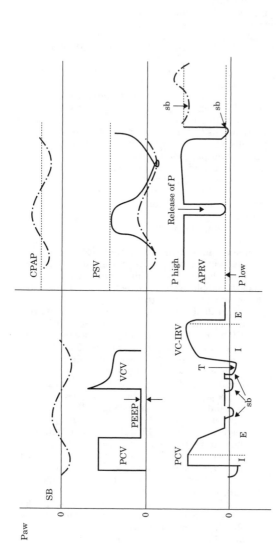

Figure 18-4. Modes of mechanical ventilation. Paw, airway pressure; SB, spontaneous breathing; PCV, pressure-controlled ventilation; PEEP, positive end-expiratory pressure; VCV, volume-controlled ventilation; VC-IRV, volume controlled-inverse ratio ventilation; I, inspirium; E, expirium; sb, spontaneous breath; T, trigger; CPAP, continuous positive airway pressure; PSV, pressure support ventilation; APRV, airway pressure release ventilation.

FRC, which decreases intrapulmonary shunting and $\dot{V}_A/\dot{Q}$ abnormalities. The application of PEEP decreases the need to give high, potentially toxic, concentrations of oxygen. On the other hand, PEEP increases Pa_{CO_2} by increasing dead space ventilation. Hemodynamically, PEEP decreases venous return, cardiac output, and systemic arterial blood pressure. These effects can be partially attenuated by hydration. The varied clinical responses of TBI patients to PEEP might be secondary to PEEP's effect on other hemodynamic and respiratory variables. The use of 10 cm H_2O of PEEP improves oxygenation but can decrease cerebral perfusion from the decrease in cardiac output. PEEP usually causes clinically inconsequential increases in ICP in patients who have severe TBI. The influence of PEEP on ICP is less prominent in patients who have stiff lungs (as with ALI/ARDS) and are presumably the ones who need PEEP the most. A PEEP of up to 30 cm H_2O has been used to treat hypoxemia with minimal adverse effect on ICP. However, because significant potentially serious increases in ICP and clinical deterioration have been observed in some TBI patients after the application of PEEP, ICP should be monitored when PEEP is used. Increases in ICP from PEEP can be reduced by elevating the head 30° and concurrently administering mannitol. The abrupt removal of PEEP might also increase ICP.

4. **Noninvasive mechanical ventilation** is contraindicated for neurosurgical patients in acute respiratory failure who do not have an endotracheal tube. This modality is useful only for patients who, in the absence of neurologic deficits, have, for example, an exacerbation of chronic obstructive pulmonary disease.

B. **Monitoring patients receiving mechanical ventilation.** The efficacy and safety of mechanical ventilation in patients is evaluated by monitoring gas exchange, airway pressure, breathing pattern, lung compliance, hemodynamic function, chest radiographs, and chest CT scans, the "gold standard" for diagnosis of lung pathology.

C. **Weaning.** Clinically stable patients should be frequently reevaluated for readiness for a trial of weaning. However, standard weaning criteria, including normal neurologic status, are not applicable to head-injured patients, in whom impaired neurologic status can delay weaning and extubation.

1. **Clinical parameters to be met before attempting weaning**
   a. Cause for instituting mechanical ventilation is sufficiently resolved.
   b. Adequate oxygenation: $PaO_2/FIO_2 \geq 150$ to 200 or hemoglobin saturation (SaO_2) of >90% on $FIO_2 \leq 0.4$ to 0.5 with PEEP ≤ 8 cm H_2O, pH ≥ 7.25.
   c. Hemodynamic stability (low-dose inotropes/vasopressors are allowed).
2. **Weaning techniques. Spontaneous breathing trial** for 30 to 120 minutes should be attempted in patients considered candidates for weaning from mechanical ventilation. The trial can be performed with a T-piece, using a low level of continuous positive pressure (5 cm H_2O) or pressure support (5 to 7 cm H_2O).

SUGGESTED READINGS

Chastre J, Fagon J-Y. Ventilator-associated pneumonia: state of the art. *Am J Respir Crit Care Med* 2002;165:867–903.

Domino KB. Pulmonary function and dysfunction in the traumatized patient. *Anesthesiol Clin North Am* 1996;14:59.

Malik AB. Mechanisms of neurogenic pulmonary edema. *Circ Res* 1985;57:1.

Pierson DJ. Tracheostomy and weaning. Weaning from mechanical ventilation. *Respir Care* 2005;50(4):526–533.

Cardiovascular Therapy

Steven J. Allen and C. Lee Parmley

I. **Basic considerations.** The crucial goal of cardiovascular therapy in perioperative neurosurgical patients is to provide sufficient metabolic substrate to the threatened central nervous system (CNS). Because glucose is usually not a problem related to cardiovascular therapy, our attention is directed to oxygen delivery. Cardiovascular therapy can affect CNS swelling and result in irreversible injury. Therefore, while maintaining oxygen delivery is important, care must be exercised not to compromise intracerebral hemodynamics.

   A. **Autoregulation** refers to the interdependence of cerebral blood flow (CBF) and mean arterial (blood) pressure (MAP). The range of MAP over which non-hypertensive patients exhibit autoregulation is 50 to 150 mm Hg. Chronically hypertensive patients have altered autoregulation and neither maintain CBF at an MAP in the low end of the normal range nor vasoconstrict when the MAP exceeds 150 mm Hg. A similar alteration of autoregulation occurs with sympathetic activation induced by shock or surgery.

   1. When autoregulation is impaired, CBF will become more dependent on the blood pressure; minor swings in MAP might have significant impact on intracerebral hemodynamics.

   2. Many conditions such as head injury and tumors are associated with either generalized or regional disruption of autoregulation.

   B. **Intracranial pressure (ICP).** The intracranial compartment is essentially a closed space, so ICP is determined by the intracranial volume, which is comprised of cerebrospinal fluid, cerebral parenchyma, and cerebral blood volume (CBV). Increases in any of these components can contribute to intracranial hypertension and result in decreased cerebral perfusion pressure (CPP).

   C. **CPP is the difference between MAP and ICP.** In most organs, venous pressure generates the back pressure that determines the pressure drop across an organ. Because venous pressure tends to be negative in the brain, parenchymal pressure (ICP) generates the back pressure for determining CPP. CPP determines CBF both globally and regionally in the CNS. Normal CBF is 50 mL/100 g brain/minute and decreases only if CPP falls from a normal value of approximately 80 mm Hg to below 50 mm Hg unless autoregulation is altered.

II. **Cerebral oxygen delivery** is a function of CBF and the quantity of oxygen carried in arterial blood (Cao_2). CBF is related to CPP, and, because blood pressure is a function of cardiac output (CO) and systemic vascular resistance

(SVR), CO becomes an important parameter to manipulate to preserve CBF and cerebral oxygen delivery. The normal awake brain consumes 3.3 mL O_2/100 g/minute, a value reduced by approximately one-third when anesthesia is being administered.

A. CO

    1. Determinants of CO. The CO is a result of four basic factors: preload, contractility, heart rate (HR), and afterload.

        a. Preload is impractical to monitor but can be best determined by measuring ventricular end-diastolic volume (EDV) by either angiography or echocardiography. Pulmonary artery occlusion pressure (PAOP) is more frequently used as a reliable estimate of left atrial preload; central venous pressure is a measure of right atrial preload. In addition to PAOP, volumetric pulmonary artery catheter (PAC) monitoring provides right ventricular EDV for preload assessment. Stroke volume variation is used to assess preload when pulse contour cardiac monitoring technology is employed.

        b. Contractility. The ejection fraction measured by either angiography or echocardiography is frequently used to assess contractility, which can also be assessed by evaluating the magnitude of the CO for a given preload condition. Right ventricular ejection fraction is available when monitoring is performed with a volumetric PAC.

        c. HR. $CO = HR \times$ stroke volume. When preload, contractility, or both limit stroke volume, an increase in HR often acts to maintain CO.

        d. Afterload. Mean aortic pressure is the afterload against which the left ventricle ejects a stroke volume. We use MAP in neuroanesthesia as a close approximation.

B. Cardiac failure occurs when CO is insufficient to deliver adequate oxygen. Typical causes include cardiomyopathies from infarction, ischemia, and chronic hypertension; dysrhythmias; increased afterload from arterial hypertension; and outflow obstruction from pulmonary embolus. Neurosurgical patients who are critically ill have additional considerations.

    1. Hypovolemia resulting in insufficient preload.

        a. Blood loss. Surgical and traumatic causes including scalp lacerations should be considered.

        b. Osmotic diuretic administration can result in intravascular volume contraction.

        c. Fluid restriction instituted to minimize cerebral swelling can lead to hypovolemia and end-organ compromise.

        d. Diabetes insipidus associated with severe traumatic brain injury (TBI) and pituitary surgery can result in hypovolemia.

2. **CNS causes**
   a. Spinal cord injury and injury to the brain stem vasomotor center can result in hypotension from decreased sympathetic tone.
   b. Neurogenic cardiomyopathy has been described in patients after they have suffered subarachnoid hemorrhage (SAH) and acute TBI. The etiology is thought to be the massive release of norepinephrine. The ensuing electrocardiographic changes are consistent with ischemia and myocardial dysfunction.
3. **Drug induced.** Occasionally, aggressive therapy with calcium-entry blocking drugs or beta-blocking drugs can result in suboptimal myocardial performance.

C. **Blood pressure**
   1. MAP = CO × SVR. CO is discussed in the preceding text.
   2. Hypotension in the presence of normal intravascular volume and cardiac function occurs because of decreases in SVR.
      a. Hypotension can be secondary to high cervical cord injury.
      b. Brain stem damage involving the vasomotor center results in hypotension. Such an insult is usually lethal.
      c. Fever and sepsis can be associated with hypotension.

III. **Drugs used in cardiovascular therapy**
A. **Guidelines for administration of vasoactive drugs**
   1. Use a calibrated pump for all infusions.
   2. Inject into the intravenous line as close to vein insertion site as possible.
   3. Avoid using systolic blood pressure as the goal of therapy because this value is prone to fluctuate from a number of causes, not all of which are related to the patient's cardiovascular condition. MAP is a more reliable variable.
   4. Potent vasoactive drugs should be administered in a graded fashion starting with a dose below one that is thought to be therapeutic.

B. **Adrenergic agonists.** See Table 19-1 for action of adrenergic receptors; see Tables 19-2 and 19-3 for relative adrenergic action and dosing recommendations. Sympathomimetic drugs appear to have little influence on the vascular tone of cerebral vessels. However, raising MAP above the upper threshold of autoregulation increases CBF. Some evidence suggests that beta-agonists can increase the cerebral metabolic rate for oxygen consumption and secondarily raise CBF.
   1. **Norepinephrine** (Levophed) has some beta activity but is used primarily as an alpha-adrenergic agonist. Its primary use is to treat refractory hypotension.

Table 19-1.   Action of adrenergic receptors

Receptor	Site	Action
α_1	Postsynaptic Vasculature Heart	Vasoconstriction
α_2	Presynaptic Peripheral and central nervous system, liver, pancreas, kidney, eye	Vasodilatation
β_1	Heart	Contractility, chronotropy
β_2	Heart	Contractility, chronotropy
	Vascular and bronchial smooth muscle	Vasodilatation Smooth muscle relaxation
Dopaminergic	Presynaptic	Smooth muscle relaxation
	Renal and splanchnic circulation, brain stem	Nausea and vomiting

2. **Epinephrine** (Adrenalin) possesses dose-related alpha and beta properties. Its primary uses are in cardiopulmonary resuscitation, anaphylaxis, and refractory hypotension. Toxicity from epinephrine is from arrhythmias and the sequelae of vasoconstriction.

Table 19-2.   Adrenergic agonist and phosphodiesterase inhibitor drugs

Name	Receptors	Dosage
Epinephrine	β_2	1–2 mcg/min
	$\beta_1 + \beta_2$	2–10 mcg/min
	α	>10 mcg/min
Norepinephrine	α, β_1	4–12 mcg/min
Dopamine	Dopaminergic	0–3 mcg/kg/min
	β	3–10 mcg/kg/min
	α	>10 mcg/kg/min
Dobutamine	β_1	2.5–10 mcg/kg/min
Phenylephrine	α, β_1 (slight)	0.1–0.5 mcg/kg/min
Ephedrine	α, β_1	5–10 mg
Isoproterenol	β_1, β_2	0.5–10 mcg/min
Amrinone	Inhibition of phosphodiesterase	0.75 mg/kg load, then 5–10 mcg/kg/min
Milrinone	Inhibition of phosphodiesterase	50–75 mg/kg load, then 0.5–0.75 mcg/kg/min

Table 19-3. **Adrenergic antagonist drugs**

Name	Receptor Blocked	Dosage
Phentolamine	α	5–10 mg
Esmolol	β	0.15–1 mg/kg, then 50–300 mcg/kg/min
Labetalol	$\beta > \alpha$	5–20 mg, then 2 mg/min
Metoprolol	β	2.5–15 mg
Propranolol	β	0.25–5 mg

    3. Dobutamine is a synthetic drug that has predominantly beta-one activity. When compared with other drugs, dobutamine tends to produce less tachycardia and elevation of pulmonary vascular pressure for the same degree of inotropic enhancement. It does not have any dopaminergic agonist action.

    4. Dopamine exhibits alpha, beta, and dopaminergic properties in a dose-related fashion. Its primary uses are to treat hypotension and provide inotropic support. Low doses inhibit renal reabsorption of sodium, resulting in a natriuresis. In high doses, dopamine's alpha properties predominate. Evidence suggests that dopamine can produce mild cerebral vasodilatation.

    5. Phenylephrine is a synthetic drug whose chief characteristic is its relative selectivity for alpha-receptors. When used to increase MAP, a baroreceptor-mediated reflex decrease in HR often occurs. Phenylephrine can be the drug of choice when the cardiac index (CI) is sufficient but MAP is below the goal.

    6. Isoproterenol is a synthetic drug that has remarkable beta selectivity. Administration is associated with tachycardia, decreased MAP, and bronchodilation.

  C. Adrenergic antagonists (Table 19-3)

    1. Esmolol is an ultrashort-acting (9 to 10 minutes' duration) beta-specific competitive antagonist. Its fast onset and short duration of action render it suitable for rapid intervention in the treatment of tachyarrhythmias in the perioperative period.

    2. Metoprolol is a cardioselective beta antagonist whose duration of action is a longer than that of esmolol. Metoprolol is most commonly used to treat angina and acute myocardial infarction but can be used intravenously in the perioperative period to control tachycardia. All beta-blocking drugs are capable of inducing bronchospasm, heart failure, or both.

    3. Labetalol blocks both alpha- and beta-receptors with more beta than alpha effects. However, a reduction in MAP usually occurs when the dose is sufficient to decrease HR. Labetalol also has a longer duration of action than either esmolol or propranolol.

4. **Propranolol** was the original clinically available beta-blocking drug. It is nonselective and has a relatively fast onset, but because the metabolism of the drug in the liver differs widely from patient to patient, dosing is variable. Curiously, propanolol shifts the hemoglobin-oxygen dissociation curve to the right.

5. **Phentolamine** specifically competes for both alpha$_1$ and alpha$_2$ receptors. Because of its duration of action, phentolamine is not frequently used as an antihypertensive in acute perioperative situations.

D. **Phosphodiesterase inhibitors.** (Information is presented in Table 19-2)

1. **Milrinone** is a nonadrenergic, nonglycosidic compound that enhances contractility and promotes pulmonary and arterial vasodilatation. It is thought to act by inhibiting phosphodiesterase, which increases the intracellular concentrations of cyclic AMP. Milrinone has little potential for causing cardiac arrhythmias but has a long half-life (hours) and can induce thrombocytopenia as well as hypotension.

E. **Vasodilators** (Table 19-4)

1. **Nicardipine** is a calcium-entry blocking drug that reliably decreases MAP when given as an intravenous infusion. It has low toxicity and a predictable response.

2. **Sodium nitroprusside** (SNP) is a potent, rapid-onset, short-acting drug that causes more arteriolar than venular vasodilatation via the release of nitric oxide. Administration of SNP is associated with the activation of the renin-angiotensin system; reflex tachycardia can interfere with blood pressure reduction. Occasionally, patients demonstrate relative resistance to SNP. They are at particular risk for developing cyanide toxicity.

3. **Nitroglycerin** (NTG) is a rapid-onset, short-acting drug that induces vasodilatation via nitric oxide. Less potent than SNP but with little toxicity,

Table 19-4. Vasodilators

Name	Dosage
Sodium nitroprusside	0.5–10 mcg/kg/min
Nitroglycerin	5–50 mcg/min
Trimethaphan	1–15 mg/min
Hydralazine	0.1–0.2 mg/kg
Nicardipine	5–15 mg/kg

NTG causes more venular than arteriolar vasodilatation.

4. **Adenosine** is an ultrafast-acting vasodilator that decreases MAP and increases CI owing to a decrease in SVR. Heart block is a potential side effect of its use.

5. **Hydralazine** is a vascular smooth muscle relaxant with no effects on contractility or chronotropy. Its use is frequently accompanied by reflex tachycardia.

F. **Vasoconstrictors**

1. **Vasopressin** (antidiuretic hormone) is a peptide with potent vasoconstricting properties, which can be useful in increasing arterial tone. It is administered as a constant infusion, and not titrated up to avoid severe complications of distal ischemia.

IV. **Goal-directed pharmacologic intervention for cardiovascular dysfunction.** The two goals of cardiovascular therapy in neurosurgical patients—adequate CPP and sufficient CO to maintain oxygen delivery—can require different drug regimens. Optimal fluid therapy should be instituted either prior to or in conjunction with drug therapy.

A. **Increasing MAP** is indicated in a number of clinical settings.

1. **Decreased SVR** from impaired sympathetic tone, sepsis, fever, or anesthetic drugs can be associated with inadequate MAP. CO can be normal or even high while CPP is too low to optimize cerebral perfusion. Norepinephrine, phenylephrine, and vasopressin are vasoconstrictor drugs that are appropriate in this setting.

2. **Increasing CPP** by raising MAP could be needed to protect cerebral perfusion after carotid endarterectomy and cerebral vasospasm. With intracerebral hemorrhage after head injury, it can be desirable to increase MAP to maintain CPP and prevent cerebral hypoperfusion if ICP cannot be controlled.

3. **Anaphylactic reactions.** Hypotension accompanying an allergic reaction is treated with epinephrine.

4. **Cardiopulmonary resuscitation.** Drugs are administered according to advanced cardiac life-support guidelines.

5. **Therapy.** MAP can be increased by administering a drug possessing vasoconstrictive properties that works by direct and/or indirect adrenergic stimulation (Table 19-2) with varying effects on HR. Pulmonary artery pressure and PAOP also tend to rise, even if no change in intravascular volume has occurred.

6. **Precautions**

a. **Myocardial risks.** Increasing MAP (afterload) in a patient who has coronary artery disease could increase myocardial oxygen demand sufficiently to outstrip delivery, causing myocardial ischemia and failure.

  b. **Left ventricular (LV) dysfunction.** Increasing MAP could decrease CO if LV dysfunction exists. Therefore, CO monitoring could be indicated during the induction of hypertension in patients suspected of having LV dysfunction.

  c. **Hypovolemia** is treated by augmentating intravascular volume rather than further masking it by the use of adrenergic drugs that only increase the risk of end-organ ischemia.

  d. **Impaired renal function.** Pharmacologically increasing MAP could cause vasoconstriction of renal vessels and could result in deterioration of renal function if perfusion is marginal.

B. Increasing CO is indicated in a number of clinical settings.

  1. **Low CO owing to cardiomyopathy** can be caused by ischemia, viral disease, chemotherapy, or drug overdose. Goals recommended for inotropic therapy include the following:

     a. MAP of ≥ 80 mm Hg.

     b. Mixed venous saturation (Sv_{O_2}) of $\geq 65\%$.

     c. CI (CO/body surface area) of ≥ 3.5 L/m^2/minute.

     d. Evidence of adequate end-organ perfusion. Monitoring urine output can be unreliable after diuretics have been administered.

  2. **Cerebral vasospasm.** Supernormal CO can reduce the risk of permanent neurologic deficit.

  3. **Therapy.** If CO is insufficient after intravascular volume has been optimized, inotropic drugs should be administered.

     a. **Beta-agonists** are the first-line drugs because their onset and duration allow rapid titration to effect. Empiric therapy is replaced by goal-directed dosing as soon as appropriate monitoring is available.

     b. **Phosphodiesterase inhibitors.** Milrinone can be used as an adjunct to enhance the increase of CO.

     c. **Digoxin** possesses mild to moderate inotropic activity. It can be given orally or intravenously and can increase CO by 10% to 20% in otherwise stable patients who have chronic heart failure.

  4. **Precautions**

     a. In doses that are high enough, all adrenergic drugs cause tachycardia; patients who have coronary artery disease are at risk for ischemia in this setting. HRs above 120 beats per minute (bpm) should be avoided.

   b. When the dose of an adrenergic drug reaches the range in which alpha activity predominates, renal perfusion can be compromised, risking renal failure.

   c. While digoxin is useful in the management of chronic cardiac failure, its onset is not immediate, nor is it easily titratable. Undocumented previous administration of digoxin, hypokalemia from diuretics, and the onset of renal failure increase the risk of digoxin toxicity.

C. Lowering MAP can be indicated in a number of clinical settings.

   1. Hypertension

   a. Unclipped aneurysm. Hypertension in the presence of an unclipped cerebral aneurysm is believed to be a significant risk factor for rebleeding.

   b. Disrupted cerebral microvascular membrane. In the presence of the disruption of the blood-brain barrier, hypertension can exacerbate the formation of vasogenic edema so that blood pressure control should be considered.

   2. Surgical exposure. Surgeons can request iatrogenic hypotension to enhance exposure, reduce risk of aneurysmal rupture, or assist with the control of bleeding.

   3. Therapy

   a. Analgesics. Clearly, the control of pain can be sufficient to return the MAP to a more acceptable level.

   b. Vasodilators. Although many vasodilator drugs are available, the patient's comorbidities and the urgency of the situation often guide the choice. Regardless, a target MAP should be chosen concomitantly with the start of therapy. In the absence of preexisting hypertension, MAP, measured at the level of the external auditory meatus, can be decreased 20% from the baseline without undue risk.

   (1) Rapid control can require the use of vasodilators such as SNP or NTG.

   (2) Drugs that have slower onset but fewer drawbacks, such as the beta-blocking drugs, nicardipine, and hydralazine, can adequately treat less urgent situations.

   4. Precautions

   a. Hypovolemia. Even small doses of vasodilators can cause dramatic hypotension in the presence of hypovolemia.

   b. Decreased intracranial compliance. Vasodilators have the potential for cerebral vascular relaxation with a resultant increase in CBV. If intracranial compliance is decreased, increases in CBV might raise ICP.

D. **Lowering HR** can be indicated in a number of clinical settings.
1. **Reduced myocardial oxygen consumption.** Tachycardia can increase myocardial oxygen demand and induce ischemia in susceptible patients.
2. **Atrial fibrillation** with a rapid ventricular response can compromise the heart's ability to deliver an adequate CO.
3. **Hypertension.** Although slowing the HR is not usually sufficient to decrease MAP by a significant degree, a smaller dose of an antihypertensive drug is subsequently required owing to the abatement of the reflex tachycardia.
4. **Therapy.** Adenosine and beta-blocking drugs, such as esmolol, metoprolol, propranolol, and labetalol, are often used as first-line drugs owing to their rapid onset and relative safety. Calcium-entry blocking drugs such as verapamil and diltiazem are also used to control ventricular rate, particularly supraventricular tachycardias.
5. **Precautions**
    a. The drugs to decrease HR have negative inotropic and vasodilatory properties that can result in both low CO and hypotension. Particular caution is necessary when beta-blocking and calcium-entry blocking drugs are combined.
    b. Some patients who have bronchospastic disease experience exacerbation of their symptoms when they receive beta-blocking drugs.
V. **Management of cardiovascular complications of neurologic disorders**
A. **Cerebral vasospasm**
1. **Pathophysiology.** *Vasospasm* is a potentially devastating complication that occurs after SAH and acute TBI. If extensive, vasospasm can decrease CBF to ischemic levels, causing permanent neurologic deficits or death. Although transcranial Doppler (TCD) is proving to be a useful diagnostic modality, vasospasm is traditionally diagnosed by angiography in which beaded narrowing of the cerebral arteries confirms the diagnosis.
2. **Monitoring.** Angiography is the gold standard for the diagnosis of vasospasm but is impractical for monitoring. TCD has the advantage of being portable, noninvasive, and amenable to regular or even continuous monitoring. TCD detects vasospasm by measuring the velocity of blood flow in a cerebral artery. Because vasospasm narrows a vessel, the velocity of blood traveling through the constriction increases.
3. **Prevention.** A statistical decrease in permanent neurologic deficits in patients at risk has been demonstrated when a cerebral-selective

calcium-entry blocking drug is used. This improve-ment is not associated with an increase in the diameter of the affected vessels.

4. **Triple-H therapy: hypervolemia, hyperten-sion, hemodilution**
    a. **Rationale.** Triple-H therapy seeks to increase blood flow through the narrowed arteries by decreasing the viscosity (hemodilution), in-creasing the driving pressure (hypertension), and expanding the blood volume (hyperv-olemia).
    b. **Invasive monitoring,** usually including pul-monary artery catheterization, is needed be-cause the knowledge of intravascular volume and the CI are of central importance. Moni-toring CO with pulse contour technology can prove sufficient.
        (1) **Fluids.** Hypervolemia is accomplished by infusion of isotonic fluids or colloids.
        (2) **Vasoactive drugs.** The two hemody-namic goals are to increase MAP and CO. Vasoactive drugs are chosen to in-crease SVR or contractility, as desired. A selective approach is achieved through the use of norepinephrine for the former and dobutamine for the latter.
    c. **Precautions.** Pulmonary edema is the pri-mary concern with triple-H therapy, even with its conscientious management. Treat-ment goals must be adjusted after pulmonary edema has been detected.
5. **Cerebral salt wasting** frequently accompanies SAH and other intracranial pathology. Urinary sodium is elevated in the presence of hypona-tremia, an electrolyte presentation seen also with the syndrome of inappropriate antidiuretic hor-mone (SIADH) secretion. With cerebral salt wast-ing, unlike SIADH, depletion of intravascular volume develops, which is undesirable when cere-bral vasospasm is a risk.

B. **Autonomic hypotension (neurogenic shock)**
    1. **Pathophysiology.** Hypotension can occur after spinal cord injury at a cervical or high thoracic level. Interruption of the sympathetic nervous system causes vasodilatation from the loss of sym-pathetic vascular tone and bradycardia because of the involvement of the cardioaccelerator nerves. Young individuals who have a high resting vagal tone, normally balanced by sympathetic activity, could experience bradycardia to the point of asys-tole.
    2. **Treatment.** Care should be taken in managing low blood pressure in patients after they suffer a spinal cord injury because they do not have intact compensatory mechanisms. They tend to

tolerate lower blood pressures without adverse sequelae as compared to neurologically intact patients.

a. Hypotension without bradycardia can be treated with careful administration of fluids if adequacy of end-organ perfusion is a concern. Urine output in the acute phase of spinal cord injury is typically low regardless of the CI or intravascular volume status.

b. If a vasoactive drug is administered, the clinician should remember that denervation hypersensitivity could result in a much larger response than expected.

c. Bradycardia can require atropine for the first 72 hours after spinal cord injury. Bradycardic episodes rarely persist to the point at which a pacemaker is needed.

C. **Carotid endarterectomy: postoperative hypotension**

1. **Pathophysiology.** Patients who have atherosclerosis sufficient to require carotid endarterectomy often have cardiovascular disease as well and are prone to instability of blood pressure, HR, and rhythm in the perioperative period. Bradycardia and dysrhythmias occur because of abnormal carotid sinus baroreceptor responses.

2. **Treatment** includes the administration of fluids to correct preexisting intravascular volume deficits: atropine if carotid sinus stimulation causes bradycardia, and either phenylephrine or dopamine to prevent end-organ compromise if hypotension persists.

D. **Carotid endarterectomy: postoperative hypertension**

1. **Pathophysiology.** Manipulation of the carotid sinus can contribute to postoperative hypertension, which is associated with a higher risk of postoperative bleeding, stroke, and death.

2. **Treatment.** Hypertension can be effectively managed by the intravenous administration of labetalol, nicardipine, hydralazine, or, if severe, SNP.

E. **Acute TBI with hypotension**

1. **Pathophysiology.** Hypotension in the patient who survives transport to the hospital after suffering a TBI is most likely the result of blood loss. TBI sufficient to damage the brain stem vasomotor center is almost always fatal.

2. **Treatment** needs to be prompt because the injured brain is particularly vulnerable to low perfusion pressure, which can already be compromised by elevated ICP.

a. As with any trauma victim suspected of having hypovolemia, intravascular volume needs to be expanded.

      b. Positive inotropic drugs or vasoconstrictors can be used for rapid restoration of the MAP to an acceptable level until intravascular volume is expanded.

F. Acute TBI with hypertension

    1. Pathophysiology

      a. Patients are commonly hypertensive after TBI because they secrete excessive catecholamines. This secretion begins within the first ten days of the traumatic event and can continue for as long as 3 months. Hypertension can be accompanied by tachycardia, tachypnea, restlessness, and diaphoresis limited to the upper body, probably from disinhibition of central sympathetic reflexes.

      b. Cushing reflex. MAP could also be elevated if ICP is approaching systemic values as a protective mechanism to maintain CPP. Original descriptions of the Cushing reflex in animals involved bradycardia, whereas tachycardia occurs more commonly in humans.

    2. Treatment. Hypertension after TBI is typically associated with elevated ICP, and there are two possible etiologies. First, with impaired autoregulation, arterial hypertension increases CBF and therefore ICP. Second, elevated ICP induces arterial hypertension via the Cushing reflex. Treatment must be cautious with concurrent monitoring of the effect on ICP.

      a. Sympathetic overactivity. Hypertension from the post-TBI syndrome is responsive to beta-blocking drugs, but large doses can be necessary to compete with the high levels of endogenous catecholamines. Beta-blocking drugs also have the benefit of improving intracranial compliance and do not cause cerebral vascular relaxation. If beta blockade does not decrease the MAP adequately, then SNP, NTG, or nicardipine can be considered. SNP and NTG can cause cerebral vascular relaxation, increasing CBV and ICP, an effect that can be ameliorated by slowly infusing the drug.

      b. Cushing reflex. If hypertension is thought to occur as a result of the Cushing reflex, attention should be directed to decreasing ICP because decreasing MAP alone can result in a critical reduction in CPP.

G. Postoperative hypertension

    1. Pathophysiology. Patients who have no prior history of hypertension can become hypertensive after a craniotomy. In the absence of intracranial hypertension, postcraniotomy hypertension should be treated to reduce the risk of cerebral swelling and bleeding in the operative site. However, if

ICP is elevated, the treatment of hypertension can decrease CPP to ischemic levels.

2. **Treatment.** Hypertension after craniotomy can be treated with analgesics and either labetalol or nicardipine with predictable results. If intracranial hypertension is suspected, management should follow that outlined in the preceding text for TBI.

SUGGESTED READINGS

Asfar P, Hauser B, Radermacher P, et al. Catecholamines and vasopressin during critical illness. *Crit Care Clin* 2006; 22:131–149.

Brigham and Women's Hospital Neurosurgery Group. Principles of cerebral oxygenation and blood flow in the neurological critical care unit. *Neurocrit Care* 2006;4:77–82.

Hill L, Zanaboni P. Vasodilators. In: Evers AS, Maze M, eds. *Anesthetic Pharmacology: Physiologic Principles and Clinical Practice. A Companion to Anesthesia.* Philadelphia, PA: Churchill Livingstone, 2004:691–702.

Kersten JR, Pagel PS, Warltier DC. Cardiovascular pharmacology of positive inotropic drugs. In: Evers AS, Maze M, eds. *Anesthetic Pharmacology: Physiologic Principles and Clinical Practice. A Companion to Anesthesia.* Philadelphia, PA: Churchill Livingstone, 2004:655–670.

Lee KH, Lukovits T, Friedman JA. "Triple-H" therapy for cerebral vasospasm following subarachnoid hemorrhage. *Neurocrit Care* 2006;4:68–76.

Rédai I, Mets B. Sympathomimetic, sympatholytic, parasympathomimetic, and parasympatholytic drugs. In: Evers AS, Maze M, eds. *Anesthetic Pharmacology: Physiologic Principles and Clinical Practice. A Companion to Anesthesia.* Philadelphia, PA: Churchill Livingstone, 2004:599–620.

Rose JC, Mayer SA. Optimizing blood pressure in neurological emergencies. *Neurocrit Care* 2004;4:287–299.

Fluid Management

Concezione Tommasino

The fluid management in patients who have central nervous system (CNS) pathology presents special challenges for anesthesiologists and intensivists. These patients often receive diuretics (e.g., mannitol, furosemide) to treat cerebral edema and to reduce intracranial hypertension. At the same time, neurosurgical patients may require large volumes of either intravenous fluid or blood as part of an initial resuscitation, treatment of cerebral vasospasm, correction of preoperative dehydration, or maintenance of intraoperative and postoperative hemodynamic stability.

Fluid restriction had been a cornerstone of the treatment of patients with CNS pathology for many years. This practice arose from the concern that the administration of fluid might exacerbate cerebral edema and intracranial hypertension. Not only has the efficacy of fluid restriction remained unproven, even after all this time, but also the consequences of fluid restriction, if pursued to the point of hypovolemia, can be devastating. A recent study of head trauma patients demonstrated that negative fluid balance (<594 mL) was associated with an adverse effect on outcome, independent of its relationship to intracranial pressure (ICP), mean arterial pressure, or cerebral perfusion pressure.

Although few human data exist concerning the impact of exogenous fluids on the injured brain to guide rational fluid management in the neurosurgical patient, it is possible to examine the factors that influence water movement into the brain and make some reasonable recommendations.

I. **Osmolality/osmolarity, colloid oncotic pressure (COP), crystalloid, and colloid.** It is important for the reader to be familiar with a number of definitions and distinctions, particularly as they apply to the brain.

   A. **Osmotic pressure.** This is the hydrostatic force acting to equalize the concentration of **water** (H_2O) on both sides of a membrane that is impermeable to substances dissolved in that water. Water moves along its concentration gradient. This means that if a solution containing 10 mosmol of sodium (Na) and 10 mosmol of chloride (Cl) are placed on one side of a semipermeable membrane with H_2O on the other, water will move "toward" the saline (NaCl) solution. The saline solution has a concentration of 20 mosmol/L, and the force driving water will be approximately 19.3 mm Hg/mosmol, or 386 mm Hg. Note that the driving force is proportional to the *gradient* across the membrane; if two solutions of equal concentration are placed across a membrane, there is no driving force. Similarly, if the membrane is permeable to the solutes (e.g., Na and Cl), this reduces the gradient and hence the osmotic forces.

B. **Osmolarity and osmolality.** *Osmolarity* describes the molar number of osmotically active particles per liter of solution. In practice, this value is typically calculated by adding up the milliequivalent (mEq) concentrations of the various ions in the solution. *Osmolality* describes the molar number of osmotically active particles per kilogram of solvent. This value is directly measured by determining either the freezing point or the vapor pressure of the solution (each of which is reduced by a dissolved solute). Note that osmotic activity of a solution demands that particles be "independent." As NaCl dissociates into Na and Cl, it creates two osmotically active particles. If electrostatic forces act to prevent dissociation of the two charged particles, osmolality is reduced. For most dilute salt solutions, osmolality is equal to or slightly less than osmolarity. For example, commercial lactated Ringer's solution has a calculated osmolarity of approximately 275 mosmol/L but a measured osmolality of approximately 254 mosmol/kg, indicating incomplete dissociation.

Calculated versus measured serum osmolality is relevant in the clinical setting. The reference method for measuring serum osmolality is the delta-cryoscopic technique. However, the technology may not be available, and/or it is not always possible to obtain an emergency measurement 24 hours a day. In such cases, osmolality can be calculated from the osmoles that are routinely measured, such as sodium, potassium, urea, and glucose. Be advised, however, that calculation of osmolality introduces a bias, overestimating osmolality in the lower ranges and underestimating it in the higher ranges.

C. **COP.** Osmolarity and osmolality are determined by the total number of dissolved "particles" in a solution regardless of their size. COP is the osmotic pressure produced by large molecules (e.g., albumin, hetastarch, dextran). This factor becomes particularly important in biological systems in which vascular membranes are often permeable to small ions but not to large molecules (typically plasma proteins). In such situations, proteins might be the only osmotically active particles. Normal COP is approximately 20 mm Hg (or equal to approximately 1 mosmol/kg).

D. **Starling's hypothesis.** In 1898, Starling published his equations describing the forces driving water across vascular membranes. The major factors that control the movement of fluids between the intravascular and extravascular spaces are the transcapillary hydrostatic gradient, the osmotic and oncotic gradients, and the relative permeability of the capillary membranes that separate these spaces. The Starling equation is as follows:

$$FM = k(P_c + \pi_i - P_i - \pi_c)$$

where FM is fluid movement, k is the filtration coefficient of the capillary wall (i.e., how leaky it is), P_c is the hydrostatic pressure in the capillaries, P_i is the hydrostatic pressure (usually negative) in the interstitial (extravascular) space, and π_i and π_c are interstitial and capillary osmotic pressures, respectively.

Fluid movement is therefore proportional to the hydrostatic pressure gradient minus the osmotic pressure gradient across a vessel wall. The magnitude of the osmotic gradient depends on the relative permeability of the vessels to solute. In the periphery (muscle, bowel, lung, etc.), the capillary endothelium has a pore size of 65 Å and is freely permeable to small molecules and ions (Na, Cl) but not to large molecules, such as proteins (Fig. 20-1). As a result, π is defined only by colloids, and the Starling equation can be simplified by saying that **fluid moves into a tissue whenever either the hydrostatic gradient increases (either intravascular pressure rises or interstitial pressure falls) or the osmotic gradient decreases.**

In normal situations, the intravascular protein concentration is higher than the interstitial concentration, acting to draw water back into the vascular space. If COP is reduced (e.g., by dilution with large amounts of isotonic crystalloid), fluid begins to accumulate in the interstitium, producing edema. This fact is familiar to all anesthesiologists who have seen marked peripheral edema in patients given many liters of crystalloid during surgery or resuscitation. By contrast, the

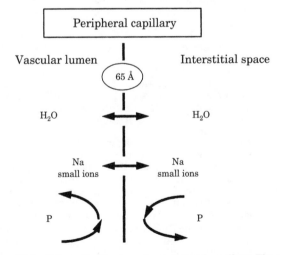

Figure 20-1. Schematic diagram of a peripheral capillary. The vessel wall is permeable to both water (H_2O) and small ions but not to proteins (P).

blood-brain barrier (BBB) is impermeable to both ions and proteins so that osmotic pressure is determined by the total osmotic gradient, of which COP contributes only a tiny fraction.

E. Interstitial clearance. Peripheral tissues have a net outward movement of fluid (i.e., the value of FM is positive). Edema is not normally present, however, because this extravasated fluid is cleared by the lymphatics. While many researchers agree that there is some lymphatic drainage of the brain, most interstitial fluid in the brain is cleared either by bulk fluid flow into the cerebrospinal fluid (CSF) spaces or via pinocytosis back into the intravascular compartment. This is a slow process and probably does not counteract rapid fluid movement into the interstitial space.

F. Hydrostatic forces and interstitial compliance. In the tissues, the net hydrostatic gradient is determined by (a) intravascular pressure and (b) interstitial tissue compliance. Normally, the direction is outward (capillary to interstitium). There is no question that in the brain (or in any organ), elevated intravascular pressure, such as that produced by either high jugular venous pressure or a head-down posture, can increase edema formation. However, an often overlooked factor that influences the pressure gradient is the interstitial compliance (i.e., the tendency of tissue to resist fluid influx). The loose interstitial space in most peripheral tissues does little to impede the influx of fluid. This explains the ease with which edema develops around, for example, the face and the eyes, even with minor hydrostatic stresses (e.g., a facedown posture).

By contrast, the interstitial space of the brain is extremely noncompliant, resisting fluid movement. As a result, minor changes in driving forces (either hydrostatic or osmotic/oncotic) do not produce measurable edema. However, a vicious cycle can develop so that, as edema forms in the brain, the interstitial matrix is disrupted, the compliance increases, and additional edema forms more easily. In contrast, the closed cranium and ICP can act to retard fluid influx. This may partially explain the exacerbation of edema formation that can occur after rapid decompression of the intracranial space.

G. Can we explain the influence of certain fluids on the brain? In contrast to capillaries elsewhere in the body, the endothelial cells in the brain are held together by continuous tight junctions to form the BBB. There are no intercellular gaps: the membranes are not fenestrated and do not have channels or chains of vesicles that form transendothelial pathways. The effective pore size of the BBB is only 7 to 9 Å, making this unique structure normally impermeable to large molecules (e.g., plasma proteins and synthetic colloids, such as hetastarch and dextrans) and relatively impermeable to many small polar solutes (Na, K, Cl) (Fig. 20-2). The

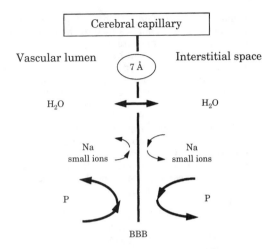

Figure 20-2. Schematic diagram of a cerebral capillary. The blood-brain barrier (BBB) is impermeable to small ions and proteins (P) but not to water (H_2O).

BBB functions as a semipermeable membrane that allows only water to move freely between the brain's interstitial space and the vasculature. This should serve to make the brain an exquisitely sensitive osmometer where water moves according to osmotic gradients.

We would then predict that **reducing serum osmolality** (e.g., by infusing water or large volumes of nonisotonic crystalloid solution) increases cerebral edema; conversely, increasing osmolality reduces brain water content. This experiment was first done in 1919 by Weed and McKibben, who showed a large and rapid increase in brain volume with the reduction of serum osmolality. Since that time, numerous studies have demonstrated the exquisite sensitivity of the brain's water content to changes in serum osmolality, in which even small changes can produce measurable changes in the brain water content. This makes sense considering that a 5 mosmol/kg gradient is equivalent to an almost 100 mm Hg force driving water (see preceding text). In fact, in experimental animals, a reduction in plasma osmolality of as little as 5% under otherwise normal conditions causes brain edema and increases ICP.

H. **What about changes in COP?** As mentioned, colloidally active molecules contribute to only a tiny fraction of the total osmolality and, when the BBB is intact, can be responsible for only a small driving force. Normal plasma COP is approximately 20 mm Hg, whereas that in the brain interstitium is approximately 0.6 mm Hg. This is equal to the force that could be generated by a change in the capillary/tissue osmotic gradient of only 1 mosmol/kg. We would therefore predict that changes in COP have only minimal effect on brain water content. This hypothesis has been tested directly in several animal experiments, which have demonstrated that normal brain water content can be altered by small changes in osmolality but not by clinically achievable changes in COP. There was also no increase in brain water content (i.e., edema) in any region with an intact BBB, even after a very large reduction (approximately 50%) in COP.

However, **what about more clinically relevant conditions, with varying degrees of BBB abnormality?** We can predict that if the BBB is made completely permeable to both small and large molecules (i.e., complete breakdown of the BBB as is common with several experimental and clinical injuries), it should be impossible to maintain any form of osmotic or oncotic gradient between the intravascular compartment and the brain interstitium. As a result, no changes in brain water content would be expected with a change in either gradient. Indeed, in several animal models resembling human brain injuries (e.g., implanted glioma and freezing lesion, which are similar to brain tumor and trauma, respectively), changes induced by a reduction in total serum osmolality were seen only in apparently normal regions of the brain relatively distant from the focus of injury. In keeping with this, several studies have shown that acute hyperosmolality (as with mannitol, urea, glycerol, hypertonic saline [HS]) reduces water content only in relatively normal brain tissue where the BBB is intact. Conversely, when the BBB is severely damaged, investigations have failed to demonstrate that reducing the COP affects cerebral edema. In the presence of mild injury to the BBB in experimental animals, a reduction in COP may potentially aggravate brain edema. Therefore, it is possible that, with a less severe injury, the BBB *may* function similarly to the peripheral tissue.

I. **Summary.** Injury to the brain interferes with the integrity of the BBB to varying degrees, depending on the severity of the damage. Regions in which there is a complete breakdown of the BBB, there will be no osmotic/oncotic gradient. Water accumulation (i.e., brain edema) occurs because of the pathologic process and cannot be directly influenced by the osmotic/oncotic gradient. In other regions where there is moderate injury to the BBB (i.e., a mild opening rendering pore size similar to the periphery), it is possible that the colloid oncotic gradient is effective as in the peripheral tissue. Finally, the BBB is normal in a significant portion of the brain. The presence of a functionally intact BBB is essential if osmotherapy is to be effective.

J. **Fluids for intravenous administration.** Table 20-1 lists a variety of solutions suitable for intravenous use.

Table 20-1. Composition of intravenous fluids

Fluid	Dextrose (g/L)	Na (mEq/L)	Cl (mEq/L)	Osmolarity[a] (mosmol/L)	Oncotic P (mm Hg)
5% Dextrose in water	50	—	—	278	—
Crystalloids:					
5% Dextrose in 0.45% saline	50	77	77	405	—
5% Dextrose in Ringer's	50	130	109	525	—
Lactated Ringer's		130	109	275	—
Plasmalyte		140	98	298	—
0.45% Saline		77	77	154	—
0.9% NS		154	154	308	—
3.0% Saline		513	513	1026	—
5.0% Saline		855	855	1711	—
7.5% Saline		1283	1283	2567	—
20% Mannitol		—	—	1098	—
Colloids:					
Plasma				295	21
Albumin (5%)				290	19
Hetastarch (6%) in NS		154	154	~310	31
Dextran (10%) 40 in NS		154	154	~310	169
Dextran (6%) 70 in NS		154	154	~310	19

[a]Osmolarity = calculated value(mosmol/L = mg ÷ molecular weight×10 × valence). NS, normal saline; —, no available data; P, pressure.

1. *Crystalloid* is the term commonly applied to solutions that do not contain any high molecular weight compound and have an oncotic pressure of zero. Crystalloids can be hyposmolar, iso-osmolar, or hyperosmolar, and may or may not contain glucose. Crystalloids can be made hyperosmolar by the inclusion of electrolytes (e.g., Na and Cl, as in HS) and low molecular weight solutes such as mannitol (molecular weight 182) or glucose (molecular weight 180).

2. *Colloid* is the term used to denote solutions that have an oncotic pressure similar to that of plasma. Some commonly administered colloids include 5% or 25% albumin, plasma, 6% hetastarch (hydroxyethyl starch, molecular weight 450), pentastarch (a low molecular weight hydroxyethyl starch, molecular weight 264), and the dextrans (molecular weights 40 and 70). Dextran and hetastarch are dissolved in normal saline so that the osmolarity of the solution is approximately 290 to 310 mosmol/L with a sodium and chloride content of approximately 154 mEq/L, which makes them hyperoncotic and hypertonic. Hetastarch should be limited and used with caution, however, because of the depletion of factor VIII and possible coagulation difficulties encountered with volumes exceeding 1,500 mL. Dextran-40 interferes with normal platelet function and is therefore not advisable for patients who have intracranial pathology other than to improve rheology as in ischemic cerebrovascular diseases. Although small volumes of hetastarch and dextran can restore normovolemia rapidly and without increasing ICP, it is unclear whether they offer any advantage over the combination of isotonic fluids and osmotic diuretics.

II. **Clinical fluid management of neurosurgical patients**
   A. **Fluid restriction.** Despite the lack of convincing experimental evidence that iso-osmolar crystalloids are detrimental, fluid restriction is widely practiced in patients who have mass lesions or cerebral edema or are at risk for intracranial hypertension. The only directly applicable data indicate that clinically acceptable restriction has little effect on edema formation. However, "modest" fluid restriction has some logic. One of the few human studies on fluid therapy in neurosurgical patients has demonstrated that patients given standard "maintenance" amounts of intravenous fluid (e.g., 2,000 mL/day of 0.45 normal saline in 5% dextrose) in the postoperative period develop a progressive reduction in serum osmolality (Fig. 20-3). On the other hand, patients given half of this volume over a period of several days (about a week) show a progressive increase in serum osmolality, which could account for dehydration of the brain (Fig. 20-3). While no CNS parameters

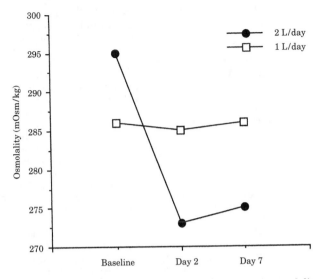

Figure 20-3.   Effect of fluid restriction (1 L/day) on serum osmolality in neurosurgical patients. (Modified by Shenkin et al., 1976).

were measured, the results suggest that usual maintenance fluids contain excess free water for the typical postoperative craniotomy patient. In this regard, fluid restriction can be viewed as "preventing" hyposmotically driven edema. However, this does not imply that even greater degrees of fluid restriction are beneficial or that the administration of a fluid mixture that does not reduce osmolality is detrimental.

B.   **Intraoperative volume replacement/resuscitation.** As a general rule, intraoperative fluids should be given at a rate sufficient to replace the urinary output and insensible losses (e.g., skin and lungs). Table 20-2 illustrates the intravascular volume expansion obtained with different types of fluids. Volume replacement with crystalloid solutions, geared to maintain the hematocrit at approximately 33%, is calculated on a 3:1 ratio (crystalloid to intraoperative blood loss) because of the larger distribution space of the crystalloids.

Table 20-2.   Volume replacement

Fluid Infused	Intravascular Volume Increase
1 L isotonic crystalloid	~250 mL
1 L 5% albumin	~500 mL
1 L hetastarch	~750 mL

The available data indicate that intravascular volume replacement and expansion will have no effect on cerebral edema as long as normal serum osmolality is maintained and cerebral hydrostatic pressure is not markedly increased (e.g., owing to true volume overload and elevated right heart pressures). Whether this is achieved with crystalloid or colloid seems irrelevant, although the **osmolality of the selected fluid is crucial**. With respect to this issue, it should also be noted that lactated Ringer's solution is not strictly isosmotic (measured osmolality 252 to 255 mosmol/kg), particularly when administered to patients whose baseline osmolality has been increased by either fluid restriction or hyperosmolar fluids (mannitol, HS, etc.).

Our recommendation is that serum osmolality be checked repeatedly with the goal of either maintaining this value or increasing it slightly. Fluid administration that results in a reduction in osmolality should be avoided. Small volumes of lactated Ringer's (1 to 3 L) are unlikely to be detrimental and can be used safely, for example, to compensate for the changes in venous capacitance that typically accompany the induction of anesthesia. If large volumes are needed (either to replace blood loss or to compensate for some other source of volume loss), a change to a more isotonic fluid such as normal saline is probably advisable. It is also important to remember that rapid infusion of a large volume of 0.9% NaCl can induce a dose-dependent hyperchloremic metabolic acidosis. Whether this acid-base abnormality is, in fact, harmful remains unclear, although animal studies suggest that hyperchloremia causes renal vasoconstriction. If large volumes are needed, a combination of isotonic crystalloids and colloids may be the best choice (Table 20-1).

These recommendations should not be interpreted, however, as a license to "give all the isotonic fluid you like." Volume *overload* can have detrimental effects on ICP by increasing either cerebral blood volume(CBV) or hydrostatically driven cerebral edema formation.

C. **Postoperative period.** In the postoperative period, the patient no longer needs large volumes of fluid. The recommendation of Shenkin to give approximately 1,000 mL/day is probably reasonable (Fig. 20-3); we would again recommend periodic measurement of serum osmolality, particularly if the patient's neurologic status deteriorates. If cerebral edema does develop, further fluid restriction is unlikely to be of value and can cause hypovolemia. Instead, treatment consists of mannitol or furosemide and maintenance of normovolemia with fluids to sustain the increased osmolality. Inducing hypovolemia so that vasopressors are required to maintain acceptable hemodynamic parameters has little advantage (and some disadvantage).

D. HS solutions. HS solutions have been evaluated for use in fluid resuscitation since the 1960s, particularly because hemodynamic improvement can be achieved with very small volumes given very quickly. Because hyperosmolality is known to reduce brain volume, HS has been used in patients who are at risk for increased ICP. In humans, acute resuscitation from hemorrhagic shock with 7.5% HS is associated with improved outcome in patients with multiple trauma and head injuries. Clinical studies suggest that HS may be better in hypotensive, brain-injured patients during transportation to the hospital.

There is no question that HS can quickly restore intravascular volume while reducing ICP through brain water reduction in uninjured brain. Additional benefit may be derived from decreases in CSF production. Unfortunately, what remains unclear is whether this approach is unique or whether the identical CNS benefit could be achieved with any resuscitation fluid that increases osmolality.

The principal disadvantage of HS is the danger of **hypernatremia**. In a recent study of neurosurgical patients undergoing elective supratentorial procedures, we have shown that equal volumes of 20% mannitol and 7.5% HS reduce brain bulk and CSF pressure to the same extent (Fig. 20-3). However, serum sodium increased during the administration of HS and peaked at more than 150 mEq/L at the conclusion of the infusion.

E. Mannitol and furosemide. Both mannitol and furosemide (and occasionally other diuretics) are used to control ICP and brain swelling in neurosurgical patients. Mannitol acts by **establishing an osmotic gradient between blood and brain** in the presence of a relatively intact BBB. This promotes removal of water from areas of normal brain. Mannitol might elevate ICP transiently from the vasodilator effects of hyperosmolality, resulting in an increase in CBV. In both dogs and humans, this phenomenon occurs neither in the presence of intracranial hypertension nor when mannitol is given at moderate rates. Mannitol may, therefore, be given to most neurosurgical patients. The exception might be patients who have significant cardiovascular disease in whom the transient volume expansion might precipitate congestive heart failure.

The other important concern is that the repeated use of mannitol may cause excessive hyperosmolality, which can be deadly. In addition, mannitol accumulates in the interstitium with repeated doses. If interstitial osmolality rises excessively, it is possible for the normal brain–blood gradient to be reversed with resultant exacerbation of the edema. Furthermore, if brain osmolality is increased, edema may be enhanced by the subsequent normalization of serum osmolality. The recommended dose of mannitol is therefore 0.25 to 1 g/kg. The smallest possible dose is selected and infused over 10 to 15 minutes.

The exact mechanism of action of **furosemide** remains controversial, although it certainly is related to the drug's ability to block Cl transportation. Furosemide and similar drugs might also act primarily by reducing cellular swelling rather than by changing the extracellular fluid volume. Several studies have demonstrated that furosemide decreases CSF production. This effect can explain the synergistic effect of mannitol and furosemide on intracranial compliance. However, the **maximal effect of furosemide compared with that of mannitol is delayed**. For this reason, mannitol probably remains the drug of choice for rapid control of ICP.

F. **Glucose-containing solutions.** Salt-free solutions containing glucose should be avoided in patients who have intracranial pathology. Free water reduces serum osmolality and increases brain water content. Furthermore, solid evidence in animals and humans indicates that **excessive glucose exacerbates neurologic damage** and can worsen the outcome from both focal and global ischemia. This happens because glucose metabolism enhances tissue acidosis in ischemic areas. The reduction of adenosine levels from hyperglycemia could also be detrimental. Adenosine inhibits the release of excitatory amino acids, which play a major role in ischemic cell damage.

Although clinical investigations have indicated a negative relationship between patients' plasma glucose on admission and outcome after stroke, cardiac arrest, and head injury, more recent studies suggest that this correlation is not necessarily one of cause and effect because the high glucose may be a concomitant of more severe CNS damage. Nor has it been possible to demonstrate that the administration of glucose to humans is detrimental. Nevertheless, withholding glucose from adult neurosurgical patients is not associated with hypoglycemia. It may therefore be prudent to withhold glucose-containing fluids from acutely injured and elective surgical patients. This *caveat* does not apply to the use of hyperalimentation in such patients, perhaps because the administration of these hyperglycemic solutions typically begins several days after the primary insult.

G. **Should insulin be administered to correct hyperglycemia in patients who have intracranial pathology?** While laboratory evidence suggests that the correction of hyperglycemia with insulin before the ischemic insult occurs improves outcome, this has not been studied in humans.

H. **Summary.** Blood sugar in neurosurgical patients should be controlled carefully to avoid both hypo- and hyperglycemia and to maintain glucose between 100 and 150 mg/dL. Glucose-containing solutions should be withheld, except in the case of neonates and patients who have diabetes in whom hypoglycemia can occur very rapidly and be detrimental.

III. **Hemodilution.** One common accompaniment of fluid administration is a reduction in the hemoglobin and hematocrit. With active blood loss, the use of asanguineous fluids can cause marked anemia. An increase in cerebral blood flow (CBF) typically accompanies this hemodilution, and physicians have long argued whether the hemodilution is beneficial, benign, or detrimental. The answer probably depends on the degree of hemodilution and on the state of the disease.

From a theoretical vantage, a hematocrit of 30% to 33% gives the optimal combination of viscosity and oxygen-carrying capacity. In the normal brain, the increase in CBF produced by hemodilution is almost certainly an active compensatory response to a decrease in arterial oxygen content; this response is essentially identical to that seen with hypoxia. With a brain injury, however, the normal CBF response to hypoxia and hemodilution is attenuated, and both conditions can contribute to secondary tissue damage.

The one situation in which hemodilution might be beneficial is the period during and immediately after a focal cerebral ischemic event. Several animal studies have shown that regional oxygen delivery may be increased (or at least better maintained) in the face of modest hemodilution to a hematocrit of approximately 30% with improvement in CBF and reduction in infarction volume. In spite of this, several clinical trials have failed to demonstrate any benefit from hemodilution in stroke patients, except in those who were polycythemic to begin with. The lack of success, however, may reflect the delay in instituting therapy or inadequate hematocrit reduction.

A. **What clinical lesson can be learned from the work on hemodilution?** Our opinion is that for elective neurosurgical patients and patients suffering from head injuries, hemodilution to a hematocrit below 30% to 35% is unlikely to be any more "beneficial" than hypoxia. Hemodilution to 30% to 35% might be better tolerated in patients who are at risk for focal ischemia. Nevertheless, active attempts to reduce the hematocrit below 30% are probably not advisable at the present time.

B. **Water and electrolyte disturbances.** Table 20-3 summarizes the principal differences among the most common water and electrolyte disturbances in patients who have intracranial pathology.

C. **Diabetes insipidus (DI).** DI is a common sequela of pituitary and hypothalamic lesions, but it can also occur with other cerebral pathology, such as head trauma, bacterial meningitis, intracranial surgery, phenytoin use, and alcohol intoxication. Patients who

Table 20-3. Principal water-electrolyte disorders

Factor	DI	SIADH	CSW
Etiology	Reduced secretion of ADH	Excessive release of ADH	Release of brain natriuretic factor
Urine			
Output	>30 mL/kg/hr		
Specific gravity	<1.002		
Sodium	<15 mEq/L	>20 mEq/L	>50 mEq/L
Osmolality vs. serum osmolality	Lower	Higher	Higher
Serum			
Sodium	Hypernatremia	Hyponatremia	Hyponatremia
Osmolality	Hyperosmolality	Hypoosmolality	
Intravascular volume	Reduced	Normal or increased	Reduced

DI, diabetes insipidus; SIADH, syndrome of inappropriate antidiuretic hormone secretion; CSW, cerebral salt wasting syndrome; ADH, antidiuretic hormone.

have markedly elevated ICP and brain death also commonly develop DI.

DI is a metabolic disorder caused by the decreased secretion of antidiuretic hormone (ADH). This results in the failure of the tubular reabsorption of water. Polyuria (>30 mL/kg/hour or, in an adult, >200 mL/hour), progressive dehydration, and hypernatremia occur subsequently. DI is present when the urine output is excessive, the urine osmolality is inappropriately low relative to serum osmolality (which is above normal because of water loss), and the urine specific gravity is <1.002.

1. **Management.** The management of DI requires restoration of normal serum sodium and carefully balancing intake and output to avoid fluid overload. The patient should receive hourly maintenance fluids plus either three-fourths of the previous hour's urine output or the previous hour's urine output minus 50 mL (Table 20-4). Half-normal saline and free water are commonly used as replacement fluids, with appropriate potassium supplementation. Serum sodium, potassium, and glucose should be checked frequently.

   If the urine output is >300 mL/hour for 2 hours, it is now standard practice to administer aqueous vasopressin, 5 to 10 international units of drug (IU), intramuscularly (i.m.) or subcutaneously (s.c.) every 6 hours or the synthetic analog of ADH, desmopressin acetate, 0.5 to 2 mcg intravenously (i.v.) every 8 hours or by nasal inhalation, 10 to 20 mcg.

D. **Syndrome of inappropriate antidiuretic hormone secretion (SIADH).** Various cerebral pathologic processes (mostly head trauma) can cause excessive release of ADH, which leads to the continued renal excretion of sodium (>20 mEq/L), despite hyponatremia and associated hypo osmolality. Urine osmolality is therefore high relative to serum osmolality. SIADH can also result from the excessive administration of free water in patients who cannot excrete free water because of excess ADH.

   1. **Management.** The mainstay of treatment of SIADH is fluid restriction to 1,000 mL/24 hours of iso-osmolar solution. If hyponatremia is severe (<110 to 115 mEq/L), the administration of hypertonic (3% to 5%) saline and furosemide might be

Table 20-4. Management of diabetes insipidus

Hourly monitoring of UO
Maintenance fluids + 75% of the previous hour's UO *or*
Maintenance fluids + the previous hour's UO − 50 mL.
If UO >300 mL/hr: vasopressin or desmopressin

UO, urinary output.

appropriate. Because rapid correction of hyponatremia has been associated with the occurrence of central pontine myelinolysis, restoring serum sodium at a rate of approximately 2 mEq/L/hour is advisable.

E. **Cerebral salt wasting syndrome (CSW).** CSW is characterized by hyponatremia, volume contraction, and high urine sodium concentration (>50 mEq/L). This syndrome is frequently seen in patients after subarachnoid hemorrhage (SAH). The causative factor seems to be the increased release of a natriuretic factor from the brain.

1. **Management.** The therapy is to reestablish normovolemia with the administration of sodium-containing solutions.

   The **distinction between SIADH and CSW is very important** because treatment of these two syndromes is quite different: fluid restriction versus fluid infusion, respectively. It should be stressed that in patients who have SAH for whom normo- to hypervolemia is advocated, fluid restriction (i.e., further volume contraction) might be especially deleterious.

IV. **Conclusion.** As neuroanesthesiologists and intensivists, we should always remember that we treat the whole patient, not only the brain. Therefore, with the exception of patients with SIADH, we should abandon the old dogma that patients who have intracranial pathology must be "run dry" and replace it with "run them isovolemic, isotonic, and iso-oncotic."

V. **Key points**
   - *Movement of water* between the normal brain and the intravascular space depends on osmotic gradients.
   - Reducing *serum osmolality* by administering free water or hypotonic crystalloid solutions (0.45% NaCl) results in edema formation in all tissues, including normal brain tissue.
   - Reduction of *COP* with maintenance of serum osmolality is associated with increased water content in many tissues, but not in the normal brain. Colloid solutions exert little influence on brain water content and ICP.
   - In the setting of *brain injury*, reducing serum osmolality increases edema and ICP. Therefore, the goal of fluid management in neurosurgery is to avoid the reduction of serum osmolality. Reduction of COP, with careful maintenance of osmolality, does not increase edema in the injured brain.
   - *Hypertonic solutions*: mannitol decreases brain water content in the normal brain and is commonly used to reduce ICP. HS decreases brain water content and ICP but can cause hypernatremia.
   - *Glucose*-containing solutions should not be used in patients who have brain pathology and should be avoided in patients at risk for cerebral ischemia.

- *Fluid restriction* minimally affects cerebral edema and, if overzealously pursued, can lead to hemodynamic instability, which is detrimental in neurosurgical patients.
- *Isotonic crystalloid solutions* are widely used to maintain and/or restore intravascular volume.

SUGGESTED READINGS

Clifton GL, Miller ER, Choi SC, et al. Fluid thresholds and outcome from severe brain injury. *Crit Care Med* 2002;30:73–45.

Drummond JC, Patel PM, Cole DJ, et al. The effect of the reduction of colloid oncotic pressure, with and without reduction of osmolality, on post-traumatic cerebral edema. *Anesthesiology* 1998;88:993–1002.

Gemma M, Cozzi S, Tommasino C, et al. 7.5% hypertonic saline versus 20% mannitol during elective neurosurgical supratentorial procedures. *J Neurosurg Anesthesiol* 1997;9:329–334.

Rudehill A, Gordon E, Ohman G, et al. Pharmacokinetics and effects of mannitol on hemodynamics, blood and cerebrospinal fluid electrolytes, and osmolality during intracranial surgery. *J Neurosurg Anesthesiol* 1993;5:4–12.

Shenkin HA, Benzier HO, Bouzarth W. Restricted fluid intake: rational management of the neurosurgical patient. *J Neurosurg* 1976;45:432–436.

Tommasino C. Fluids and the neurosurgical patient. *Anesthesiol Clin North America* 2002;20:329–346.

Vialet R, Lèone M, Albanèse J, et al. Calculated serum osmolality can lead to systematic bias compared to direct measurement. *J Neurosurg Anesthesiol* 2005;17:106–109.

Zornow MH, Scheller MS, Todd MM, et al. Acute cerebral effects of isotonic crystalloid and colloid solutions following cryogenic brain injury in the rabbit. *Anesthesiology* 1988;69:180–184.

Nutritional Support in the Critically Ill Patient

John M. Taylor and Linda Liu

The goals of nutritional support in patients who are critically ill are to provide protein and caloric replacement while attenuating a negative nitrogen balance. It is estimated that 50% of hospitalized patients and 60% to 80% of patients in the intensive care unit (ICU) are malnourished. Delays in the initiation of nutritional support may result in muscle and gastrointestinal (GI) atrophy, inability to be weaned from ventilatory support, heart failure, impaired immunity, and an increase in the incidence of sepsis, length of hospital stay, and morbidity and mortality.

There is no doubt that effective nutritional support coupled with appropriate monitoring improves patient outcome. Since the early 1980s, the importance of nutritional support in patients who have severe neurologic injury has been appreciated. Recent studies have also documented the same nutritional and metabolic requirements in patients who have acute ischemic injury and other critical neurologic illnesses. Compelling evidence now exists that strict glycemic control in critically ill patients reduces morbidity and mortality.

I. **Pathophysiology.** The effects of elective operations, trauma, and critical illness activate the neural and endocrine systems. The resultant increase in sympathetic outflow leads to lipolysis, proteolysis, and decreased glucose uptake owing to the antagonism of insulin by growth hormone and epinephrine. This sympathetic surge increases energy expenditure (EE), tissue catabolism, and mobilization of protein, fat, and carbohydrates. Immobility and delays in the administration of nutritional support exacerbate these effects of increased sympathetic outflow. Other untoward effects include hyperglycemia, poor wound healing, decreased serum proteins, increased carbon dioxide (CO_2) production, release of inflammatory mediators, and depressed immune function.

After neurologic injury, the ensuing state of cardiac hyperdynamism increases oxygen consumption and caloric requirements. Studies using indirect calorimetry demonstrate that patients with severe head injury are hypermetabolic and hypercatabolic. The resting energy expenditure (REE) can increase 40% to 165%. This increase has been demonstrated in patients who are treated both with and without steroids. In addition, delayed gastric emptying, bacterial translocation, and altered vascular permeability with resultant intestinal edema and malabsorption also occur.

A. **Patients with neurologic injury.** Patients who have head injury exhibit changes consistent with hypermetabolism, hypercatabolism, hyperglycemia, suppressed immunity, and a generalized inflammatory response. Nutritional support should satisfy these physiologic demands.

B. **Patients who have suffered a stroke.** These patients also exhibit hypermetabolic physiology. Although it has been suggested that protein supplementation beyond normal nutritional support after stroke may improve outcome, recent trials have not supported this strategy.

C. **Patients who are obese.** Recent estimates indicate that approximately 40% of adults in the United States are overweight. Patients who are obese are more likely to manifest comorbid medical conditions including hypertension, coronary artery disease, diabetes mellitus, pulmonary disease, and gout. Critical illness is likely to result in protein malnutrition, inhibition of lipolysis, and preferential use of carbohydrate substrate for gluconeogenesis. It has been suggested that patients who have actual body weight (ABW) in excess of 125% of ideal body weight (IBW) may benefit from diets that are hypocaloric and high protein in structure. The goal for obese patients is to provide adequate protein intake to meet but not exceed metabolic demands. Ideally, the nutritional supplementation will contain enough protein to keep the patient in a positive nitrogen balance, but sufficient relative calorie deficit to encourage a net increase in lean body mass (LBM) and a loss of total body fat.

II. **Nutritional assessment.** Delivery of appropriate metabolic support begins with an assessment of the patient's nutritional status. It is important to identify patients who present with subtle signs of deficiencies in caloric, protein, vitamin, or trace metal intake. These patients should be considered candidates for earlier and more aggressive support.

A. **Definitions.** The malnourished state exists when intake does not meet nutritional demands. When approximately 10% of LBM is lost, moderate protein energy malnutrition exists. A loss of 20% of LBM indicates severe protein malnutrition and describes a severely underweight patient. When more than 35% of LBM is lost, it is likely that irreversible changes leading to death have occurred.

B. **History.** In most cases, a history of recent unintentional weight loss (5% LBM in 1 month or 10% LBM in 6 months) raises the possibility of malnutrition. A careful social history may demonstrate vitamin or mineral deficiencies associated with alcoholism or other substance abuse. Patients who have renal failure lose amino acids, vitamins, and trace metals during dialysis. Patients who have cancer may have deficiencies owing either to the underlying disease or to chemotherapy (e.g., methotrexate). Other risk factors for malnutrition include age >75 years, homelessness, nothing by mouth for more than 3 days, major surgery, corticosteroid administration, renal dialysis, malabsorption syndromes, and chronic disease states, especially cancer, stroke, and acquired immunodeficiency disease.

C. **Physical examination.** Caloric intake can be assessed by the amount of fat in the extremities, buttocks, and buccal fat pad. The adequacy of protein intake can be evaluated from the bulk of the extremity muscles, grip strength, and size of the temporal muscle. Vitamin deficiencies may manifest themselves as changes in skin texture and hair quality and texture, cheilosis, glossitis, or loss of vibration and position sense. Examination of the head and neck may reveal xerostomia, malocclusion, odynophagia, dysphagia, esophagitis, or other findings suggestive of difficulty with eating.

D. **Anthropometrics.** Measurements are used to estimate the stores of body fat and protein. Body fat is approximated by the thickness of the triceps skin fold (TSF), and protein status is estimated by the mid-arm muscle circumference (MAMC).

MAMC = mid-arm circumference − fat

MAMC = mid-arm circumference − (0.314 × TSF)

These data are then compared with normal values to determine the patient's nutritional status. Two possibly incorrect assumptions are that body fat is uniformly distributed and that population standards apply to patients who are critically ill. In fact, anthropometric measurements are generally invalid in patients who are critically ill owing to anasarca. Adjustments in the estimations can be based on IBW calculated from the measurements of height and weight.

E. **Biochemical measurements.** Various biochemical and metabolic measurements have been studied as potential indices of nutritional status. Although many of these tests have significant value in assessing either stable patients who are scheduled for elective surgery or those well on the way to recovery, their applicability to patients who are critically ill has not been demonstrated. Trends between the same patient's measurements taken on different days can be used if other factors are relatively stable.

1. **Plasma proteins.** Plasma protein levels depend on hepatic synthetic function and the availability of substrate. Unfortunately, a decrease in level is not specific because the biologic half-life, the catabolic rate, and a variety of nonnutritional factors can alter plasma protein levels. For example, expansion of the extracellular fluid compartment results in a reduction in albumin

concentration. In addition, some serum protein levels decrease promptly in response to trauma, sepsis, or severe illness as a result of fluid shifts, alterations in capillary permeability, and changes in rates of synthesis and degradation. Liver disease, nephrotic syndrome, eclampsia, and protein-losing enteropathies are additional causes of hypoproteinemia.

a. **Albumin** has a half-life of approximately 18 days. It is the most commonly used test to diagnose protein-calorie undernutrition. Depending on measured albumin alone, however, can lead to delays in treating nutritional deficits because plasma levels can be maintained for a long time owing to the long half-life. In critical illness, albumin may also remain low until the remission of the inflammatory response despite adequate nutritional intake. Serum albumin levels have been shown to be good predictors of sepsis and major infection in surgical patients. However, serum albumin has not been correlated with either morbidity or mortality in the setting of severe neurologic injury.

b. **Transferrin** has a half-life of approximately 8 days. Therefore, transferrin levels reflect acute changes in nutritional status more accurately than albumin. Low serum transferrin is indicative of protein malnutrition. Iron deficiency, pregnancy, and hypoxia stimulate synthesis of transferrin whereas chronic infection, sepsis, and iron overload decrease transferrin levels.

c. **Thyroxine-binding prealbumin and retinol-binding protein (RBP)** have a half-life of 2 to 3 days and 8 to 12 hours, respectively. RBP complexes with prealbumin in the circulation. The resultant compounds are much more sensitive to short-term alterations in protein and total caloric intake; low levels can return to normal after only 3 days of adequate nutritional support. While serum levels of the RBP-prealbumin complex reflect acute changes in nutritional status and indicate the adequacy of nutritional supplementation, many nonnutritional factors can affect these levels as well. Infection and trauma depress prealbumin levels. Stress and vitamin A deficiency decrease the concentration of RBP; renal failure can cause erroneous elevation of RBP. The short half-lives and the myriad of factors influencing their serum concentrations have limited the clinical significance and usefulness of these proteins.

2. **Immunologic functions.** Total lymphocyte count (TLC) and reactivity to skin test antigens are immunologic functions that can assess nutritional status, but they are not routinely used in patients who are critically ill. Any stressful situation, especially any disease process that requires a stay in the ICU, can depress cellular immunity, leading to a nonspecific test result.

III. **Estimation of energy requirements.** Because all of the previously mentioned tests measure nutritional status indirectly, other more sensitive and specific techniques have been developed to assess nutritional status.

A. **Predictive equations**

1. **Harris-Benedict equation.** REE is the energy requirement at rest and can be estimated using the Harris-Benedict equation as follows:

Women: REE (kcal/day) $= 65 + 9.6W + 1.8H - 4.7A$

Men: REE (kcal/day) $= 66 + 13.7W + 5H - 6.8A$

where $W = $ ABW in kilograms or IBW in kilograms if the patient is edematous; $H = $ height in centimeters; and $A = $ age in years. If the patient is obese, an adjusted IBW should be used as follows:

Adjusted IBW $= $ IBW $+ 0.25$ (ABW $- $ IBW)

2. **Adjustments to REE.** EE can vary greatly from daily resting energy requirement in active subjects. Hospitalized patients typically require 30 kcal/kg/day in the absence of severe illness or obesity. Fever increases the REE by approximately 10% above baseline for each degree Celsius rise in temperature. Brain injury induces a hyperdynamic state. Elevated EE is usually associated with total body surface area burns of 20% to 40%. Figure 21-1 shows the EE as the percentage above normal for several disease states. A common practice is to adjust the estimated REE for the state of hypermetabolism that characterizes patients who are critically ill. Usual correction factors are as follows:
Fever: REE $\times 1.1$ (for each 1°C above normal)
Mild stress: REE $\times 1.2 - 1.3$
Moderate stress: REE $\times 1.4 - 1.5$
Severe stress: REE $\times 1.6 - 1.8$

3. Using predictive equations in patients who are critically ill has a potential limitation. The Harris-Benedict equation was determined using healthy volunteers as test subjects. The validity of applying this equation to patients who are critically ill has been questioned.

B. **Indirect calorimetry.** Indirect calorimetry relies on the measurement of oxygen consumption (V_{O_2}) and the production of carbon dioxide (V_{CO_2}). The oxygen consumed in a given period of time is the amount required for oxidation of carbohydrate, fat, and protein.

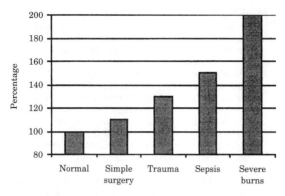

Figure 21-1. Energy expenditure as a percentage above normal in several disease states.

Simultaneously, CO_2 is produced from the oxidation of carbohydrate, fat, and protein. If the patient inspires a known concentration of O_2 and CO_2, measurements of Vo_2 and Vco_2 can be made. A metabolic computer can then calculate the REE and the respiratory quotient (RQ). Normal RQ is 0.8. An elevated RQ indicates overfeeding or excess carbohydrate in the diet.

Usually, measurements taken over a minimum period of 20 to 30 minutes generate better baseline values. Indirect calorimetry can be performed only on patients who have fraction of inspired oxygen (Fio_2) requirements of 50% or less. To account for sedation, ICU activity, dietary-induced thermogenesis, anabolism, and the work of breathing, an extra percentage is added to the measured EE. Examples of usual correction factors are as follows:
Thermogenesis: 5% to 10%
ICU activity: 10%
Anabolism: 5% to 10%
Sedation: 0% to 30%
1. REE can be calculated using indirect calorimetry:

$$REE \ (kcal/day) = (3.9 \times [Vo_2] + 1.1 \times [Vco_2]) \times 1.44$$

C. The Fick equation and mixed venous oxygen content (Cvo_2). The 24-hour EE for an ICU patient is approximately 7 times the Vo_2, calculated using measured arterial oxygen content (Cao_2), mixed venous oxygen content (Cvo_2), and the cardiac output (CO). The arterial oxygen saturation (Sao_2) and mixed venous oxygen saturation (Svo_2) should be measured at the same time that CO is measured.

$$Cao_2 - Cvo_2 = Hb \ (g/dL) \times 1.39 \times (Sao_2 - Svo_2)$$

$$Vo_2 \ (mL/minute) = (Cao_2 - Cvo_2) \times 10 \times CO \ (L/minute)$$

$$24\text{-hour EE} \ (kcal/day) = 7 \times Vo_2$$

These "spot" measurements should be performed for several days in succession to establish an accurate trend.

IV. Estimation of protein requirements. The daily protein requirements are usually estimated first and measured later.

A. **Predictive equations.** The goal of protein supplementation is to decrease the degree of loss of LBM because there are no protein stores in the body. Approximate protein requirements can be estimated on the basis of the patient's weight, degree of illness, and extent of organ system failure. High-dose steroids, which are often given to patients after neurologic insult, also increase protein requirements because of catabolism.

Normal protein requirement: 0.8 to 1 g protein/kg/day

Mild stress requirements: 1 to 1.2 g protein/kg/day

Moderate stress requirements: 1.2 to 1.4 g protein/kg/day

Severe stress requirements: 1.4 to 1.6 g protein/kg/day

Patients in renal failure on hemodialysis: 1.2 g protein/kg/day

Patients who have encephalopathy: 0.8 g protein/kg/day

1. Studies of patients with head injury receiving 1 to 1.5 g protein/kg/day have still reported negative nitrogen balances. Current recommendations are to provide 2 g protein/kg/day if renal function is normal and to reassess the nitrogen balance in a few days.

2. Postsurgical patients typically require 2 g protein/kg/day.

B. **Nitrogen balance.** Nitrogen balance is used to assess the adequacy of caloric and/or protein intake and whether the anabolic state has been achieved as a result of nutritional therapy.

Nitrogen balance equals nitrogen intake minus nitrogen output. Total nitrogen output equals urine urea nitrogen from a 24-hour urine collection and 2 to 4 g/day of nonurinary losses. In patients who are critically ill, this may be as much as 6 g/day owing to blood loss, increased mucosal sloughing, and increased fecal nitrogen loss from diarrhea. Because protein is 16% nitrogen, each gram of urinary nitrogen represents 6.25 g of degraded protein.

$$\text{Nitrogen balance} = (\text{protein intake}/6.25)$$

$$-(\text{urine urea nitrogen} + [2 \text{ or } 4])$$

Measurements of nitrogen balance may not be reliable in patients who have renal and hepatic failure owing to altered protein synthesis and clearance. For patients who are in renal failure, the creatinine (Cr) clearance must be >50 mL/minute to achieve a valid result.

V. Macronutrients

A. **Carbohydrates.** As long as the diet provides adequate energy and protein, there is no specific requirement for dietary carbohydrate, but current recommendations are to provide 50% to 60% of total calories as carbohydrates. Much of this is used by the central nervous system, which relies on glucose as its primary fuel source.

B. **Fat.** The goals of lipid supplementation include providing for essential fatty acids, promoting nitrogen sparing, and offering a balanced approach to fulfilling energy requirements. Increased fat decreases the incidence of hepatic steatosis and the production of CO_2 from a high-carbohydrate diet. Lipid oxidation as an energy source is increased in the patient who is critically ill. The recommendation is therefore to provide 30% to 40% of the total calories as lipid. A minimum of 3% of the kilocalories delivered as fat should be linoleic acid to prevent a deficiency of essential fatty acids.

C. **Protein.** The goal of protein supplementation is to provide substrate for cellular protein synthesis and the maintenance of LBM. Protein requirements increase if excessive losses from the GI tract, skin, or draining wounds occur. It is often difficult to achieve positive balance in patients who are critically ill, but the effort to minimize negative nitrogen balance should be made.

D. **Fluid.** Nonhospitalized patients consume approximately 1 mL of free water/kcal ingested. With a normal diet, this is approximately 30 to 50 mL/kg of body weight per day. Patients who are hospitalized typically require 30 to 35 mL/kg/day. The patients' underlying medical condition and comorbidities must be considered when replacing fluids. Patients should be adequately volume resuscitated before initiating parenteral nutrition.

When calculating free water replacement in patients receiving enteral nutrition, it is important to remember to subtract the free water in the enteral formula from the total daily volume of free water.

VI. **Micronutrients.** Because the response to injury is characterized by greatly increased energy demands and clinical malnutrition, appropriate nutritional support might prevent the multisystem organ failure that often occurs in patients who are critically ill. The gut is now being seen as an important metabolic organ that has a critical need for certain substrates. Clinical trials are being conducted to evaluate diets enriched with immunomodulatory components. Although the use of these components has been advocated, currently their benefits remain controversial.

A. **Vitamins.** Vitamins are involved in metabolism, wound healing, and immune function. They are essential and cannot be synthesized by the body. The 12 essential vitamins that should be supplied daily are divided into fat- and water-soluble categories. Recommended dietary allowances of vitamins are listed in Table 21-1.

**Table 21-1. Recommended dietary allowance
of vitamins for a healthy 25- to 50-year-old man**

Vitamin	Amount	Vitamin	Amount
Vitamin A	1,000 mcg	Vitamin D	5 mcg
Vitamin E	10 mg	Vitamin K	80 mcg
Vitamin C	60 mg	Thiamine	1.5 mg
Riboflavin	1.7 mg	Niacin	19 mg
Vitamin B_6	2 mg	Folate	200 mcg
Vitamin B_{12}	2 mcg		

B. Trace nutrients. Deficiencies in the nine essential
trace elements can lead to problems in several organ
systems including insulin resistance, myopathy, increased susceptibility to infections, and pancytopenia.
Recommended dietary allowances of trace elements
are listed in Table 21-2.

For patients in renal failure, zinc and chromium
should be either reduced or omitted because they are
excreted in the urine. Similarly, in the presence of
biliary tract obstruction, the intake of copper and
manganese is either reduced or omitted because both
are excreted primarily in the bile.

Decreased serum zinc levels and increased urinary
zinc losses have been reported after a head injury,
although the mechanism and clinical significance are
unknown. No other specific changes in vitamin and
mineral metabolism have been identified after neurologic injury.

1. Glutamine. The primary fuel for the intestine,
glutamine is important in maintaining intestinal structure and function, preventing mucosal
atrophy during starvation, decreasing bacterial
translocation, and stimulating the intestinal immune system in sepsis and stress. Glutamine may
also decrease intestinal injury during ischemia by
preserving the level of glutathione in the gut.

**Table 21-2. Recommended dietary allowance
of trace elements for a healthy 25- to 50-year-old
man**

Element	Oral	Intravenous
Zinc	10–15 mg	2.5–4.0 mg
Chromium	50–290 mcg	10–15 mcg
Copper	1.2–3 mg	0.5–1.5 mg
Manganese	0.7–5 mg	0.15–0.8 mg
Selenium	50–200 mcg	40–120 mcg
Molybdenum		200 mcg

2. **Arginine.** Arginine improves wound healing, stimulates immune function by increasing the production of natural killer and helper T cells, and enhances intestinal absorption and proliferation. Arginine is also responsible for the synthesis of nitric oxide, which maintains the integrity of microvascular structure in the gut after injury.

3. **Omega-3 fatty acids.** The omega-6 fatty acids have been shown to impair the immune response by generating degradation products that suppress T cell and macrophage activity. Replacement of dietary omega-6 fatty acids with omega-3 fatty acids might down regulate several aspects of the inflammatory response and thereby improve immune function. A few reports have indicated, however, that omega-3 fatty acids may interfere with wound healing. Balance should therefore be maintained between the two fatty acids.

4. **Dietary nucleotides.** Dietary nucleotides are important for intestinal structure and function. In animals, the addition of dietary nucleotides to total parenteral nutrition (TPN) diminishes the intestinal mucosal atrophy. Ribonucleic acid nucleotides have also been shown to stimulate the immune system by promoting the development of T lymphocytes.

5. **Growth hormone.** In patients who are critically ill, growth hormone has beneficial anabolic effects. It is associated with the mobilization of fat stores as an energy source and the enhancement of whole-body protein stores in trauma patients. TLC and serum albumin and transferrin levels have also increased after the administration of growth hormone. Intestinal function is also enhanced directly by the binding of growth hormone to growth hormone receptors in the gut and indirectly by the growth hormone's stimulation of insulin-like growth factor.

6. **Anabolic steroids.** Anabolic steroids are sometimes used as a replacement for growth hormone because of their beneficial effect on the deposition of lean tissue. They cause less hyperglycemia than growth hormone and also cost substantially less.

VII. **Timing and route of feeding.** Although some patients can safely tolerate protein and calorie deprivation for several days, nutritional support should not be delayed in patients who are critically ill and are not expected to have any oral intake for a prolonged period. Nutritional support should also be administered promptly to patients who will have huge caloric requirements from burns, sepsis, trauma, or head injury. The decision as to which route (enteral or parenteral) to use involves assessing the functional capacity of the gut. It is important to remember that enteral feeding and parenteral feeding are not mutually exclusive; combinations are often appropriate. Each has specific advantages and complications, but overall, it appears that early nutritional support is more important than the route chosen.

A.   Enteral feeding. If the GI tract is functional, enteral feeding is preferred because it is easier, safer, and less expensive. Auscultation of the abdomen for bowel sounds as an indication of bowel function can be misleading. The absence of bowel sounds does not mean the absence of bowel function. If no air is present, there will be no bowel sounds, but the small bowel will likely still have peristalsis and absorptive function. Contraindications for the use of tube feedings include ileus, intestinal obstruction, and the need for total bowel rest. Studies in animals have shown that villus atrophy increases intestinal permeability, and bacterial translocation occurs after parental nutrition and gut disuse. Although this has yet to be demonstrated in humans, the occurrence of the sequence has been extrapolated from clinical cases in which bacteria from the gut have been cultured in patients who are critically ill and had no clear focus of abdominal infection.

   1.   Types of formulas. The selection of an enteral formula is based on the patient's digestive capacity and specific nutritional needs. Table 21-3 lists some enteral formulas and their nutritional components.

      a.   Polymeric contains intact nutrients and requires normal digestion and absorption.

      b.   Fiber enriched is frequently used in patients who have diarrhea or constipation.

      c.   Calorically dense is used in patients who have cardiac, renal, or hepatic failure and when fluid restriction is required.

      d.   Elemental contains one or more partially digested macronutrients and is used in patients who have compromised GI function.

      e.   Modular is composed of individual nutrient modules to produce a formula customized to meet a patient's specific needs. These formulations have increased caloric and protein concentrations. They can also be used to modify a preexisting commercial formula to add to the caloric and/or protein density.

      f.   There has been a great deal of interest in the immunomodulating potential of nutrients such as omega-3 fatty acids, branched-chain amino acids, nucleotides, arginine, and glutamine. While these nutrients do change the intermediate metabolic pathways that affect cellular survival *in vitro*, thus far randomized trials have not demonstrated any difference in length of hospital stay, morbidity, or mortality.

Table 21-3. Enteral formulas and their components

Product	Formula type	kcal/mL	mosmol	Composition per liter (g)		
				Protein	Fat	CHO
Osmolite	Polymeric	1.06	300	37	38	145
Osmolite HN Plus		1.2	360	56	39	158
Jevity	Fiber-enriched	1.06	300	44	36	151
Jevity Plus		1.2	450	56	39	175
Glucerna		1	375	42	56	94
Two Cal HN	Calorically dense	2	690	84	91	217
Peptamen	Peptide-based (semielemental)	1	270	40	39	127
Peptamen VHP		1	300	62	39	104
Crucial		1.5	490	94	68	135
Vivonex Plus	Elemental	1	650	45	6.7	189

CHO, carbohydrate.

2. **Routes of enteral feeding**
   a. **Gastric.** Gastric feeding can be established either by the insertion of a feeding tube through the nose to the stomach or by the surgical insertion ("open" or laparoscopically) of a gastrostomy tube. This method takes advantage of the reservoir capacity of the stomach, but many patients, especially those who have elevated intracranial pressure, might not tolerate this owing to delayed gastric emptying, impaired gag reflex, and/or gastric atony.
   b. **Duodenal.** The proposed advantage is that there is reduced risk of reflux and aspiration, but, unfortunately, there is no evidence to support this hypothesis. Patients can still aspirate, even with jejunal feeds. Feedings given into the duodenum must be as continuous infusions because large boluses are not tolerated.
   c. **Percutaneous enteral tubes.** Gastric (percutaneous endoscopic gastrostomy [PEG]) and jejunal (percutaneous endoscopic jejunostomy [PEJ]) tubes can be inserted percutaneously under either fluoroscopic or endoscopic guidance. PEG tubes allow enteral feeding of patients who have dysphagia or altered mental status. PEJ tubes allow enteral nutrition with a reduction in gastric residuals. Neither PEG nor PEJ feeding prevents aspiration.
3. **Initiation and advancement.** Before initiating enteral feeding, proper placement of the enteral tube should be ascertained radiographically. An abdominal radiograph is performed to locate the distalmost portion of the enteral tube.
   a. Isotonic solutions can be started slowly at full strength and then the rate advanced as tolerated until the goal rate is achieved. Hypertonic solutions should be diluted to isotonicity and the concentration advanced to full strength before the infusion rate is increased. These strategies help guard against diarrhea and electrolyte disturbances.
   b. Enteral feeding through the stomach (nasogastric or PEG) is typically advanced while monitoring gastric residuals. Patients requiring intensive care often have delayed gastric emptying and gastric distention, which predispose them to aspiration. Enteral feeding may begin at 10 to 15 mL/hour; and the rate is increased by 10 to 15 mL/hour every 8 hours until a predetermined goal rate is reached. If the feeds are delivered to the stomach, gastric residuals should be checked every 6 hours and infusions held for residuals of >200 mL.

  c. Emesis, gross abdominal distention with absent bowel sounds, and radiographic evidence of bowel obstruction necessitate alterations in feeding.

 4. **Complications of enteral feeding**

  a. **Mechanical.** Misplaced nasal feeding tubes might end up in the bronchus or in the brain in patients who have fractures of the cribriform plate. There is also a higher incidence of epistaxis and sinusitis because the tube passes through the nares.

  b. **GI.** Nausea and vomiting might occur from postinjury ileus and gastric atony. Diarrhea can be a problem because of the concentration, osmolarity, or volume of the administration of the tube feeds; the presence of lactose, fat, or gluten; low residue; or bacterial contamination. Diarrhea may also be caused by either the lack of fiber or an intestinal obstruction and may lead to either free water deficits or dehydration.

  c. **Pulmonary.** Pulmonary aspiration is probably the most common serious, potentially fatal complication of enteral nutrition. The reported incidence is highly variable (0% to 95%), depending on the population of patients studied and the definition of aspiration because chemical evidence of aspiration is more common than clinically diagnosed aspiration pneumonia. The presence of tube feeds in the pulmonary secretions can be detected by checking for glucose or adding food coloring to the feeds and checking the secretions for a color change.

  d. **Metabolic.** Osmolarity and volume status must be carefully monitored to avoid hyperosmolarity and volume overload. Electrolyte imbalance (e.g., hyponatremia) is common, especially in patients who have a head injury and are at risk for the syndrome of inappropriate antidiuretic hormone secretion (SIADH) or diabetes insipidus. Hypophosphatemia, hypokalemia, and hypomagnesemia occur commonly when feeding is begun again.

B. **Parenteral feeding.** TPN should be initiated when gut failure is demonstrated. Before initiating parenteral nutrition, the patient's total energy requirements, total protein requirements, daily fluid requirements, and the proportion of calories to be delivered as fat must be determined.

 1. **Parenteral solutions.** There are three elemental nutrients in parenteral nutrition.

  a. **Dextrose** is available in concentrations ranging from 10% to 70%. The higher the percentage of dextrose, the higher the osmolarity and the greater the need for central access. Only solutions with <10% dextrose are considered safe for peripheral venous administration because solutions with an osmolarity of >900 mOsm/L can cause either sclerosis or phlebitis.

b. **Amino acids** provide for protein requirement.

c. **Fat emulsions** are rich in linoleic acid. The infusions are given over several hours, and the rate of infusion should be adjusted for patients receiving propofol for sedation. Propofol is in a fat emulsion and provides the equivalent of 1.1 kcal/mL of fat calories.

d. **Additives** such as electrolytes, vitamins, and trace elements are added directly to the dextrose and amino acid infusion.

2. **Routes of parenteral feeding.** Intravenous calories can be given peripherally or centrally.

a. **Peripheral access** for administration of TPN should be used only for short-term nutritional support. The hyperosmolarity and low pH of TPN predispose small veins to thrombophlebitis. It is also difficult to provide the necessary caloric requirements by way of this route owing to the limitations imposed by dextrose (maximum 10%) and amino acid concentrations. Long peripheral lines that extend into a central vein can be used as a central line and do not have the same limitations from the dextrose and amino acid concentrations.

b. **Central access** should be used when longer periods of parenteral feeding are necessary or if the patient is seriously ill.

3. **Initiation and advancement.** Parenteral nutrition is usually started at a slow rate of infusion and then the rate is advanced every 12 to 24 hours until the goal rate is achieved. When the infusion is discontinued, the rate should be tapered so that hypoglycemia does not result from the increase in insulin production stimulated by the parenteral nutrition.

4. **Complications**

a. **Mechanical.** Significant venous thrombosis, which can usually be diagnosed by ultrasound or the injection of radiopaque contrast, requires the removal of the catheter and heparinization. Catheter infections must always be suspected. Meticulous catheter care, a high index of suspicion, and a low threshold for removal are essential.

b. **GI.** Elevated transaminases are common at the beginning of the administration of TPN, but they should not persist for long. Fatty liver might develop from the excess carbohydrates or total calories in the diet. Cholelithiasis or gall bladder sludge might be secondary to changes in bile composition as well as the decreased frequency of gallbladder contractions. These usually resolve after enteral alimentation has been initiated.

   c. **Metabolic.** Elevations in glucose can occur early from relative insulin resistance and might require an infusion of insulin. Hypercapnia can result from refeeding a malnourished patient who cannot adequately increase minute ventilation. Decreasing the daily calories or replacing dextrose with fat can reduce carbon dioxide production. Any electrolyte abnormality can occur, so that daily adjustments must be made in conjunction with the laboratory results. Suggested laboratory monitoring guidelines are listed in Table 21-4. Vitamin K is the most common vitamin deficiency, because it is not contained in multivitamin preparations.

C. **Monitoring.** While receiving enteral or parenteral nutrition, the patient must be monitored for changes in body composition, blood chemistry, blood glucose, triglycerides, and protein synthesis.

Table 21-4. Suggested monitoring guidelines for enteral and parental nutrition

Schedule	Enteral	Parenteral
Baseline	Electrolytes, BUN, Cr, Ca, Mg, PO$_4$, glucose, albumin	Electrolytes, BUN, Cr, Ca, Mg, PO$_4$, glucose, liver function tests, triglycerides, cholesterol, albumin
Daily	Intake and output, weight	Intake and output, weight
Daily until stable; then 2 to 3 times/week	Electrolytes, BUN, Cr, glucose	Electrolytes, BUN, Cr, glucose
Every other day until stable; then 1 to 2 times/week	Ca, Mg, PO$_4$	Ca, Mg, PO$_4$
Every 10–14 days	Albumin	Liver function tests, albumin, triglycerides
Weekly	PT, prealbumin	PT, prealbumin

BUN, blood urea nitrogen; PT, prothrombin time; Cr, creatinine; PO$_4$, phosphate.

1. Daily weight and the total volume of the patient's intake and output need to be monitored in addition to assessing other markers of hydration and volume status.

2. Electrolytes (Na, K, Cl, Mg, Phosphate, and Ca) and markers of renal function (blood urea nitrogen and creatinine) should be monitored routinely.

3. Intensive glycemic therapy in patients who are critically ill has been shown to reduce morbidity and mortality to a significant extent. Maintaining blood glucose levels of 80 to 110 mg/dL in all patients who are critically ill, regardless of preexisting diabetes mellitus, resulted in a relative morbidity and mortality risk reduction of approximately 40%. Recent studies also suggest that tight glycemic control in patients who have isolated severe brain injury may reduce secondary central and peripheral neurologic injury.

4. Hypertriglyceridemia is a potential complication of sedation with continuous infusion of propofol because of the lipid carrier solution. Escalating or preexisting elevated triglyceride levels may predispose patients to pancreatitis and therefore necessitate alternate sedation strategies.

D. **Refeeding syndrome.** Patients who are severely malnourished could have a physiologic response to carbohydrate utilization. During starvation, insulin production decreases in the absence of carbohydrates. Protein and fat are preferentially used to meet metabolic demands. As a result, intracellular electrolytes are depleted, especially phosphate. When carbohydrates are administered, insulin causes electrolyte and fluid shifts. This results in hypokalemia, hypomagnesemia, hypophosphatemia, and fluid retention. Without phosphate, adenosine triphosphate cannot be generated. In the most severe cases, arrhythmias, heart failure, respiratory failure, seizures, or death may occur. Prolonged fasting, prolonged intravenous hydration, chronic malnutrition, chronic alcoholism, and anorexia nervosa are a few of the risk factors for the refeeding syndrome. Closely monitoring electrolytes and vital signs can prevent a potentially fatal complication of refeeding patients who are severely malnourished.

SUGGESTED READINGS

Baudowin S, Evans T. Nutrition in the critically ill. In: Hall J, Schmidt G, Wod L, eds. *Principles of Critical Care*, 2nd ed. New York, NY: McGraw-Hill, 1998:205–220.

Dennis MS, Lewis SC, Warlow C, FOOD Trial Collaboration. Routine oral nutritional supplementation for stroke patients in hospital (FOOD): a multicenter randomized controlled trial. *Lancet* 2005;365(9461):755–763.

Dickerson RN. Hypocaloric feeding of obese patients in the intensive care unit. *Curr Opin Clin Nutr Metab Care* 2005;8:189–196.

Heyland DK. Nutritional support in the critically ill patients. A critical review of the evidence. *Curr Opin Clin Nutr Metab Care* 1998;14:423–440.

Jeremitsky E, Omert LA, Dunham CM, et al. The impact of hyperglycemia on patients with severe brain injury. *J Trauma* 2005;58:47–50.

Marik P, Varon J. The obese patient in the ICU. *Chest* 1998;113:492–498.

Slone DS. Nutritional support of the critically ill and injured patient. *Crit Care Clin* 2004;20:135–157.

Van den Berghe G, Wouters P, Weekers F, et al. Intensive insulin therapy in the critically ill patients. *N Engl J Med* 2001;345:1359–1367.

Traumatic Brain Injury, Stroke, and Brain Death

Seth Manoach and Jean G. Charchaflieh

I. **Impact of traumatic brain injury (TBI).** Each year in the United States, approximately 52,000 people die and 80,000 people suffer permanent disability as the result of TBI. The death and disability result from the impact itself (primary injury), and from subsequent changes in cerebral substrate delivery (secondary injury [Table 22-1]). In patients with severe head injury (Glasgow Coma Scale [GCS] score ≤8), the presence of hypotension (systolic blood pressure [SBP] <90 mm Hg) or hypoxia (partial pressure of arterial oxygen [PaO$_2$] , 60 mm Hg) at the time of admission is associated with increased mortality (75% when both hypotension and hypoxia were present) and poorer functional outcomes. Intracranial complications such as edema, hemorrhage, and vasospasm contribute to a reduction in cerebral blood flow (CBF) to almost 50% of the pretrauma level during the first day after TBI. Patients who have sustained either moderate or severe TBI are therefore treated in an intensive care unit (ICU) to prevent and treat secondary brain injury.

A. **Brain Trauma Foundation (BTF) clinical practice guidelines.** The BTF has developed evidence-based clinical practice guidelines that it revises periodically as new data become available. Recent studies suggest that the following ICU protocols based on BTF guidelines can decrease morbidity, mortality, and the cost of care.

1. **Initial resuscitation.** Patients who have TBI should be treated at a designated trauma center that has neurosurgical coverage or transferred to such a center after initial stabilization. The management of TBI begins with the treatment of associated injuries that may cause hypoxia, hypoventilation, and shock. This is best accomplished by using a systemic approach such as the Advanced Trauma Life Support (ATLS) Algorithm, which consists of primary and secondary surveys of the patient.

a. **Primary survey**

(1) To the extent possible, a brief history and examination are performed. The history is obtained according to the AMPLE mnemonic (**a**llergies, **m**edications, **p**ast medical history, **l**ast meal, **e**vent). Examination and immediate resuscitation are performed according to the

Table 22-1. Systemic complications contributing to secondary injury

Minutes to hours after initial impact:
  Hypoxia
  Hypercarbia
  Hypotension
  Anemia
  Hyperglycemia
Hours to days after initial impact:
  Seizures
  Infection/sepsis
  Hyperthermia
  Electrolyte disturbances
  Coagulation abnormalities

ABCDE mnemonic (**a**irway, **b**reathing, **c**irculation, **d**isability, **e**xposure).

(2) In the setting of TBI, **airway management** is performed with particular attention to changes in mean arterial pressure (MAP), intracranial pressure (ICP), and partial pressures of arterial carbon dioxide ($Paco_2$) and of oxygen (Pao_2).

  (a) Indications for **intubation** include inability to protect the airway, difficulty with either oxygenation or ventilation, shock, GCS score <9, or rapid neurologic deterioration.

  (b) Manual **in-line stabilization** of the head and neck is maintained during intubation to minimize the risk of cervical spinal cord injury in all patients in whom cervical spine injury has not been ruled out. A series of collaborative studies by a team of neurosurgeons, anesthesiologists, and radiologists has questioned this practice. Studies using fluoroscopy in cadaver models of injury found that spinal stabilization maneuvers during laryngoscopy and intubation were not helpful and may have worsened subluxation at the injury site. These results have not yet been replicated in other models or by other investigators, and as a result, manual in-line stabilization remains standard of care.

(c) **Rapid sequence induction** and intubation are performed in patients who have full stomachs, using direct laryngoscopy when this is thought to be feasible.

(d) Using these special precautions, direct laryngoscopy is considered the fastest and safest way to intubate the trachea of most patients including those who have a possible fracture of the cervical spine.

(e) Flexible **fiberoptic intubation** may be useful in patients who have difficult airways and unstable cervical spine fractures. This technique may be limited, however, in patients who are unstable or agitated or have either blood or particulate matter in the airway or significant trauma to it.

(f) Laryngeal mask airways (LMAs), including the intubating LMA, are useful backup techniques for ventilation and intubation.

(g) **Surgical airway techniques**, such as cricothyroidotomy and tracheotomy, are also backup methods for intubation and, in rare cases, the first line of management.

(h) Lidocaine, 1.5 mg/kg, given intravenously (i.v.) 1.5 minutes before intubation has been shown to blunt the increase in ICP in response to airway manipulation.

(i) The induction drugs propofol and thiopental decrease ICP, CBF, and the cerebral metabolic rate for oxygen consumption (CMR_{O_2}) and have anticonvulsantt effects. However, the associated decrease in MAP may be deleterious in patients after TBI. Etomidate, 0.3 mg/kg, may be a better choice because it produces similar decreases in ICP, CBF, and CMR_{O_2} without a significant decrease in MAP.

(j) **Muscle relaxants** facilitate tracheal intubation and decrease the risk of straining.

  (i) The depolarizing muscle relaxant succinylcholine, 1.5 mg/kg, which has the fastest onset of action among the currently available muscle relaxants (30 to

45 seconds), has been shown in animal studies to increase ICP. However, results in human studies have been inconsistent, and a controlled study in patients with brain injury demonstrated that the effects of succinylcholine on ICP were not significantly different from those of normal saline. Succinylcholine is contraindicated, however, 24 hours after TBI associated with spinal cord, crush, or burn injury owing to the risk of hyperkalemia.

(ii) Nondepolarizing neuromuscular blocking drugs (NDNMB) including rocuronium, 1 mg/kg, and mivacurium, 0.2 mg/kg, do not increase ICP and are associated with fewer side effects than succinylcholine. However, they have a slower onset of action (60 to 90 seconds).

(iii) The risks and benefits of each muscle relaxant should be carefully considered for the specific patient and situation.

(k) Endotracheal intubation must be confirmed by a CO_2 detection method such as colorimetric or continuous capnography in addition to physical examination.

(l) Chest radiographs are useful for confirming endotracheal tube (ET) position as well as associated chest pathology such as pneumothorax, lung contusion, and pulmonary edema.

(3) **Breathing** considerations include the following:

(a) **Supplemental high-flow oxygen** is provided to all patients to prevent hypoxia (Pao_2 <90 mm Hg). In patients who are mechanically ventilated, the benefit of positive end-expiratory pressure (PEEP) in improving oxygenation must be weighed against its potential effects on ICP and CBF. In patients who are euvolemic, PEEP of 5 to 10 cm H_2O is not likely to increase ICP. In patients who are hypovolemic,

PEEP >10 cm H_2O may reduce CBF.

(b) **Positive pressure ventilation** is provided as needed to maintain adequate ventilation and oxygenation. $Paco_2$ should be maintained at near normal levels of 35 to 40 mm Hg. Hyperventilation to a $Paco_2$ of 25 to 30 mm Hg decreases ICP, but its routine use is not recommended because it can also reduce CBF to ischemic levels. Hyperventilation should be used only when rapid reduction in ICP is necessary to prevent either neurologic deterioration or impending herniation.

(c) **Sedation and analgesia** are provided to patients who are conscious and mechanically ventilated. The ideal sedative drug for treating TBI would have a rapid onset and offset, anticonvulsant properties, and favorable effects on cerebral perfusion pressure (CPP), the difference between MAP and ICP. Short-acting sedative drugs, such as propofol, 10 to 50 mcg/kg/minute, and dexmedetomidine, load 1 mcg/kg over 10 minutes and then 0.2 to 0.7 mcg/kg/hour for <24 hours, have rapid onset and offset, which allows prompt awakening for neurologic assessment. The associated decrease in MAP, however, may be detrimental to CPP. Furthermore, dexmedetomidine-induced sedation in volunteers has been found to decrease regional and global CBF in excess of the accompanying fall in $CMRo_2$. Benzodiazepines such as lorazepam, 1 to 2 mg over 5 minutes repeated as necessary, are longer acting and may interfere with intermittent neurologic examination but cause less hypotension. Analgesia can be provided with opioids such as fentanyl, 0.5 to 1 mcg/kg, and morphine, 0.05 to 0.1 mg/kg, with particular attention to their respiratory and neurologic depressant effects. All the drugs may also be administered by continuous infusion.

(4) **Circulation.** Life-threatening hypovolemic or cardiogenic shock should be identified and controlled or definitively

Table 22-2. Signs and symptoms of increased intracranial pressure

Headache

Nausea, vomiting

Papilledema

Unilateral pupillary dilatation

Oculomotor or abducens palsy

Depressed level of consciousness

Irregular breathing

Midline shift (0.5 cm) or encroachment of expanding brain on cerebral ventricles (CT scan or MRI)

CT, computed tomography; MRI, magnetic resonance imaging.

treated (e.g., by the release of tension pneumothorax). SBP should be maintained at or above 90 mm Hg through the use of intravenous fluids, vasoactive drugs, or both, to maintain CPP.

(5) **Disability.** When not absolutely contraindicated by the need for immediate intubation, the initial **neurologic disability assessment** should be performed before the administration of sedative or neuromuscular blocking drugs. Neurologic status is assessed by using the GCS and looking for signs and symptoms of increased ICP (Table 22-2) and brain herniation. The GCS, a quantitative measure of neurologic status with good interevaluator agreement and an estimate of progress and prognosis, defines neurologic impairment in terms of eye opening and verbal and motor responses (Table 22-3). The total score is 15. The scores indicate the following:

Severe head injury, ≤8, persisting for 6 or more hours.

Moderate injury, 9 to 12.

Mild injury, 13 to 15.

In addition, pupillary response and the presence of lateralizing signs and spinal motor and sensory levels are carefully noted. Signs of **transtentorial brain herniation** include unilateral pupillary dilatation, sudden neurologic deterioration, contralateral hemiparesis, coma, hypertension, and bradycardia. Emergency therapy includes reassessment and treatment of extracranial

Table 22-3. Glasgow Coma Scale

Eye opening:	Spontaneous	4
	To verbal command	3
	To pain	2
	None	1
Best verbal response:	Oriented, conversing	5
	Disoriented, conversing	4
	Inappropriate words	3
	Incomprehensible sounds	2
	None	1
Best motor response:	Obeys verbal commands	6
	Localizes pain	5
	Flexion/withdrawal	4
	Flexion/abnormal (decorticate)	3
	Extension (decerebrate)	2
	None	1
	Total:	3–15

insults such as hypoxia and shock, elevation of the head of the bed (HOB) (up to 30°), infusion of mannitol, **brief** hyperventilation, and surgical decompression.

(6) **Exposure.** The patient is fully undressed and examined for any associated injuries, while precautions are taken to avoid hypothermia.

b. **Secondary survey.** The secondary survey includes a more complete history and physical examination as well as laboratory and ancillary testing to diagnose the extent of TBI and associated injuries.

(1) Indicated investigations include radiologic examination of the chest and pelvis, complete metabolic panel, complete blood count, prothrombin time (PT) and partial thromboplastin time (PTT), urinalysis, ethanol level, urine drug screen, and blood type and screen.

(2) Unless contraindicated by the need for emergency laparotomy or thoracotomy to prevent death from exsanguination, all patients who have sustained TBI should have a noncontrast computed tomographic (CT) scan of the head and cervical spine as soon as possible. In addition, CT scan of the abdomen is often necessary.

(3) If immediate laparotomy, thoracotomy, or interventional procedure is required,

the concurrent placement of an intraventricular catheter to monitor ICP should be discussed with a neurosurgeon.

(4) Plans for initial operative or nonoperative management should be based on the results of the primary and secondary survey. Epidural and subdural hematomas that exert significant mass effect have better outcomes after prompt surgical intervention than do other injury-related lesions.

2. **Critical care management after the initial resuscitation includes the following:**
   a. **ICP monitoring and treatment**
      (1) Indications for insertion of an ICP monitor include an abnormal CT scan and a GCS score of 3 to 8 after adequate resuscitation of shock and hypoxia or a normal CT scan and a GCS of 3 to 8 accompanied by two or more of the following: age >40 years, posturing, or SBP of <90 mm Hg.
      (2) ICP monitoring using an intraventricular catheter is preferred because it provides dependable readings and allows therapeutic drainage of cerebrospinal fluid (CSF).
      (3) Treatment to decrease ICP is usually initiated at ICP levels of 20 to 25 mm Hg. The aim is to maintain CPP >70 mm Hg. The CPP should be correlated with the patient's neurologic examination, overall physiologic status, and state of CBF autoregulation. Loss of autoregulation causes the CBF to depend on the MAP, which increases the risk of cerebral ischemia when the MAP falls and of hyperemia when the MAP rises. The BTF suggests maintaining a CPP of >70 mm Hg in patients whose autoregulation may be impaired because this level has been associated with improved outcome. Results of a recent study suggest that patients who have defective autoregulation, as evidenced by an increase in ICP >2 mm Hg in response to a 15 mm Hg increase in MAP (ICP/MAP slope >0.13), benefit from lowering the ICP treatment threshold to 20 mm Hg and the target CPP to 50 to 60 mm Hg. Patients whose autoregulation is intact (ICP/MAP slope <0.13) benefit from ICP treatment thresholds of 25 to 30 mm Hg and CPP >70 mm Hg.
      (4) If an ICP monitor is not in place, treatment to decrease ICP should be initiated

when either neurologic deterioration occurs or signs of brain herniation are present.

(5) Treatment of intracranial hypertension includes elevation of the head 15° to 30°, control of seizure activity, ventilation to a low-normal Pa_{CO_2} of 35 mm Hg, maintenance of normal body temperature, release of any obstruction to jugular venous outflow (e.g., tape placed circumferentially to secure the endotracheal tube), assurance of optimal fluid resuscitation and overall physiologic homeostasis, and the provision of sedation and pharmacologic muscle relaxation as needed. If these measures fail to decrease ICP, additional therapies are provided in a first- and second-tier stepwise manner.

(a) First-tier therapy involves the following:

(i) Incremental **CSF drainage** via an intraventricular catheter.

(ii) Diuresis with mannitol, 0.25 to 1.5 mg/kg over 10 minutes; recent data support the upper end of that range. Mannitol lowers ICP by deceasing brain edema and improving CBF. However, mannitol-induced diuresis may cause hypotension, especially in the early resuscitative phase when invasive monitoring is not yet in place and the extent of associated injuries is unknown. Therefore, either euvolemia or mild hypervolemia is maintained during mannitol therapy and serum osmolarity is monitored and maintained below 320 mOsm/L.

(iii) Moderate hyperventilation to a Pa_{CO_2} of 35 to 40 mm Hg also decreases ICP by reducing CBF. Hyperventilation should therefore be used briefly to treat either acute neurologic deterioration or increased ICP refractory to CSF drainage and mannitol administration.

(b) Second-tier therapy involves the following:

(i) Aggressive hyperventilation to a $Paco_2$ <30 mm Hg may be required for increased ICP refractory to first-tier therapy. When aggressive hyperventilation is used, monitoring of either jugular venous oxygen saturation (Sjo_2) or cerebral tissue oxygenation is recommended to assess the effect of decreased CBF on cerebral oxygen metabolism. The Sjo_2 percentages indicate the following:

40% or less is consistent with ischemic levels of CBF.

40% to 60% is consistent with hypoperfusion.

60% to 75% is within normal range.

75% to 90% is consistent with hyperperfusion.

90% or more indicates cessation of flow and brain death.

Changes in Sjo_2 in response to therapeutic interventions provide a useful guide to the adequacy and appropriateness of these interventions and the need for further or alternative treatment.

(ii) High-dose barbiturate therapy decreases ICP by decreasing CBF in parallel with cerebral metabolism. It is reserved for patients who are hemodynamically stable, salvageable, and have increased ICP refractory to first-tier therapy. Treatment is typically provided in the form of pentobarbital with a loading dose of 10 mg/kg over 30 minutes followed by boluses of 5 mg/kg/hour for 3 hours and then an infusion of 1 to 3 mg/kg/hour. The infusion rate is titrated to achieve electroencephalographic (EEG) burst suppression using bedside monitoring. Complications include myocardial depression and hypotension.

(iii) **Decompressive craniectomy** has been shown to decrease ICP and improve certain physiologic parameters but not overall patient outcome.

b. **Blood pressure monitoring** involves the following:

(1) The insertion of an arterial catheter allows direct, accurate, real-time measurements of MAP and regular arterial blood-gas sampling.

(2) Adequate MAP is achieved by infusing isotonic fluids to maintain either euvolemia or mild hypervolemia. If hypotension persists despite adequate volume resuscitation, vasoactive medications are added. The need for vasoactive drugs should prompt consideration of occult bleeding and other critical illnesses such as sepsis, cardiac dysfunction, neurogenic shock, and adrenal insufficiency.

c. **Monitoring intravascular volume** includes the following:

(1) Insertion of a central venous catheter that allows continuous measurement of central venous pressure (CVP), which is an indicator of intravascular volume.

(2) Insertion of an indwelling urinary catheter that facilitates measurement of urinary volume and content. The volume of urine is an additional indicator of volume status and, with urine and serum composition, facilitates the diagnosis of conditions of altered urinary output associated with TBI such as diabetes insipidus (DI), the syndrome of inappropriate antidiuretic hormone (SIADH) secretion, cerebral salt wasting syndrome, and the hyperosmolar state.

(3) Insertion of a pulmonary artery catheter that allows the measurement of pulmonary vascular pressure and calculation of cardiac output. Recent studies have questioned the benefit of pulmonary artery catheters in the management of critically ill patients.

d. **Seizure prophylaxis** is recommended during the first week after TBI, particularly in high-risk patients such as those who have GCS scores <10; cortical contusion; depressed skull fracture; subdural, epidural, or intracerebral hematoma; penetrating head trauma;

or seizures occurring within the first 24 hours after injury. This prophylaxis reduces the risk of seizures in the first week after injury but has not been demonstrated to improve outcome. The drug of choice is phenytoin, loading dose 15 mg/kg i.v., over 20 minutes followed by 5 to 7 mg/kg/day, or fosphenytoin, loading dose phenytoin equivalent (PE) 15 to 20 mg/kg i.v., and then 4 to 6 PE mg/kg/day. Adverse effects of phenytoin include fever and rash.

e. **Nutritional support** is required to facilitate recovery and should be initiated as soon as possible. By 1 week after injury, 15% of total calories should come from protein. Enteral feeding is preferred, and jejunal placement of the feeding tube protects against aspiration and gastric intolerance. Stress-ulcer prophylaxis should be provided using H_2 antagonists such as famotidine, 20 mg every 12 hours, or proton-pump inhibitors such as pantoprazole, 40 mg daily.

f. **Hyperglycemia** has been shown in animal studies to exacerbate neurologic outcome after brain injury. Prospective randomized trials in patients who are critically ill have demonstrated that patients who receive intensive insulin therapy to achieve glucose levels of 80 to 100 mg/dL had better outcomes than control patients who had glucose levels of 180 to 200 mg/dL. Retrospective data of patients with TBI suggest that early hyperglycemia is associated with poor outcomes and that nutritional support does not increase serum glucose concentration. Hyperglycemia (>200 mg/dL) must be avoided; euglycemia (80 to 110 mg/dL) may be optimal if it can be achieved without significant risk of hypoglycemic episodes.

g. **Fever** increases ICP and cerebral metabolism and may worsen outcome after TBI. Fever should be treated with cooling blankets, acetaminophen, and evaluation for infection or pharmacologic causes (e.g., phenytoin). Studies of the protective effects of hypothermia in TBI have been inconclusive. A major trial reported in 1997 demonstrated significant outcome improvements at 3 and 6 months from injury in patients admitted with GCS scores between 5 and 7. A similar trial published in 2001 was stopped after interim analysis concluded that the probability of demonstrating a significant benefit was <1%. Studies of therapeutic hypothermia in TBI are ongoing.

    h. **Steroids** have not been shown to provide any benefit to patients with TBI. A recent randomized, controlled trial suggested that they might actually increase mortality.

    i. **Drugs** designed to reduce oxidative damage, antagonize N-methyl D-aspartate (NMDA) receptors, or mitigate neurotoxicity through other mechanisms have had encouraging results in animal studies but have not been demonstrated in human trials. Drugs currently being developed or investigated in clinical trials include cannabinoids, novel NMDA and/or amino-hydroxy-methyl-isoxalone propionic acid (AMPA) antagonists, and immune modulators.

    j. **Prophylaxis** against deep venous thrombosis (DVT) with pneumatic compression devices should be initiated as soon as possible after the patient's admission to the ICU.

II. Stroke
A. Ischemic stroke

1. **Pathophysiology.** Ischemic stroke may result from cardioembolic, large-vessel atherothrombotic, or small-vessel pathology (e.g., lacunar infarct). Lacunar infarcts often occur in the basal ganglia and brain stem; they may remain subclinical or may produce dementia through multiple repeated events.

2. **Diagnosis.** The clinical presentation of ischemic stroke consists mainly of focal neurologic deficits. Headache and decreased level of consciousness are more likely to accompany hemorrhagic stroke. A noncontrast CT scan of the head differentiates between the two. The differential diagnosis of stroke includes migraine, postictal deficit, hypoglycemia, metabolic derangements, infection, and, when accompanied by chest or back pain, aortic dissection.

3. **Treatment**

    a. **Intravenous thrombolytic therapy** with recombinant tissue plasminogen activator (rTPA) has been shown to benefit patients after ischemic stroke. The randomized, double-blinded, placebo-controlled trial conducted by the National Institute of Neurologic Disorders and Stroke (NINDS) found that rTPA administered within 3 hours of the onset of symptoms resulted in a 12% absolute and 32% relative improvement in outcome. Patients who receive rTPA are more likely to have either minimal or no disability 3 months after a stroke. Patients in the treatment group experienced a 10-fold increased incidence of symptomatic intracranial hemorrhage (ICH) (6.4% vs. 0.6%), but there was no significant difference in mortality. A Cochrane review of this and other thrombolysis trials for ischemic stroke found that thrombolytic therapy reduced the combined endpoint of death or dependence and that rTPA may have advantages over the other thrombolytic agents.

(1) **Treatment criteria.** To minimize the risk of ICH and other complications, patients who receive rTPA for stroke must meet the stringent criteria derived from the NINDS and subsequent trials. Absolute and relative contraindications to the administration of rTPA must be carefully considered. There is some disagreement as to the importance of the different relative contraindications, so the risks and benefits of rTPA must be weighed in all cases.

(a) **Medical history criteria**

(i) Patients must be >18 years of age.

(ii) Patients must receive therapy within 3 hours of the onset of symptoms. Patients who cannot precisely recall the onset of symptoms (e.g., those who fell asleep >3 hours before possible drug administration and awakened with symptoms) are ineligible.

(iii) Patients should not have symptoms that suggest aneurysmal subarachnoid hemorrhage (SAH).

(iv) Patients should not have had seizures at the onset of the event.

(v) Patients must not have had another stroke, serious head trauma, or intracranial or intraspinal surgery within the past 3 months.

(vi) Patients should not have a history of ICH or bleeding from either an SAH or arteriovenous malformation.

(vii) Patients should not be taking oral anticoagulants (e.g., warfarin), have received heparin within the last 48 hours, or have coagulation abnormalities.

(viii) Relative contraindications include a major operation or trauma within the last 2 weeks, gastrointestinal or genitourinary hemorrhage within the last 3 weeks, arterial puncture at a non-compressible site within the last week, lumbar puncture within the last 3 weeks, myocardial infarction (MI) within last 3 months, or post-MI pericarditis.

(b) **Clinical examination criteria**

  (i) Patients who have minor or rapidly resolving deficits are ineligible.

  (ii) Patients should have an SBP of <185 mm Hg and diastolic blood pressure (DBP) of <110 mm Hg. A trial of nitroglycerin, 1 to 2 inches of paste; labetalol, 10 to 20 mg i.v. push over 1 to 2 minutes repeated once in 10 minutes, or enalapril, 0.625 to 1.25 mg i.v. over 5 minutes may be administered to lower blood pressure. Patients should not receive thrombolysis if these measures do not keep blood pressure below 185/110 mm Hg.

(c) **Laboratory criteria**

  (i) Platelets must be >100,000/mm^3.

  (ii) PT must be <15 seconds (international normalized ratio <1.7) with a normal PTT.

  (iii) Relative contraindication is serum glucose below 50 or above 400 mg/dL. Hypoglycemia as the etiology of the neurologic deficit must be strongly considered, especially if improvement ensues after the administration of glucose.

(d) **Radiographic criteria**

  (i) Noncontrast CT scan should demonstrate no evidence of either ICH or mass lesion.

  (ii) Review of NINDS patients who developed symptomatic ICH after thrombolysis demonstrated that the risk of developing ICH was doubled for patients who had evidence of baseline edema on their initial CT scan.

(e) Additional relative contraindications include:

(i) Pregnancy

(ii) Marked lethargy or coma

(iii) Clinical or CT-scan evidence of infarction involving >one-third of the middle cerebral artery territory, which is predictive of a significantly higher incidence of ICH.

(2) **Mode of administration**

(a) If all the above criteria are met and consent is obtained, rTPA, 0.9 mg/kg, is given intravenously with 10% as a bolus and 90% as an infusion administered over 1 hour.

(b) The drug should be administered in the emergency department if transfer to the ICU will delay therapy.

(c) During therapy, patients are monitored for evidence of ICH and neurologic deterioration.

(d) After therapy, patients are admitted to the ICU for monitoring of neurologic status and blood pressure over the next 24 to 48 hours.

(e) Blood pressure should be checked every 15 minutes for the first 2 hours and every 30 minutes thereafter.

(i) Patients with SBP of >180 mm Hg or DBP of >110 mm Hg should be treated with either labetalol, 10 mg i.v., repeated or doubled every 10 minutes to a total dose of 150 mg followed by an infusion of 1 to 8 mg/minute, if necessary, or enalapril, 0.625 to 1.25 mg i.v. over 5 minutes.

(ii) Patients with severe refractory hypertension (DBP of >140 mm Hg) are treated with nitroprusside, i.v. infusion of 0.5 to 3 mcg/kg/minute, to reduce the MAP by 10% to 20%.

(f) Anticoagulants and antiplatelet drugs are contraindicated for 24 hours after rTPA administration.

(g) Because the criteria for administration of rTPA are so strict, relatively few stroke patients are eligible to receive therapy. Means of increasing the application of this beneficial therapy include:

(i) Public health campaigns emphasizing the urgency of stroke treatment and comparing stroke to heart attack (i.e., "brain attack") to increase public awareness of the need for earlier presentation to hospitals.

(ii) Organization of stroke teams that integrate prehospital, emergency department, neurologic, critical care, laboratory, and radiology staff to facilitate rapid patient evaluation and prompt securing of crucial laboratory and radiographic data.

(3) **Future developments.** Current diagnostic and therapeutic techniques under investigation that seek to lengthen the therapeutic window for rTPA administration, increase the efficacy of rTPA, and improve salvage rates include:

(a) Use of magnetic resonance imaging to identify patients who have salvageable brain tissue and low risk of ICH so that rTPA may be administered beyond the 3-hour window.

(b) Direct intra-arterial administration of thrombolytic drugs.

(c) Intra-arterial mechanical disruption of thromboembolic occlusion.

(d) Ultrasonographic enhancement of thrombolytic therapy.

(e) Use of different thrombolytic agents or dosing regimens, or both.

b. **Nonthrombolytic therapy.** The principles of care for patients after ischemic stroke who are not candidates for rTPA emphasize the optimization of CBF, prevention of secondary brain injury, infarct extension, hemorrhagic conversion, and poststroke complications (e.g., pulmonary embolus and aspiration pneumonia), early mobilization and rehabilitation, and attention to psychiatric and social consequences of stroke, including depression and the need for assistance with daily activities.

(1) Airway management, hemodynamic monitoring, and treatment of increased ICP are provided as outlined in the preceding text.

(2) **Antihypertensive therapy** is generally avoided because, after ischemic stroke, patients tend to have long-term changes in CBF autoregulation so that optimal CBF occurs at higher MAP ranges than for healthy (normotensive) individuals. As a result, aggressive antihypertensive therapy may exacerbate ischemia by decreasing CBF. A generally accepted cutoff for the administration of antihypertensive therapies is SBP >220 mm Hg, DBP >120 mm Hg, or MAP >130 mm Hg. The treatment protocol outlined in the preceding text is recommended.

(3) In the absence of hemorrhage on a CT scan, **antiplatelet therapy** is initiated in the form of aspirin starting with 325 mg by mouth followed by 81 to 160 mg daily.

(4) Multiple studies have failed to show a benefit to heparin administration, although anticoagulation is usually initiated when atrial fibrillation is present.

(5) **Hyperglycemia** worsens neurologic outcome. Therefore, euglycemia (80 to 110 mg/dL) is beneficial if it can be achieved without substantially increasing the risk of hypoglycemia.

(6) **Seizures** are treated with phenytoin, loading dose 15 mg/kg i.v. over 20 minutes followed by 5 to 7 mg/kg/day, or fosphenytoin, loading dose PE 15 to 20 mg/kg i.v., and then 4 to 6 PE mg/kg/day.

(7) **DVT prophylaxis** is provided using pneumatic compression or low-molecular-weight heparin such as enoxaparin, 0.5 mg/kg subcutaneously twice a day.

(8) After the evaluation of airway reflexes and adequacy of swallowing, **nutrition** is provided via a suitable route.

(9) Although **elevation of the HOB to 30°** is often prescribed to facilitate venous drainage and prevent aspiration, some evidence indicates that positioning the HOB at 15° for patients who have normal ICP improves CBF and neurologic function.

(10) **Rehabilitation** and **psychiatric evaluation** are essential. Depression often complicates cerebrovascular accidents. Treatment of depression and other psychiatric comorbidities facilitates rehabilitation and improves functional status.

B. **Hemorrhagic stroke or intracranial hemorrhage (ICH)**

1. **Pathophysiology.** Hemorrhagic stroke is caused primarily by hypertensive cerebrovascular disease, and occurs most commonly in the subcortical regions of the brain. Cortical ICH often results from amyloid angiopathy, which is increasing in incidence as the population ages. Hemorrhagic stroke is devastating; only 30% of patients are able to live independently 6 months after the event. Mass effect from the post-ICH hematoma has traditionally been thought to play a major role in the pathophysiology of ICH. Recent animal data indicate, however, that the most important pathophysiologic process may be the dissection of the hematoma along tissue planes followed by neurotoxicity and cerebral edema from blood proteins and their breakdown products. Early enlargement of the hematoma occurs in approximately 40% of ICH patients and significantly worsens prognosis.

2. **Diagnosis.** Hemorrhagic stroke typically presents with headache, nausea, and vomiting as well as seizures and focal neurologic deficits. Larger hemorrhagic strokes cause lethargy, stupor, and coma.

3. **Treatment** includes rapid assessment to detect treatable conditions that may mimic hemorrhagic stroke; support of airway, breathing, and circulation; seizure control; noncontrast CT scan of the head; reversal of iatrogenic and spontaneous coagulopathy; consideration of recombinant activated factor VII (rFVIIa) therapy; and general neurointensive care.

   a. **Treatable conditions** that may mimic ICH include:

      (1) Hypoglycemia and other metabolic abnormalities, including disorders of sodium and calcium homeostasis.

      (2) Meningitis, encephalitis, sepsis, SAH, and shock.

      (3) Toxins, including illicit drugs, ethanol, environmental and occupational agents, and prescription medications administered either by the patient or a physician.

      (4) Many of these conditions can be detected by simple bedside tests and are easily treated. Hypoglycemic patients should receive glucose, 25 g i.v. Thiamine, 100 mg i.v., and naloxone, 1 mg i.v., may be initiated to patients who are suspected of either ethanol or opiate abuse.

   b. **Support of the airway, breathing, and circulation (ABC)** is provided as outlined in the preceding text.

   c. **Coagulopathy** must be corrected as rapidly as possible. Fresh frozen plasma (FFP), 15 mL/

kg i.v., rapidly reverses coagulopathy. Because this can require an infusion of a liter or more of FFP, volume status must be carefully monitored. Long-term correction of coagulopathy can be achieved by administering vitamin K, 5 mg intramuscular (i.m.) or i.v. daily for 3 days. Intravenous administration effects more rapid correction but may cause anaphylaxis. Patients who have ICH related to rTPA administration may also be treated with FFP, although there are no data on efficacy to support any specific therapy.

d. **Seizures** are treated with lorazepam, 2 mg i.v.; phenytoin, loading dose 15 mg/kg i.v. over 20 minutes followed by 5 to 7 mg/kg/day, or fosphenytoin, loading dose PE 15 to 20 mg/kg i.v., and then 4 to 6 PE mg/kg/day. The American Heart Association (AHA) recommends that seizure prophylaxis with phenytoin be given for 1 month to all patients after ICH.

e. **Euvolemia** is maintained with an intravenous infusion of isotonic solution. Hypotonic fluids may exacerbate cerebral edema, and glucose-containing solutions are not used unless patients are hypoglycemic.

f. **Treatment of elevated blood pressure** has not been shown to benefit patients who suffered ICH. Concerns about exacerbating hemorrhage must be weighed against the possibility that antihypertensive drugs may reduce CBF and worsen ischemia. As with patients after ischemic stroke, many patients who have had an hemorrhagic stroke have altered autoregulation of CBF and require a higher MAP to maintain adequate CBF. In general, an MAP of 130 mm Hg is considered to be a trigger for treating hypertension. Either labetalol or enalapril may be used as described in the preceding text to reduce MAP by approximately 10% to 15%.

g. **A recent randomized, placebo-controlled trial** indicated that the administration of rFVIIa, 80 to 160 mcg/kg i.v., within 4 hours of the onset of symptoms of hemorrhagic stroke limits expansion of the hematoma and decreases the incidence of death and severe disability at 3 months. Contraindications include thrombotic and vaso-occlusive disease. Research to refine the doses and indications for this therapy is in progress.

h. **Normothermia** is maintained.

i. Indications for placement of an intraventricular catheter for **ICP monitoring** and therapeutic CSF drainage include intraventricular hemorrhage and hydrocephalus. ICP monitoring may also be instituted in patients who are either deteriorating or comatose but are thought to be salvageable. Prophylactic antibiotics, microbiologic monitoring, and weekly dressing changes have been recommended to decrease the risk of catheter infection.

   j. Multiple trials in patients above 45 years of age have failed to demonstrate benefit from craniotomy and evacuation of an intracerebral hematoma. **Indications for operation** that have traditionally been accepted or may be inferred from recent trials include cerebellar hematomas >3 cm^2 or accompanied by neurologic deterioration, large accessible cortical hematomas (<1 cm from cortical surface), and neurologic deterioration. Younger patients are more likely to benefit from surgery than older patients.

   k. Trials of minimally invasive techniques using endoscopic evacuation of hematomas have been inconclusive, although it is possible that refinements in equipment and technique will result in improved outcome.

   l. Pneumatic compressive devices are recommended for DVT prophylaxis.

   m. Nutritional support and stress-ulcer prophylaxis are provided using H_2 antagonists such as famotidine, 20 mg i.v., every 12 hours, or proton-pump inhibitors such as pantoprazole, 40 mg i.v. daily.

   n. Steroids are contraindicated for patients with ICH.

   o. Critical care issues such as the maintenance of CPP, treatment of elevated ICP, role of barbiturate therapy, and medical complications of ICH were discussed in the preceding text.

III. Brain death and organ donation

   A. The importance of brain death and organ donation. *Brain death* is accepted as a legal definition of death in the United States and most other countries. Diagnosing brain death allows the discontinuation of artificial support of vital functions that maintain certain biologic functions in a brain-dead person. This diagnosis decreases the ambiguity and emotional suffering for family members, decreases the waste of medical resources, and allows for organ donation. Appropriate counseling of family members is essential in helping them understand and accept the reality of death despite the apparent maintenance of certain aspects of life through artificial means. Coordinators of organ procurement organizations (OPOs) assist in this process by counseling family members, clarifying legal issues, helping in the consent process, providing advice about care for the brain-dead organ donor, and arranging organ harvest. This process shifts the focus of care from resuscitation to organ preservation for harvesting and transplantation.

B. Physiology of brain death. Brain death entails the cessation of CBF with resultant loss of brain function. The final common pathway for brain death is the loss of cerebral perfusion with the cessation of brain stem activity. The process proceeds in a rostral to caudal direction. Loss of blood flow to the medulla is often accompanied by a catecholamine surge that results in increased MAP, followed by hemodynamic instability and even frank hypotension. This process is followed by metabolic derangements from ischemia or infarction of the pituitary gland. The most important consequence of pituitary dysfunction is central DI, requiring the replacement of antidiuretic hormone for the maintenance of sodium and fluid balance.

C. Diagnosis of brain death

    1. Brain death is clinically marked by complete unresponsiveness, apnea, and loss of brain stem reflexes. Cessation of cortical function often precedes brain stem death but is not sufficient for diagnosis because patients may retain brain stem function indefinitely. Brain death can be diagnosed only when the cause of the coma has been identified (e.g., TBI, ICH, SAH) and conditions that mimic brain death have been ruled out clinically. These conditions include the locked-in syndrome, severe hypothermia, severe intoxication (including anesthetic and neuromuscular blocking drugs), and Guillain-Barré syndrome with peripheral and cranial nerve involvement. Brain death is diagnosed clinically; the need for confirmation with ancillary tests is based on patient status and age. Spinal reflexes are often maintained and do not contradict the diagnosis of brain death. Demonstration of the absence of brain stem reflexes and confirmation of apnea are central to the diagnosis (Table 22-4).

    2. The apnea test is performed as follows:

        a. The patient is **preoxygenated** with 100% oxygen.

        b. Apneic oxygenation is provided at 15 L/minute through a catheter placed in the ET tube to the level of the carina.

        c. The patient is disconnected from the ventilator and observed for spontaneous ventilation.

        d. Pa_{CO_2} typically rises at 3 mm Hg/minute of apnea. In the United States, apnea in the presence of a rise of Pa_{CO_2} to 60 mm Hg or an increase of 20 mm Hg from baseline is considered confirmatory. The United Kingdom Code of Practice recommends a 10-minute apnea test.

Table 22-4. Clinical criteria for brain death in adults and children

Coma

Absence of motor responses

Absence of pupillary responses to light and pupils at midposition
with respect to dilatation (4–6 mm)

Absence of corneal reflexes

Absence of caloric responses

Absence of gag reflex

Absence of coughing in response to tracheal suctioning

Absence of sucking and rooting reflexes

Absence of respiratory drive at a $PaCO_2$ of 60 mm Hg or 20 mm Hg
above normal base-line values[a]

Interval between two evaluations, according to patient's age

    Term to 2 mo old, 48 hr

    >2 mo to 1 y old, 24 hr

    >1 y to <18 y old, 12 hr

    >18 y old, interval optional

Confirmatory test

    Term to 2 mo old, 2 confirmatory tests

    >2 mo to 1 y old, 1 confirmatory test

    >1 y to <18 y old, optional

    >18 y old, optional

[a] $PaCO_2$ denotes the partial pressure of arterial carbon dioxide tension.

      3. **Confirmatory testing** for brain death includes:
        a. **Isoelectric EEG**
        b. **Absence of cerebral perfusion** as demonstrated by cerebral angiography, technetium 99 scanning, or transcranial Doppler ultrasonography
    D. **Care of the brain-dead organ donor.** This should be done in coordination with the local OPO coordinator.
      1. **Exclusion criteria for organ donation** may vary by organ and by geographic region. This should be discussed with the OPO coordinator. In general, absolute contraindications include human immunodeficiency virus (HIV) disease, metastatic cancer, sepsis, and prion disease.
      2. **Screening tests for organ donors include:**
        a. HIV, hepatitis B, hepatitis C, cytomegalovirus (CMV), Epstein-Barr virus (EBV), and human T-cell lymphoma/leukemia virus-1 (HTLV-1) serology
        b. ABO and human lymphocyte antigen (HLA) typing
        c. Blood, sputum, and urine cultures

   d. Complete blood count, metabolic panel, urinalysis, arterial blood gas
   e. Organ-specific tests as requested by the OPO
3. **Perioperative monitoring** includes electrocardiogram, pulse oximetry, temperature, urine output, invasive arterial blood pressure, and central venous and/or pulmonary artery pressures. Because the process of organ harvest requires sequential vessel ligation, the arterial catheter should be inserted in the left arm, and the central venous or pulmonary artery catheterization should be performed on the right.
4. **Optimal physiologic goals** for organ donors include:
   a. MAP 60 to 80 mm Hg; SBP >90 mm Hg
   b. CVP 8 to 12 mm Hg; pulmonary artery wedge pressure 10 to 15 mm Hg
   c. Heart rate 60 to 100 beats/minute
   d. Cardiac index >2.1 L/minute/m^2
   e. Urine output 1 to 2 mL/kg/hour, with volume replacement generally 50 mL/hour more than urine output
   f. Temperature maintained between 97° and 100° F using warming or cooling blankets
5. **Therapeutic maneuvers** include the following:
   a. **Antiarrhythmic drugs** for the treatment of arrhythmia.
   b. **Isoproterenol or cardiac pacing** for the treatment of severe bradycardia.
   c. **Isotonic intravenous fluids** to maintain targeted blood pressure and CVP.
   d. **If hypotension persists** after achieving CVP of 10 mm Hg, vasoactive drugs are used as follows:
      (1) Dopamine, 5 to 15 mcg/kg/minutes, for hypotension with normal or elevated cardiac output.
      (2) Dobutamine, 5 to 10 mcg/kg/minutes, is added for hypotension with decreased cardiac output. Dobutamine may cause hypotension through its beta-agonist effects and tachydysrhythmia, particularly when combined with dopamine.
      (3) Phenylephrine, 100 mcg loading dose followed by an infusion of 50 to 150 mcg/minute, may be added to dobutamine to counteract its beta-agonist effects.
      (4) Dobutamine, 5 to 10 mcg/kg/minute, is the drug of choice for patients who have decreased cardiac output and increased systemic vascular resistance.
   e. **DI** involves increased urine output (>7 mL/kg/hour), decreased urine-specific gravity (<1.010), decreased urine osmolarity (less than serum osmolarity), hypernatremia

($>$150 mEq/L), and serum hyperosmolarity ($>$295 mOsm/L). Treatment includes the infusion of dextrose 5% in water (D_5W) to replace free-water deficits and maintain serum Na at $<$155 mEq/L and the administration of vasopressin, 1 unit i.v., bolus followed by 0.5 to 4 units/hour, to maintain urine output between 1 and 2 mL/kg/hour.

f. Insulin infusion, 2 to 7 units/hour, may be needed to maintain serum glucose between 80 and 160 mg/dL. Replacement to maintain potassium (K) at $>$4 mEq/L may be needed with insulin infusions.

g. Triiodothyronine, 4 mcg i.v. bolus followed by 3 mcg/hour, is administered to maintain euthyroid status.

h. Mechanical ventilation should be performed with the aim of minimizing lung injury.

    (1) Ventilation rate is set to maintain normocapnia. Triggered breaths may result from cardiac activity and may be confused with spontaneous ventilation.

    (2) Tidal volume is set at 6 to 8 mL/kg. Pressure-controlled ventilation may be used as an alternative to minimize barotrauma.

    (3) PEEP is kept as close to 5 mm Hg as possible.

    (4) The fraction of inspired oxygen (FIO_2) is reduced to the minimum value necessary to maintain PaO_2 at $>$90 mm Hg. The target FIO_2 is $<$40%.

i. Hypokalemia, hypophosphatemia, and hypocalcemia are common electrolyte abnormalities that must be monitored and corrected.

j. Packed red blood cells are transfused to maintain hemoglobin at $\geq$9 g/dL.

k. FFP and platelets are transfused to correct coagulopathy and bleeding disorders.

l. The OPO coordinator usually recommends methylprednisolone, 15 mg/kg i.v., as well as an antibiotic regimen.

6. Organ harvesting is typically performed by different teams that represent various potential recipients. The OPO coordinates the process which includes steps designed to minimize warm ischemia time for each organ. Muscle relaxants are often used to facilitate organ harvest and prevent reflex movements. After opening the thoracoabdominal cavity, the bowel is retracted, organ attachments are incised, and major vessels are cannulated for infusion of cold organ-preservation solution. The aorta is then cross-clamped, preservative solution is infused, and the organs are removed. Mechanical ventilation is terminated after the preservative solution is administered and cardioplegia occurs.

E. **Non-heart beating donors (NHBDs).** NHBDs are non-brain-dead patients who have irreversible disease processes from whom resuscitative care is withdrawn either because of advanced directives or upon request of the next of kin. Organ harvesting is initiated immediately after death. Success rates for renal transplants from NHBDs are similar to those for kidneys harvested from brain-dead donors. Livers and lungs may also be suitable. Corneas, bones, skin, and heart valves are all relatively durable and can be donated up to 24 hours after death. Physicians should consult with hospital ethicists, risk-management staff, and the local OPO when the withdrawal of resuscitative care from a potential NHBD is being considered.

SUGGESTED READINGS

Andrews PJD. Critical care management of acute ischemic stroke. *Curr Opin Crit Care* 2004;10:110–115.

Brain Trauma Foundation. *Management and prognosis of severe traumatic brain injury*, www.braintrauma.org/guidelines Accessed, 2006.

Broderick JP, Adams HP, Barsan W, et al. Guidelines for the management of spontaneous intracerebral hemorrhage: a statement for healthcare professionals from a special writing group of the stroke council, American Heart Association. *Stroke* 1999;30:905–915.

Chestnut RM, Marshall LF, Klaubner MR, et al. The role of secondary brain injury in determining outcome from severe head injury. *J Trauma* 1993;34:216–222.

Clifton GL, Miller ER, Choi SC, et al. Lack of effect of induction of hypothermia after acute brain injury. *N Engl J Med* 2001;344:544–563.

Cruz J, Minoja G, Okuchi K. Major clinical and physiologic benefits of early high doses of mannitol for intraparenchymal temporal lobe hemorrhages with abnormal pupillary widening: a randomized trial. *Neurosurgery* 2002;51:628–638.

Edwards P, Arango M, Balica L. Final results of MRC CRASH, a randomised placebo-controlled trial of intravenous corticosteroid in adults with head injury-outcomes at 6 months. *Lancet* 2005;365:1957–1959.

Fakhry SM, Trask AL, Waller MA, et al. Management of brain-injured patients by an evidence-based protocol improves outcomes and decreases hospital charges. *J Trauma* 2005;56:492–500.

Haltiner AM, Newell DW, Temkin NR, et al. Side effects and mortality associated with the use of phenytoin for early posttraumatic seizure prophylaxis. *J Neurosurg* 1999;91:588–592.

Howells T, Elf K, Jones PA, et al. Pressure reactivity as a guide in the treatment of cerebral perfusion pressure in patients with brain trauma. *J Neurosurg* 2005;102:311–317.

Hutchinson PJ, Kirkpatrick PJ. Decompressive craniectomy after head injury. *Curr Opin Crit Care* 2004;10:101–104.

Intensive Care Society Working Group on Organ and Tissue Donation. *Guidelines for adult organ and tissue donation*, www.ics.ac.uk/downloads/Standards/Master%20ICS%20Guidelines%20all%20sections%20(Nov04).PDF

Jeremitsky E, Omert LA, Dunham CM, et al. The impact of hyperglycemia on patients with severe brain injury. *J Trauma* 2005;58:47–50.

Kovarik WD, Mayberg TS, Lam AM, et al. Succinylcholine does not change intracranial pressure, cerebral blood flow velocity, or the electroencephalogram in patients with neurologic injury. *Anesth Analg* 1994;78:469–473.

Marion DW, Puccio A, Wisniewski SR, et al. Effect of hyperventilation on extracellular concentrations of glutamate, lactate, pyruvate, and local cerebral blood flow in patients with severe traumatic brain injury. *Crit Care Med* 2002;30:2619–2625.

Mayer SA, Brun NC, Begtrup K, et al. Recombinant activated factor VII for acute intracerebral hemorrhage. *N Engl J Med* 2005;352:777–785.

Mendelow A, Gregson BA, Fernandes HM, et al. Early surgery versus initial conservative treatment in patients with spontaneous intracerebral hematomas in the International Surgical Trial in Intracerebral Haemorrhage (STICH): a randomised trial. *The Lancet* 2005;365:387–397.

Mielke O, Wardlaw J, Liu M. Thrombolysis (different doses, routes of administration and agents) for acute ischaemic stroke. *Cochrane Database Syst Rev* 2004(4): CD000514.

Nakano T, Ohkuma H. Surgery versus conservative treatment for intracerebral haemorrhage - is there an end to the long controversy? *The Lancet* 2005;365:361–362.

Ramos HC, Lopez R. Critical care management of the brain-dead organ donor. *Curr Opin Organ Transplant* 2002;7:70–75.

The National Institute of Neurological Disorders and Stroke r-TPA Stroke Study Group. Tissue plasminogen activator for acute ischemic stroke. *N Engl J Med* 1995;333:1581–1587.

Tuhrim S. Management of stroke and transient ischemic attack. *Mt Sinai J Med* 2002;69:121–130.

Wardlaw JM, del Zoppo G, Yamaguchi T, et al. Thrombolysis for acute ischaemic stroke. *Cochrane Database Syst Rev* 2003;(3):CD000213.

Wijdicks EFM. The diagnosis of brain death. *N Engl J Med* 2001;344:1215–1221.

Wojner-Alexandrov AW, Garami Z, Chernyshev OY, et al. Flat positioning improves blood flow velocity in acute ischemic stroke. *Neurology* 2005;64:1354–1357.

Index

Note: Page numbers followed by *f* indicate figures; those followed by *t* indicate tables.

When I left the meeting, I had the definite impression that I had found the same game as with the seals: management reducing criteria and accepting more and more errors that weren't designed into the device, while the engineers are screaming from below, "HELP!" and "This is a RED ALERT!"

The next evening, on my way home in the airplane, I was having dinner. After I finished buttering my roll, I took the little piece of thin cardboard that the butter pat comes on, and bent it around in a U shape so there were two edges facing me. I held it up and started blowing on it, and pretty soon I got it to make a noise like a whistle.

Back in California, I got some more information on the shuttle engine and its probability of failure. I went to Rocketdyne and talked to engineers who were building the engines. I also talked to consultants for the engine. In fact one of them, Mr. Covert, was on the commission. I also found out that a Caltech professor had been a consultant for Rocketdyne. He was very friendly and informative, and told me about all the problems the engine had, and what he thought the probability of failure was.

I went to JPL and met a fellow who had just written a report for NASA on the methods used by the FAA* and the military to certify their gas turbine and rocket engines. We spent the whole day going back and forth over how to determine the probability of failure in a machine. I learned a lot of new names—like "Weibull," a particular mathematical distribution that makes a certain shape on a graph. He said that the

---

* Federal Aviation Administration.

original safety rules for the shuttle were very similar to those of the FAA, but that NASA had modified them as they began to get problems.

It turned out that NASA's Marshall Space Center in Huntsville designed the engine, Rocketdyne built them, Lockheed wrote the instructions, and NASA's Kennedy Space Center installed them! It may be a genius system of organization, but it was a complete fuzdazzle, as far as I was concerned. It got me terribly confused. I didn't know whether I was talking to the Marshall man, the Rocketdyne man, the Lockheed man, or the Kennedy man! So in the middle of all this, I got lost. In fact, all during this time—in March and April—I was running back and forth so much between California, Alabama, Houston, Florida, and Washington, D.C., that I often didn't know what day it was, or where I was.

After all this investigating on my own, I thought I'd write up a little report on the engine for the other commissioners. But when I looked at my notes on the testing schedules, there was some confusion: there would be talk about "engine #12" and how long "the engine" flew. But no engine ever was like that: it would be repaired all the time. After each flight, technicians would inspect the engines and see how many cracked blades there were on the rotor, how many splits there were in the casing, and so on. Then they'd repair "the engine" by putting on a new casing, a new rotor, or new bearings—they would replace lots of parts. So I would read that a particular engine had rotor #2009, which had run for 27 minutes in flight such-and-such, and casing #4091, which had run for 53 minutes in flights such-and-such and so-and-so. It was all mixed up.

When I finished my report, I wanted to check it. So the next time I was at Marshall, I said I wanted to talk to the engineers about a few very technical problems, just to check the details—I didn't need any management there.

This time, to my surprise, nobody came but the three engineers I had talked to before, and we straightened everything out.

When I was about to leave, one of them said, "You know that question you asked us last time—with the papers? We felt that was a loaded question. It wasn't fair."

I said, "Yes, you're quite right. It *was* a loaded question. I had an idea of what would happen."

The guy says, "I would like to revise my answer. I want to say that I cannot quantify it." (This guy was the one who had the most detailed answer before.)

I said, "That's fine. But do you agree that the chance of failure is 1 in 100,000?"

"Well, uh, no, I don't. I just don't want to answer."

Then one of the other guys says, "I said it was 1 in 300, and I still say it's 1 in 300, but I don't want to tell you how I got my number."

I said, "It's okay. You don't have to."

AN INFLAMED APPENDIX

All during this time, I had the impression that somewhere along the line the whole commission would
come together again so we could talk to each other
about what we had found out.

In order to aid such a discussion, I thought I'd write little
reports along the way: I wrote about my work with the ice crew
(analyzing the pictures and the faulty temperature readings);
I wrote about my conversations with Mr. Lamberth and the
assembly workers; and I even wrote about the piece of paper
that said "Let's go for it." All these little reports I sent to Al
Keel, the executive officer, to give to the other commissioners.

Now, this particular adventure—investigating the lack of
communication between the managers and the engineers
who were working on the engine—I also wrote about, on my
little IBM PC at home. I was kind of tired, so I didn't have the
control I wanted—it wasn't written with the same care as my
other reports. But since I was writing it only as a report to
the other commissioners, I didn't change the language before
I sent it on to Dr. Keel. I simply attached a note that said "I

think the other commissioners would be interested in this, but you can do with it what you want—it's a little strong at the end."

He thanked me, and said he sent my report to everybody.

Then I went to the Johnson Space Center, in Houston, to look into the avionics. Sally Ride's group was there, investigating safety matters in connection with the astronauts' experiences. Sally introduced me to the software engineers, and they gave me a tour of the training facilities for the astronauts.

It's really quite wonderful. There are different kinds of simulators with varying degrees of sophistication that the astronauts practice on. One of them is just like the real thing: you climb up, you get in; at the windows, computers are producing pictures. When the pilot moves the controls, the view out of the windows changes.

This particular simulator had the double purpose of teaching the astronauts and checking the computers. In the back of the crew area, there were trays full of cables running down through the cargo bay to somewhere in the back, where instruments simulated signals from the engines—pressures, fuel flow rates, and so on. (The cables were accessible because the technicians were checking for "cross talk"—interferences in the signals going back and forth.)

The shuttle itself is operated essentially by computer. Once it's lit up and starts to go, nobody inside does anything, because there's tremendous acceleration. When the shuttle reaches a certain altitude, the computers adjust the engine thrust down for a little while, and as the air thins out, the computers adjust the thrust up again. About a minute later, the two solid rocket boosters fall away, and a few minutes after that, the main fuel tank falls away; each operation is controlled by the computers.

The shuttle gets into orbit automatically—the astronauts just sit in their seats.

The shuttle's computers don't have enough memory to hold all the programs for the whole flight. After the shuttle gets into orbit, the astronauts take out some tapes and load in the program for the next phase of the flight—there are as many as six in all. Near the end of the flight, the astronauts load in the program for coming down.

The shuttle has four computers on board, all running the same programs. All four are normally in agreement. If one computer is out of agreement, the flight can still continue. If only two computers agree, the flight has to be curtailed and the shuttle brought back immediately.

For even more safety, there's a fifth computer—located away from the other four computers, with its wires going on different paths—which has only the program for going up and the program for coming down. (Both programs can barely fit into its memory.) If something happens to the other computers, this fifth computer can bring the shuttle back down. It's never had to be used.

The most dramatic thing is the landing. Once the astronauts know where they're supposed to land, they push one of three buttons—marked Edwards, White Sands, and Kennedy—which tells the computer where the shuttle's going to land. Then some small rockets slow the shuttle down a little, and get it into the atmosphere at just the right angle. That's the dangerous part, where all the tiles heat up.

During this time, the astronauts can't see anything, and everything's changing so fast that the descent has to be done automatically. At around 35,000 feet the shuttle slows down to less than the speed of sound, and the steering can be done manually, if necessary. But at 4000 feet something happens that is not done by the computer: the pilot pushes a button to lower the landing wheels.

I found that very odd—a kind of silliness having to do with the psychology of the pilots: they're heroes in the eyes of the public; everybody has the idea that they're steering the shuttle around, whereas the truth is they don't have to do anything until they push that button to lower the landing gear. They can't stand the idea that they really have nothing to do.

I thought it would be safer if the computer would lower the landing wheels, in case the astronauts were unconscious for some reason. The software engineers agreed, and added that putting down the landing wheels at the wrong time is very dangerous.

The engineers told me that ground control can send up the signal to lower the landing wheels, but this backup gave them some pause: what happens if the pilot is half-conscious, and thinks the wheels should go down at a certain time, and the controller on the ground knows it's the wrong time? It's much better to have the whole thing done by computer.

The pilots also used to control the brakes. But there was lots of trouble: if you braked too much at the beginning, you'd have no more brake-pad material left when you reached the end of the runway—and you're still moving! So the software engineers were asked to design a computer program to control the braking. At first the astronauts objected to the change, but now they're very delighted because the automatic braking works so well.

Although there's a lot of good software being written at Johnson, the computers on the shuttle are so obsolete that the manufacturers don't make them anymore. The memories in them are the old kind, made with little ferrite cores that have wires going through them. In the meantime we've developed much better hardware: the memory chips of today are much, much smaller; they have much greater capacity; and they're much more reliable. They have internal error-correcting codes that automatically keep the memory good. With today's computers we can design separate program modules so that changing the payload doesn't require so much program rewriting.

Because of the huge investment in the flight simulators and all the other hardware, to start all over again and replace the millions of lines of code that they've already built up would be very costly.

I learned how the software engineers developed the avionics for the shuttle. One group would design the software programs, in pieces. After that, the parts would be put together into huge programs, and tested by an independent group.

After both groups thought all the bugs had been worked out, they would have a simulation of an entire flight, in which every part of the shuttle system is tested. In such cases, they had a principle: this simulation is not just an exercise to check if the programs are all right; it is a *real flight*—if anything fails now, it's extremely serious, as if the astronauts were really on board and in trouble. Your reputation is on the line.

In the many years they had been doing this, they had had only six failures at the level of flight simulation, and not one in an actual flight.

So the computer people looked like they knew what they were doing: they knew the computer business was vital to the shuttle but potentially dangerous, and they were being extremely careful. They were writing programs that operate a very complex machine in an environment where conditions are changing drastically—programs which measure those changes, are flexible in their responses, and maintain high safety and accuracy. I would say that in some ways they were once in the forefront of how to ensure quality in robotic or interactive computer systems, but because of the obsolete hardware, it's no longer true today.

I didn't investigate the avionics as extensively as I did the engines, so I might have been getting a little bit of a sales talk, but I don't think so. The engineers and the managers communicated well with each other, and they were all very careful not to change their criteria for safety.

I told the software engineers I thought their system and their attitude were very good.

One guy muttered something about higher-ups in NASA wanting to cut back on testing to save money: "They keep saying we always pass the tests, so what's the use of having so many?"

Before I left Houston, I continued my surreptitious investigation of the rumor that the White House had put pressure on NASA to launch the shuttle. Houston is the center of communication, so I went over to the telemetry people and asked about their switching system. I went through the same stuff as I did in Florida—and they were just as nice to me—but this time I found out that if they wanted to tie in the shuttle to the Congress, the White House, or to anywhere, they need a three-minute warning—not three months, not three days, not three hours—three minutes. Therefore they can do it whenever they want, and nothing has to be written down in advance. So that was a blind alley.

I talked to a *New York Times* reporter about this rumor one time. I asked him, "How do you find out if things like this are true?"

He says, "One of the things I thought to do was to go down and talk to the people who run the switching system. I tried that, but I wasn't able to come up with anything."

During the first half of April, General Kutyna's group received the final results of the tests NASA was making at Marshall. NASA included its own interpretations of the results, but we thought we should write everything over again in our own way. (The only exceptions were when a test didn't show anything.)

General Kutyna set up a whole system at Marshall for writing our group's report. It lasted about two days. Before we could get anywhere, we got a message from Mr. Rogers: "Come back to Washington. You shouldn't do the writing down there."

So we went back to Washington, and General Kutyna gave me an office in the Pentagon. It was fine, but there was no secretary, so I couldn't work fast.

Bill Graham had always been very cooperative, so I called him up. He arranged for me to use a guy's office—the guy was out of town—and his secretary. She was very, very helpful: she could write up something as fast as I could say it, and then she'd revamp it, correcting my mistakes. We worked very hard for about two or three days, and got large pieces of the report written that way. It worked very well.

Neil Armstrong, who was in our group, is extremely good at writing. He would look at my work and immediately find every weak spot, just like that—he was right every time—and I was very impressed.

Each group was writing a chapter or two of the main report. Our group wrote some of the stuff in "Chapter 3: The Accident," but our main work was "Chapter 4: The Cause of the Accident." One result of this system, however, was that we never had a meeting to discuss what each of our groups found out—to comment on each other's findings from our different perspectives. Instead, we did what they call "wordsmithing"—or what Mr. Hotz later called "tombstone engraving"—correcting punctuation, refining phrases, and so on. We never had a *real* discussion of ideas, except incidentally in the course of this wordsmithing.

For example, a question would come up: "Should this sentence about the engines be worded this way or that way?"

I would try to get a little discussion started. "From my own experiences, I got the impression that the engines aren't as good as you're saying here . . ."

So they'd say, "Then we'll use the more conservative wording here," and they'd go on to the next sentence. Perhaps that's a very efficient way to get a report out quickly, but we spent meeting after meeting doing this wordsmithing.

Every once in a while we'd interrupt that to discuss the typography and the color of the cover. And after each discussion, we were asked to vote. I thought it would be most efficient to vote for the same color we had decided on in the meeting before, but it turned out I was always in the minority! We finally chose red. (It came out blue.)

One time I was talking to Sally Ride about something I mentioned in my report on the engines, and she didn't seem to know about it. I said, "Didn't you see my report?"

She says, "No, I didn't get a copy."

So I go over to Keel's office and say, "Sally tells me she didn't get a copy of my report."

He looks surprised, and turns to his secretary. "Please make a copy of Dr. Feynman's report for Dr. Ride."

Then I discover Mr. Acheson hasn't seen it.

"Make a copy and give it to Mr. Acheson."

I finally caught on, so I said, "Dr. Keel, I don't think anybody has seen my report."

So he says to his secretary, "Please make a copy for all the commissioners and give it to them."

Then I said to him, "I appreciate how much work you're doing, and that it's difficult to keep everything in mind. But I thought you told me that you showed my report to everybody."

He says, "Yes, well, I meant all of the staff."

I later discovered, by talking to people on the staff, that they hadn't seen it either.

When the other commissioners finally got to see my report, most of them thought it was very good, and it ought to be in the commission report somewhere.

Encouraged by that, I kept bringing up my report. "I'd like to have a meeting to discuss what to do with it," I kept saying.

"We'll have a meeting about it next week" was the standard answer. (We were too busy wordsmithing and voting on the color of the cover.)

Gradually I realized that the way my report was written, it would require a lot of wordsmithing—and we were running out of time. Then somebody suggested that my report could go in as an appendix. That way, it wouldn't have to be word-smithed to fit in with anything else.

But some of the commissioners felt strongly that my report should go in the main report somehow: "The appendices won't come out until months later, so nobody will read your report if it's an appendix," they said.

I thought I'd compromise, however, and let it go in as an appendix.

But now there was a new problem: my report, which I had written on my word processor at home, would have to be con-verted from the IBM format to the big document system the commission was using. They had a way of doing that with an optical scanning device.

I had to go to a little bit of trouble to find the right guy to do it. Then, it didn't get done right away. When I asked what happened, the guy said he couldn't find the copy I had given him. So I had to give him another copy.

A few days later, I finished writing my report about the avionics, and I wanted to combine it with my report on the engines. So I took the avionics report to the guy and I said, "I'd like to put this in with my other report."

Then I needed to see a copy of my new report for some rea-son, but the guy gave me an old copy, before the avionics was added. "Where's the new one with the avionics?" I said.

"I can't find it"—and so on. I don't remember all the details, but it seemed my report was always missing or half-cooked. It could easily have been mistakes, but there were too many of them. It was quite a struggle, nursing my report along.

Then, in the last couple of days, when the main report is ready to be sent to the printer, Dr. Keel wants my report to be wordsmithed too, even though it's going in as an appendix. So I took it to the regular editor there, a capable man named Hansen, and he fixed it up without changing the sense of it. Then it was put back into the machine as "Version #23"—there were revisions and revisions.

(By the way: *everything* had 23 versions. It has been noted that computers, which are supposed to increase the speed at which we do things, have not increased the speed at which we write reports: we used to make only three versions—because they're so hard to type—and now we make 23 versions!)

The next day I noticed Keel working on my report: he had put all kinds of big circles around whole sections, with X's through them; there were all kinds of thoughts left out. He explained, "This part doesn't have to go in because it says more or less what we said in the main report."

I tried to explain that it's much easier to get the logic if all the ideas are together, instead of everything being distributed in little pieces all over the main report. "After all," I said, "it's only gonna be an appendix. It won't make any difference if there's a little repetition."

Dr. Keel put back something here and there when I asked him to, but there was still so much missing that my report wasn't anything like it was before.

THE TENTH RECOMMENDATION

S ometime in May, at one of our last meetings, we got around to making a list of possible recommendations. Somebody would say, "Maybe one of the things we should discuss is the establishment of a safety board."

"Okay, we'll put that down."

I'm thinking, "At last! We're going to have a discussion!"

But it turns out that this tentative list of topics *becomes* the recommendations—that there be a safety board, that there be a this, that there be a that. The only discussion was about which recommendation we should write first, which one should come second, and so forth.

There were many things I wanted to discuss further. For example, in regard to a safety board, one could ask: "Wouldn't such a committee just add another layer to an already overgrown bureaucracy?"

There had been safety boards before. In 1967, after the Apollo accident, the investigating committee at the time invented a special panel for safety. It worked for a while, but it didn't last.

We didn't discuss why the earlier safety boards were no longer effective; instead, we just made up more safety boards: we called them the "Independent Solid Rocket Motor Design Oversight Committee," the "Shuttle Transportation System Safety Advisory Panel," and the "Office of Safety, Reliability, and Quality Assurance." We decided who would oversee each safety board, but we didn't discuss whether the safety boards created by our commission had any better chance of working, whether we could fix the existing boards so they *would* work, or whether we should have them at all.

I'm not as sure about a lot of things as everybody else. Things need to be thought out a little bit, and we weren't doing enough *thinking* together. Quick decisions on important matters are not very good—and at the speed we were going, we were bound to make some impractical recommendations.

We ended up rearranging the list of possible recommendations and wordsmithing them a little, and then we voted yes or no. It was an odd way of doing things, and I wasn't used to it. In fact, I got the feeling we were being railroaded: things were being decided, somehow, a little out of our control.

At any rate, in our last meeting, we agreed to nine recommendations. Many of the commissioners went home after that meeting, but I was going to New York a few days later, so I stayed in Washington.

The next day, I happened to be standing around in Mr. Rogers's office with Neil Armstrong and another commissioner when Rogers says, "I thought we should have a tenth recommendation. Everything in our report is so negative; I think we need something positive at the end to balance it."

He shows me a piece of paper. It says,

> The Commission strongly recommends that NASA con-
> tinue to receive the support of the Administration and
> the nation. The agency constitutes a national resource
> and plays a critical role in space exploration and devel-
> opment. It also provides a symbol of national pride and
> technological leadership. The Commission applauds
> NASA's spectacular achievements of the past and antic-
> ipates impressive achievements to come. The findings
> and recommendations presented in this report are
> intended to contribute to the future NASA successes
> that the nation both expects and requires as the 21st cen-
> tury approaches.

In our four months of work as a commission, we had never
discussed a policy question like that, so I felt there was no reason to put it in. And although I'm not saying I disagreed with
it, it wasn't obvious that it was true, either. I said, "I think this
tenth recommendation is inappropriate."

I think I heard Armstrong say, "Well, if somebody's not in
favor of it, I think we shouldn't put it in."

But Rogers kept working on me. We argued back and forth a
little bit, but then I had to catch my flight to New York.

While I was in the airplane, I thought about this tenth recommendation some more. I wanted to lay out my arguments
carefully on paper, so when I got to my hotel in New York, I
wrote Rogers a letter. At the end I wrote, "This recommendation reminds me of the NASA flight reviews: 'There are critical
problems, but never mind—keep on flying!'"

It was Saturday, and I wanted Mr. Rogers to read my letter

before Monday. So I called up his secretary—everybody was working seven days a week to get the report out in time—and I said, "I'd like to dictate a letter to you; is that all right?"

She says, "Sure! To save you some money, let me call you right back." She calls me back, I dictate the letter, and she hands it directly to Rogers.

When I came back on Monday, Mr. Rogers said, "Dr. Feynman, I've read your letter, and I agree with everything it says. But you've been out-voted."

"Out-voted? How was I out-voted, when there was no meeting?"

Keel was there, too. He says, "We called everybody, and they all agree with the recommendation. They all voted for it."

"I don't think that's fair!" I protested. "If I could have presented my arguments to the other commissioners, I don't think I'd have been out-voted." I didn't know what to do, so I said, "I'd like to make a copy of it."

When I came back, Keel says, "We just remembered that we didn't talk to Hotz about it, because he was in a meeting. We forgot to get his vote."

I didn't know what to make of that, but I found out later that Mr. Hotz was in the building, not far from the copy machine.

Later, I talked to David Acheson about the tenth recommendation. He explained, "It doesn't really mean anything; it's only motherhood and apple pie."

I said, "Well, if it doesn't mean anything, it's not necessary, then."

"If this were a commission for the National Academy of Sciences, your objections would be proper. But don't forget," he says, "this is a presidential commission. We should say something for the President."

"I don't understand the difference," I said. *"Why can't I be careful and scientific when I'm writing a report to the President?"*

Being naive doesn't always work: my argument had no effect. Acheson kept telling me I was making a big thing out of nothing, and I kept saying it weakened our report and it shouldn't go in.

So that's where it ended up: "The Commission strongly recommends that NASA continue to receive the support of the Administration and the nation . . ."—all this "motherhood and apple pie" stuff to "balance" the report.

While I was flying home, I thought to myself, "It's funny that the only part of the report that was *genuinely* balanced was my own report: I said negative things about the engine, and positive things about the avionics. And I had to struggle with them to get it in, even as a lousy appendix!"

I thought about the tenth recommendation. All the other recommendations were based on evidence we had found, but this one had no evidence whatsoever. I could see the white-wash dripping down. It was *obviously* a mistake! It would make our report look bad. I was very disturbed.

When I got home, I talked to Joan, my sister. I told her about the tenth recommendation, and how I had been "out-voted."

"Did you call any of the other commissioners and talk to them yourself?" she said.

"Well, I talked to Acheson, but he was for it."

"Any others?"

"Uh, no." So I called up three other commissioners—I'll call them A, B, and C.

I call A, who says, *"What* tenth recommendation?"

I call B, who says, "Tenth recommendation? What are you talking about?"

I call C, who says, "Don't you remember, you dope? I was in the office when Rogers first told us, and I don't see anything wrong with it."

It appeared that the only people who knew about the tenth recommendation were the people who were in the office when Rogers told us. I didn't bother to make any more telephone calls. After all, it's enough—I didn't feel that I had to open all the safes to check that the combination is the same!*

Then I told Joan about my report—how it was so emasculated, even though it was going in as an appendix.

She says, "Well, if they do that to your report, what have you accomplished, being on the commission? What's the result of all your work?"

"Aha!"

I sent a telegram to Mr. Rogers:

PLEASE TAKE MY SIGNATURE OFF THE REPORT UNLESS TWO THINGS OCCUR: 1) THERE IS NO TENTH RECOMMEN- DATION, AND 2) MY REPORT APPEARS WITHOUT MODIFI- CATION FROM VERSION #23.

(I knew by this time I had to define everything carefully.)

In order to get the number of the version I wanted, I called Mr. Hotz, who was in charge of the documentation system and publishing the report. He sent me Version #23, so I had something definite to publish on my own, if worse came to worst.

---

* This refers to "Safecracker Meets Safecracker," another story told in *"Surely You're Joking, Mr. Feynman!"*

The result of this telegram was that Rogers and Keel tried to negotiate with me. They asked General Kutyna to be the intermediary, because they knew he was a friend of mine. What a *good* friend of mine he was, they didn't know.

Kutyna says, "Hello, Professor, I just wanted to tell you that I think you're doing very well. But I've been given the job of trying to talk you out of it, so I'm going to give you the arguments."

"Fear not!" I said. "I'm not gonna change my mind. Just give me the arguments, and fear not."

The first argument was that if I don't accept the tenth recommendation, they won't accept my report, even as an appendix.

I didn't worry about that one, because I could always put out my report myself.

All the arguments were like that: none of them was very good, and none of them had any effect. I had thought through carefully what I was doing, so I just stuck to my guns.

Then Kutyna suggested a compromise: they were willing to go along with my report as I wrote it, except for one sentence near the end.

I looked at the sentence and I realized that I had already made my point in the previous paragraph. Repeating the point amounted to polemics; removing the phrase made my report much better. I accepted the compromise.

Then I offered a compromise on the tenth recommendation: "If they want to say something nice about NASA at the end, just don't call it a recommendation, so people will know that it's not in the same class as the other recommendations: call it a 'concluding thought' if you want. And to avoid confusion, don't use the words 'strongly recommends.' Just say 'urges'— 'The Commission urges that NASA continue to receive the support of the Administration and the nation.' All the other stuff can stay the same."

A little bit later, Keel calls me up: "Can we say '*strongly urges*'?"

"No. Just 'urges'."

"Okay," he said. And that was the final decision.

MEET THE PRESS

I put my name on the main report, my own report got in as an appendix, and everything was all right. In early June we went back to Washington and gave our report to the President in a ceremony held in the Rose Garden. That was on a Thursday. The report was not to be released to the public until the following Monday, so the President could study it.

Meanwhile, the newspaper reporters were working like demons: they knew our report was finished and they were trying to scoop each other to find out what was in it. I knew they would be calling me up day and night, and I was afraid I would say something about a technical matter that would give them a hint.

Reporters are very clever and persistent. They'll say, "We heard such-and-such—is it true?" And pretty soon, what you're thinking you didn't tell them shows up in the newspaper!

I was determined not to say a word about the report until it was made public, on Monday. A friend of mine convinced me to go on the "MacNeil/Lehrer Newshour," so I said yes for Monday evening's show.

I also had my secretary set up a press conference for Tuesday at Caltech. I said, "Tell the reporters who want to talk to me that I haven't any comment on anything: any questions they have, I'll be glad to answer on Tuesday at my press conference."

Over the weekend, while I was still in Washington, it leaked somehow that I had threatened to take my name off the report. Some paper in Miami started it, and soon the story was running all over about this argument between me and Rogers. When the reporters who were used to covering Washington heard "Mr. Feynman has nothing to say; he'll answer all your questions at his press conference on Tuesday," it sounded suspicious—as though the argument was still on,

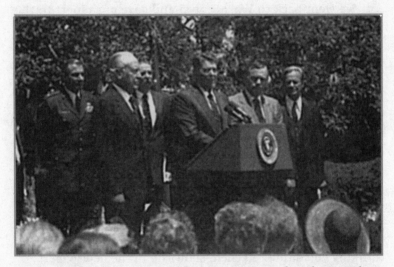

Figure 18. The Commission Report was presented to the President in the Rose Garden at the White House. Visible, from left to right, are General Kutyna, William Rogers, Eugene Covert, President Reagan, Neil Armstrong, and Richard Feynman. (© PETE SOUZA, THE WHITE HOUSE.)

and I was going to have this press conference on Tuesday to explain why I took my name off the report.

But I didn't know anything about it. I isolated myself from the press so much that I wasn't even reading the newspapers.

On Sunday night, the commission had a goodbye dinner arranged by Mr. Rogers at some club. After we finished eating, I said to General Kutyna, "I can't stay around anymore. I have to leave a little early."

He says, "What can be so important?"

I didn't want to say.

He comes outside with me, to see what this "important" something is. It's a bright red sports car with two beautiful blonds inside, waiting to whisk me away.

I get in the car. We're about to speed off, leaving General

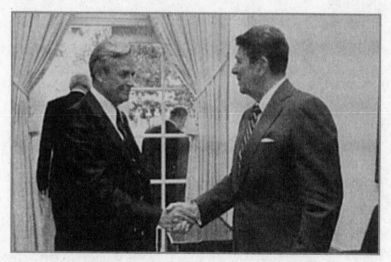

Figure 19. At the reception. (© PETE SOUZA, THE WHITE HOUSE.)

Kutyna standing there scratching his head, when one of the blonds says, "Oh! General Kutyna! I'm Ms. So-and-so. I interviewed you on the phone a few weeks ago."

So he caught on. They were reporters from the "MacNeil/ Lehrer Newshour."

They were very nice, and we talked about this and that for the show Monday night. Somewhere along the line I told them I was going to have my own press conference on Tuesday, and I was going to give out my report—even though it was going to appear as an appendix three months later. They said my report sounded interesting, and they'd like to see it. By this time we're all very friendly, so I gave them a copy.

They dropped me off at my cousin's house, where I was staying. I told Frances about the show, and how I gave the reporters a copy of my report. Frances puts her hands to her head, horrified.

I said, "Yes, that was a dumb mistake, wasn't it! I'd better call 'em up and tell 'em not to use it."

I could tell by the way Frances shook her head that it wasn't gonna be so easy!

I call one of them up: "I'm sorry, but I made a mistake: I shouldn't have given my report to you, so I'd prefer you didn't use it."

"We're in the news business, Dr. Feynman. The goal of the news business is to get news, and your report is newsworthy. It would be completely against our instincts and practice not to use it."

"I know, but I'm naive about these things. I simply made a mistake. It's not fair to the other reporters who will be at the press conference on Tuesday. After all, would you like it if you came to a press conference and the guy had mistakenly given his report to somebody else? I think you can understand that."

"I'll talk to my colleague and call you back."

Two hours later, they call back—they're both on the line— and they try to explain to me why they should use it: "In the news business, it's customary that whenever we get a document from somebody the way we did from you, it means we can use it."

"I appreciate that there are conventions in the news business, but I don't know anything about these things, so as a courtesy to me, please don't use it."

It went back and forth a little more like that. Then another "We'll call you back," and another long delay. I could tell from the long delays that they were having a lot of trouble with this problem.

I was in a very good fettle, for some reason. I had already lost, and I knew what I needed, so I could focus easily. I had no difficulty admitting complete idiocy—which is usually the case when I deal with the world—and I didn't think there was any law of nature which said I had to give in. I just kept going, and didn't waver at all.

It went late into the night: one o'clock, two o'clock, we're still working on it. "Dr. Feynman, it's very unprofessional to give someone a story and then retract it. This is not the way people behave in Washington."

"It's obvious I don't know anything about Washington. But this is the way *I* behave—like a fool. I'm sorry, but it was simply an error, so as a courtesy, please don't use it."

Then, somewhere along the line, one of them says, "If we

go ahead and use your report, does that mean you won't go on the show?"

"*You* said it; *I* didn't."

"We'll call you back."

Another delay.

Actually, I hadn't decided whether I'd refuse to go on the show, because I kept thinking it was possible I could undo my mistake. When I thought about it, I didn't think I could legitimately play that card. But when one of them made the mistake of proposing the possibility, I said, "*You* said it; *I* didn't"—very cold—as if to say, "I'm not threatening you, but you can figure it out for yourself, honey!"

They called me back, and said they wouldn't use my report.

When I went on the show, I never got the impression that any of the questions were based on my report. Mr. Lehrer did ask me whether there had been any problems between me and Mr. Rogers, but I weaseled: I said there had been no problems.

After the show was over, the two reporters told me they thought the show went fine without my report. We left good friends.

I flew back to California that night, and had my press conference on Tuesday at Caltech. A large number of reporters came. A few asked questions about my report, but most of them were interested in the rumor that I had threatened to take my name off the commission report. I found myself telling them over and over that I had no problem with Mr. Rogers.

AFTERTHOUGHTS

Now that I've had more time to think about it, I still like Mr. Rogers, and I still feel that everything's okay. It's my judgment that he's a fine man. Over the course of the commission I got to appreciate his talents and his abilities, and I have great respect for him. Mr. Rogers has a very good, smooth way about him, so I reserve in my head the possibility—not as a suspicion, but as an unknown—that I like him because he knew how to make me like him. I prefer to assume he's a genuinely fine fellow, and that he is the way he appears. But I was in Washington long enough to know that I can't tell.

I'm not exactly sure what Mr. Rogers thinks of me. He gives me the impression that, in spite of my being such a pain in the ass to him in the beginning, he likes me very much. I may be wrong, but if he feels the way I feel toward him, it's good.

Mr. Rogers, being a lawyer, had a difficult job to run a commission investigating what was essentially a technical question. With Dr. Keel's help, I think the technical part of it was handled well. But it struck me that there were several fishinesses associated with the big cheeses at NASA.

Every time we talked to higher level managers, they kept saying they didn't know anything about the problems below them. We're getting this kind of thing again in the Iran-Contra hearings, but at that time, this kind of situation was new to me: either the guys at the top didn't know, in which case they should have known, or they did know, in which case they're lying to us.

When we learned that Mr. Mulloy had put pressure on Thiokol to launch, we heard time after time that the next level up at NASA knew nothing about it. You'd think Mr. Mulloy would have notified a higher-up during this big discussion, saying something like, "There's a question as to whether we should fly tomorrow morning, and there's been some objection by the Thiokol engineers, but we've decided to fly anyway—what do you think?" But instead, Mulloy said something like, "All the questions have been resolved." There seemed to be some reason why guys at the lower level didn't bring problems up to the next level.

I invented a theory which I have discussed with a considerable number of people, and many people have explained to me why it's wrong. But I don't remember their explanations, so I cannot resist telling you what I think led to this lack of communication in NASA.

When NASA was trying to go to the moon, there was a great deal of enthusiasm: it was a goal everyone was anxious to achieve. They didn't know if they could do it, but they were all working together.

I have this idea because I worked at Los Alamos, and I experienced the tension and the pressure of everybody working together to make the atomic bomb. When somebody's having a problem—say, with the detonator—everybody knows that it's a big problem, they're thinking of ways to beat it, they're making suggestions, and when they hear about the solution they're excited, because that means their work is now useful: if the detonator didn't work, the bomb wouldn't work.

I figured the same thing had gone on at NASA in the early days: if the space suit didn't work, they couldn't go to the moon. So everybody's interested in everybody else's problems.

But then, when the moon project was over, NASA had all these people together: there's a big organization in Houston and a big organization in Huntsville, not to mention at Kennedy, in Florida. You don't want to fire people and send them out in the street when you're done with a big project, so the problem is, what to do?

You have to convince Congress that there exists a project that only NASA can do. In order to do so, it is necessary—at least it was *apparently* necessary in this case—to exaggerate: to exaggerate how economical the shuttle would be, to exaggerate how often it could fly, to exaggerate how safe it would be, to exaggerate the big scientific facts that would be discovered. "The shuttle can make so-and-so many flights and it'll cost such-and-such; we went to the moon, so we can *do* it!"

Meanwhile, I would guess, the engineers at the bottom are saying, "No, no! We can't make that many flights. If we had to make that many flights, it would mean such-and-such!" And, "No, we can't do it for that amount of money, because that would mean we'd have to do thus-and-so!"

Well, the guys who are trying to get Congress to okay their projects don't want to hear such talk. It's better if they don't hear, so they can be more "honest"—they don't want to be in the position of lying to Congress! So pretty soon the attitudes begin to change: information from the bottom which is disagreeable—"We're having a problem with the seals; we should fix it before we fly again"—is suppressed by big cheeses and middle managers who say, "If you tell me about the seals problems, we'll have to ground the shuttle and fix it." Or, "No, no, keep on flying, because otherwise, it'll look bad," or "Don't tell me; I don't want to hear about it."

Maybe they don't say explicitly "Don't tell me," but they discourage communication, which amounts to the same thing. It's not a question of what has been written down, or who should tell what to whom; it's a question of whether, when you *do* tell somebody about some problem, they're *delighted* to hear about it and they say "Tell me more" and "Have you tried such-and-such?" or they say "Well, see what you can do about it"—which is a completely different atmosphere. If you try once or twice to communicate and get pushed back, pretty soon you decide, "To hell with it."

So that's my theory: because of the exaggeration at the top being inconsistent with the reality at the bottom, communication got slowed up and ultimately jammed. That's how it's possible that the higher-ups didn't know.

The other possibility is that the higher-ups did know, and they just *said* they didn't know.

I looked up a former director of NASA—I don't remember his name now—who is the head of some company in California. I thought I'd go and talk to him when I was on one of my breaks at home, and say, "They all *say* they haven't heard. Does that make any sense? How does someone go about investigating them?"

He never returned my calls. Perhaps he didn't want to talk to the commissioner investigating higher-ups; maybe he had had enough of NASA, and didn't want to get involved. And because I was busy with so many other things, I didn't push it.

There were all kinds of questions we didn't investigate. One was this mystery of Mr. Beggs, the former director of NASA who was removed from his job pending an investigation that had nothing to do with the shuttle; he was replaced by Graham shortly before the accident. Nevertheless, it turned out that, every day, Beggs came to his old office. People came in to see him, although he never talked to Graham. What was he doing? Was there some activity still being directed by Beggs?

From time to time I would try to get Mr. Rogers interested in investigating such fishinesses. I said, "We have lawyers on the commission, we have company managers, we have very fine people with a large range of experiences. We have people who know how to get an answer out of a guy when he doesn't want to say something. I don't know how to do that. If a guy tells me the probability of failure is 1 in 10^5, I know he's full of crap—but I don't know what's natural in a bureaucratic system. We oughta get some of the big shots together and ask them questions: just like we asked the second-level managers like Mr. Mulloy, we should ask the first level."

He would say, "Yes, well, I think so."

Mr. Rogers told me later that he wrote a letter to each of the big shots, but they replied that they didn't have anything they wanted to say to us.

There was also the question of pressure from the White House.

It was the President's idea to put a teacher in space, as a symbol of the nation's commitment to education. He had proposed the idea a year before, in his State of the Union address. Now, one year later, the State of the Union speech was coming up again. It would be perfect to have the teacher in space, talking to the President and the Congress. All the circumstantial evidence was very strong.

I talked to a number of people about it, and heard various opinions, but I finally concluded that there was no pressure from the White House.

First of all, the man who pressured Thiokol to change its position, Mr. Mulloy, was a second-level manager. Ahead of time, nobody could predict what might get in the way of a launch. If you imagine Mulloy was told "Make sure the shuttle flies tomorrow, because the President wants it," you'd have to imagine that *everybody else* at his level had to be told—and there are a lot of people at his level. To tell that many people would make it sure to leak out. So that way of putting on pressure was very unlikely.

By the time the commission was over, I understood much better the character of operations in Washington and in NASA. I learned, by seeing how they worked, that the people in a big system like NASA *know* what has to be done—*without* being told.

There was *already* a big pressure to keep the shuttle flying. NASA had a flight schedule they were trying to meet, just to show the capabilities of NASA—never mind whether the president was going to give a speech that night or not. So I don't believe there was any direct activity or any special effort from the White House. There was no need to do it, so I don't believe it was done.

I could give you an analog of that. You know those signs that appear in the back windows of automobiles—those little yellow diamonds that say BABY ON BOARD, and things like that? You don't have to *tell* me there's a baby on board; I'm gonna drive carefully *anyway!* What am I supposed to do when I see there's a baby on board: act differently? As if I'm suddenly gonna drive more carefully and not hit the car because there's a baby on board, when all I'm trying to do is not hit it anyway!

So NASA was trying to get the shuttle up anyway: you don't have to say there's a baby on board, or there's a teacher on board, or it's important to get this one up for the President.

Now that I've talked to some people about my experiences on the commission, I think I understand a few things that I didn't understand so well earlier. One of them has to do with what I said to Dr. Keel that upset him so much. Recently I was talking to a man who spent a lot of time in Washington, and I asked him a particular question which, if he didn't take it right, could be considered a grave insult. I would like to explain the question, because it seems to me to be a real possibility of what I said to Dr. Keel.

The only way to have real success in science, the field I'm familiar with, is to describe the evidence very carefully without regard to the way you feel it should be. If you have a theory, you must try to explain what's good and what's bad about it equally. In science, you learn a kind of standard integrity and honesty.

In other fields, such as business, it's different. For example, almost every advertisement you see is obviously designed, in some way or another, to fool the customer: the print that they don't want you to read is small; the statements are written in an obscure way. It is obvious to anybody that the product is not being presented in a scientific and balanced way. Therefore, in the selling business, there's a lack of integrity.

My father had the spirit and integrity of a scientist, but he was a salesman. I remember asking him the question "How can a man of integrity be a salesman?"

He said to me, "Frankly, many salesmen in the business are not straightforward—they think it's a better way to sell. But I've tried being straightforward, and I find it has its advantages. In fact, I wouldn't do it any other way. If the customer thinks at all, he'll realize he has had some bad experience with another salesman, but hasn't had that kind of experience with you. So in the end, several customers will stay with you for a long time and appreciate it."

My father was not a big, successful, famous salesman; he was the sales manager for a medium-sized uniform company. He was successful, but not enormously so.

When I see a congressman giving his opinion on something, I always wonder if it represents his *real* opinion or if it represents an opinion that he's designed in order to be elected. It seems to be a central problem for politicians. So I often wonder: what is the relation of integrity to working in the government?

Now, Dr. Keel started out by telling me that he had a degree in physics. I always assume that everybody in physics has integrity—perhaps I'm naive about that—so I must have asked him a question I often think about: "How can a man of integrity get along in Washington?"

It's very easy to read that question another way: "Since you're getting along in Washington, you can't be a man of integrity!"

Another thing I understand better now has to do with where the idea came from that cold affects the O-rings. It was General Kutyna who called me up and said, "I was working on my carburetor, and I was thinking: what is the effect of cold on the O-rings?"

Well, it turns out that one of NASA's own astronauts told him there was information, somewhere in the works of NASA, that the O-rings had no resilience whatever at low temperatures—and NASA wasn't saying anything about it.

But General Kutyna had the career of that astronaut to worry about, so the *real* question the General was thinking about while he was working on his carburetor was, "How can I get this information out without jeopardizing my astronaut friend?" His solution was to get the professor excited about it, and his plan worked perfectly.

APPENDIX F:
PERSONAL OBSERVATIONS
ON THE RELIABILITY
OF THE SHUTTLE

Introduction

It appears that there are enormous differences of opinion as to the probability of a failure with loss of vehicle and of human life.* The estimates range from roughly 1 in 100 to 1 in 100,000. The higher figures come from working engineers, and the very low figures come from management. What are the causes and consequences of this lack of agreement? Since 1 part in 100,000 would imply that one could launch a shuttle each day for 300 years expecting to lose only one, we could properly ask, "What is the cause of management's fantastic faith in the machinery?"

We have also found that certification criteria used in flight readiness reviews often develop a gradually decreasing strict-

---

* Leighton's note: The version printed as Appendix F in the commission report does not appear to have been edited for spelling or grammar, so I took it upon myself—perhaps improperly—to smooth it out a little bit.

ness. The argument that the same risk was flown before without failure is often accepted as an argument for the safety of accepting it again. Because of this, obvious weaknesses are accepted again and again—sometimes without a sufficiently serious attempt to remedy them, sometimes without a flight delay because of their continued presence.

There are several sources of information: there are published criteria for certification, including a history of modifications in the form of waivers and deviations; in addition, the records of the flight readiness reviews for each flight document the arguments used to accept the risks of the flight. Information was obtained from direct testimony and reports of the range safety officer, Louis J. Ullian, with respect to the history of success of solid fuel rockets. There was a further study by him (as chairman of the Launch Abort Safety Panel, LASP) in an attempt to determine the risks involved in possible accidents leading to radioactive contamination from attempting to fly a plutonium power supply (called a radioactive thermal generator, or RTG) on future planetary missions. The NASA study of the same question is also available. For the history of the space shuttle main engines, interviews with management and engineers at Marshall, and informal interviews with engineers at Rocketdyne, were made. An independent (Caltech) mechanical engineer who consulted for NASA about engines was also interviewed informally. A visit to Johnson was made to gather information on the reliability of the avionics (computers, sensors, and effectors). Finally, there is the report "A Review of Certification Practices Potentially Applicable to Man-rated Reusable Rocket Engines," prepared at the Jet Propulsion Laboratory by N. Moore et al. in February 1986 for NASA Headquarters, Office of Space Flight. It deals with the methods used by the FAA and the military to certify their gas turbine and rocket engines. These authors were also interviewed informally.

Solid Rocket Boosters (SRB)

An estimate of the reliability of solid-fuel rocket boosters (SRBs) was made by the range safety officer by studying the experience of all previous rocket flights. Out of a total of nearly 2900 flights, 121 failed (1 in 25). This includes, however, what may be called "early errors"—rockets flown for the first few times in which design errors are discovered and fixed. A more reasonable figure for the mature rockets might be 1 in 50. With special care in selecting parts and in inspection, a figure below 1 in 100 might be achieved, but 1 in 1000 is probably not attainable with today's technology. (Since there are two rockets on the shuttle, these rocket failure rates must be doubled to get shuttle failure rates due to SRB failure.)

NASA officials argue that the figure is much lower. They point out that "since the shuttle is a manned vehicle, the probability of mission success is necessarily very close to 1.0." It is not very clear what this phrase means. Does it mean it *is* close to 1 or that it *ought to be* close to 1? They go on to explain, "Historically, this extremely high degree of mission success has given rise to a difference in philosophy between manned space flight programs and unmanned programs; i.e., numerical probability usage versus engineering judgment." (These quotations are from "Space Shuttle Data for Planetary Mission RTG Safety Analysis," pages 3-1 and 3-2, February 15, 1985, NASA, JSC.) It is true that if the probability of failure was as low as 1 in 100,000 it would take an inordinate number of tests to determine it: you would get nothing but a string of perfect flights with no precise figure—other than that the probability is likely less than the number of such flights in the string so far. But if the real probability is not so small, flights would show troubles, near failures, and possibly actual failures with a reasonable number of trials, and standard statistical methods could give a reasonable estimate. In fact, previous NASA experience had shown, on occasion, just such difficulties, near accidents, and even accidents, all giving warning that the probability of flight failure was not so very small.

Another inconsistency in the argument not to determine reliability through historical experience (as the range safety officer did) is NASA's appeal to history: "Historically, this high degree of mission success . . ." Finally, if we are to replace standard numerical probability usage with engineering judgment, why do we find such an enormous disparity between the management estimate and the judgment of the engineers? It would appear that, for whatever purpose—be it for internal or external consumption—the management of NASA exaggerates the reliability of its product to the point of fantasy.

The history of the certification and flight readiness reviews will not be repeated here (see other parts of the commission report), but the phenomenon of accepting seals that had shown erosion and blowby in previous flights is very clear. The *Challenger* flight is an excellent example: there are several references to previous flights; the acceptance and success of these flights are taken as evidence of safety. But erosion and blowby are not what the design expected. They are warnings that something is wrong. The equipment is not operating as expected, and therefore there is a danger that it can operate with even wider deviations in this unexpected and not thoroughly understood way. The fact that this danger did not lead to a catastrophe before is no guarantee that it will not the next time, unless it is completely understood. When playing Russian roulette, the fact that the first shot got off safely is of little comfort for the next. The origin and consequences of the erosion and blowby were not understood. Erosion and blowby did not occur equally on all flights or in all joints: sometimes there was more, sometimes less. Why not sometime, when whatever conditions determined it were right, wouldn't there be still more, leading to catastrophe?

In spite of these variations from case to case, officials behaved as if they understood them, giving apparently logical arguments to each other—often citing the "success" of previous flights. For example, in determining if flight 51-L was safe to fly in the face of ring erosion in flight 51-C, it was noted that the erosion depth was only one-third of the radius. It had been noted in an experiment cutting the ring that cutting it as deep as one radius was necessary before the ring failed. Instead of being very concerned that variations of poorly understood conditions might reasonably create a deeper erosion this time, it was asserted there was "a safety factor of three."

This is a strange use of the engineer's term "safety factor." If a bridge is built to withstand a certain load without the beams permanently deforming, cracking, or breaking, it may be designed for the materials used to actually stand up under three times the load. This "safety factor" is to allow for uncertain excesses of load, or unknown extra loads, or weaknesses in the material that might have unexpected flaws, et cetera. But if the expected load comes on to the new bridge and a crack appears in a beam, this is a failure of the design. There was no safety factor at all, even though the bridge did not actually collapse because the crack only went one-third of the way through the beam. The O-rings of the solid rocket boosters were not designed to erode. Erosion was a clue that something was wrong. Erosion was not something from which safety could be inferred.

There was no way, without full understanding, that one could have confidence that conditions the next time might not produce erosion three times more severe than the time before. Nevertheless, officials fooled themselves into thinking they had such understanding and confidence, in spite of the peculiar variations from case to case. A mathematical model was made to calculate erosion. This was a model based not on physical understanding but on empirical curve fitting. Specifically, it was supposed that a stream of hot gas impinged on the O-ring material, and the heat was determined at the point of stagnation (so far, with reasonable physical, thermodynamical laws). But to determine how much rubber eroded, it was assumed that the erosion varied as the .58 power of heat, the .58 being determined by a nearest fit. At any rate, adjusting some other numbers, it was determined that the model agreed with the erosion (to a depth of one-third the radius of the ring). There is nothing so wrong with this analysis as believing the answer! Uncertainties appear everywhere in the model. How strong the gas stream might be was unpredictable; it depended on holes formed in the putty. Blowby showed that the ring might fail, even though it was only partially eroded. The empirical formula was known to be uncertain, for the curve did not go directly through the very data points by which it was determined. There was a cloud of points, some twice above and some twice below the fitted curve, so erosions twice those predicted were reasonable from that cause alone. Similar uncertainties surrounded the other constants in the formula, et cetera, et cetera. When using a mathematical model, careful attention must be given to the uncertainties in the model.

Space Shuttle Main Engines (SSME)

During the flight of the 51-L the three space shuttle main engines all worked perfectly, even beginning to shut down in the last moments as the fuel supply began to fail. The question arises, however, as to whether—had the engines failed, and we were to investigate them in as much detail as we did the solid rocket booster—we would find a similar lack of attention to faults and deteriorating safety criteria. In other words, were the organization weaknesses that contributed to the accident confined to the solid rocket booster sector, or were they a more general characteristic of NASA? To that end the space shuttle main engines and the avionics were both investigated. No similar study of the orbiter or the external tank was made.

The engine is a much more complicated structure than the solid rocket booster, and a great deal more detailed engineering goes into it. Generally, the engineering seems to be of high quality, and apparently considerable attention is paid to deficiencies and faults found in engine operation.

The usual way that such engines are designed (for military or civilian aircraft) may be called the component system, or bottom-up design. First it is necessary to thoroughly understand the properties and limitations of the materials to be used (turbine blades, for example), and tests are begun in experimental rigs to determine those. With this knowledge, larger component parts (such as bearings) are designed and tested individually. As deficiencies and design errors are noted they are corrected and verified with further testing. Since one tests only parts at a time, these tests and modifications are not overly expensive. Finally one works up to the final design of the entire engine, to the necessary specifications. There is a good chance, by this time, that the engine will generally succeed, or that any failures are easily isolated and analyzed because the failure modes, limitations of materials, et cetera, are so well understood. There is a very good chance that the modifications to get around final difficulties in the engine are not very hard to make, for most of the serious problems have already been discovered and dealt with in the earlier, less expensive stages of the process.

The space shuttle main engine was handled in a different manner—top down, we might say. The engine was designed and put together all at once with relatively little detailed pre-liminary study of the materials and components. But now, when troubles are found in bearings, turbine blades, coolant pipes, et cetera, it is more expensive and difficult to discover the causes and make changes. For example, cracks have been found in the turbine blades of the high-pressure oxygen turbopump. Are they caused by flaws in the material, the effect of the oxy-gen atmosphere on the properties of the material, the thermal stresses of startup or shutdown, the vibration and stresses of steady running, or mainly at some resonance at certain speeds, or something else? How long can we run from crack initiation to crack failure, and how does this depend on power level? Using the completed engine as a test bed to resolve such questions is extremely expensive. One does not wish to lose entire engines in order to find out where and how failure occurs. Yet, an accu-rate knowledge of this information is essential to acquiring a confidence in the engine reliability in use. Without detailed understanding, confidence cannot be attained.

A further disadvantage of the top-down method is that if an understanding of a fault is obtained, a simple fix—such as a new shape for the turbine housing—may be impossible to implement without a redesign of the entire engine.

The space shuttle main engine is a very remarkable machine. It has a greater ratio of thrust to weight than any previous engine. It is built at the edge of—sometimes outside of—previous engineering experience. Therefore, as expected, many different kinds of flaws and difficulties have turned up. Because, unfortunately, it was built in a top-down manner, the flaws are difficult to find and to fix. The design aim of an engine lifetime of 55 mission equivalents (27,000 seconds of operation, either in missions of 500 seconds each or on a test stand) has not been obtained. The engine now requires very frequent maintenance and replacement of important parts such as turbopumps, bearings, sheet metal housings, et cetera. The high-pressure fuel turbopump had to be replaced every three or four mission equivalents (although this may have been fixed now) and the high-pressure oxygen turbopump every five or six. This was, at most, 10 percent of the original design specifications. But our main concern here is the determination of reliability.

In a total of 250,000 seconds of operation, the main engines have failed seriously perhaps 16 times. Engineers pay close attention to these failings and try to remedy them as quickly as possible by test studies on special rigs experimentally designed for the flaw in question, by careful inspection of the engine for suggestive clues (like cracks), and by considerable study and analysis. In this way, in spite of the difficulties of top-down design, through hard work many of the problems have apparently been solved.

A list of some of the problems (and their status) follows:

Turbine blade cracks in high-pressure fuel turbopumps (HPFTP). (May have been solved.)

Turbine blade cracks in high-pressure oxygen fuel turbopumps (HPOTP). (Not solved.)

Augmented spark igniter (ASI) line rupture. (Probably solved.)

Purge check valve failure. (Probably solved.)

ASI chamber erosion. (Probably solved.)

HPFTP turbine sheet metal cracking. (Probably solved.)

HPFTP coolant liner failure. (Probably solved.)

Main combustion chamber outlet elbow failure. (Probably solved.)

Main combustion chamber inlet elbow weld offset. (Probably solved.)

HPOTP subsynchronous whirl. (Probably solved.)

Flight acceleration safety cutoff system (partial failure in a redundant system). (Probably solved.)

Bearing spalling. (Partially solved.)

A vibration at 4000 hertz making some engines inoperable. (Not solved.)

Many of these apparently solved problems were the early difficulties of a new design: 13 of them occurred in the first 125,000 seconds and only 3 in the second 125,000 seconds. Naturally, one can never be sure that all the bugs are out; for some, the fix may not have addressed the true cause. Thus it is not unreasonable to guess there may be at least one surprise in the next 250,000 seconds, a probability of $\frac{1}{500}$ per engine per mission. On a mission there are three engines, but it is possible that some accidents would be self-contained and affect only one engine. (The shuttle can abort its mission with only two engines.) Therefore, let us say that the unknown surprises do not, in and of themselves, permit us to guess that the probability of mission failure due to the space shuttle main engines is less than $\frac{1}{500}$. To this we must add the chance of failure from known, but as yet unsolved, problems. These we discuss below.

(Engineers at Rocketdyne, the manufacturer, estimate the total probability as $\frac{1}{10,000}$. Engineers at Marshall estimate it as $\frac{1}{300}$, while NASA management, to whom these engineers report, claims it is $\frac{1}{100,000}$. An independent engineer consulting for NASA thought 1 or 2 per 100 a reasonable estimate.)

The history of the certification principles for these engines is confusing and difficult to explain. Initially the rule seems to have been that two sample engines must each have had twice the time operating without failure, as the operating time of the engine to be certified (rule of 2x). At least that is the FAA practice, and NASA seems to have adopted it originally, expecting the certified time to be 10 missions (hence 20 missions for each sample). Obviously, the best engines to use for comparison would be those of greatest total operating time (flight plus test), the so-called fleet leaders. But what if a third sample engine and several others fail in a short time? Surely we will not be safe because two were unusual in lasting longer. The short time might be more representative of the real possibilities, and in the spirit of the safety factor of

2, we should only operate at half the time of the short-lived samples.

The slow shift toward a decreasing safety factor can be seen in many examples. We take that of the HPFTP turbine blades. First of all the idea of testing an entire engine was abandoned. Each engine has had many important parts (such as the turbopumps themselves) replaced at frequent intervals, so the rule of 2x must be shifted from engines to components. Thus we accept an HPFTP for a given certification time if two samples have each run successfully for twice that time (and, of course, as a practical matter, no longer insisting that this time be as long as 10 missions). But what is "successfully"? The FAA calls a turbine blade crack a failure, in order to really provide a safety factor greater than 2 in practice. There is some time that an engine can run between the time a crack originally starts and the time it has grown large enough to fracture. (The FAA is contemplating new rules that take this extra safety time into account, but will accept them only if it is very carefully analyzed through known models within a known range of experience and with materials thoroughly tested. None of these conditions applies to the space shuttle main engines.)

Cracks were found in many second-stage HPFTP turbine blades. In one case three were found after 1900 seconds, while in another they were not found after 4200 seconds, although usually these longer runs showed cracks. To follow this story further we must realize that the stress depends a great deal on the power level. The *Challenger* flight, as well as previous flights, was at a level called 104 percent of rated power during most of the time the engines were operating. Judging from some material data, it is supposed that at 104 percent of rated power, the time to crack is about twice that at 109 percent, or full power level (FPL). Future flights were to be at 109 percent because of heavier payloads, and many tests were made at this level. Therefore, dividing time at 104 percent by 2, we obtain units called equivalent full power level (EFPL). (Obviously, some uncertainty is introduced by that, but it has not been studied.) The earliest cracks mentioned above occurred at 1375 seconds EFPL.

Now the certification rule becomes "limit all second-stage blades to a maximum of 1375 seconds EFPL." If one objects that the safety factor of 2 is lost, it is pointed out that the one turbine ran for 3800 seconds EFPL without cracks, and half of this is 1900 so we are being more conservative. We have fooled ourselves in three ways. First, we have only one sample, and it is not the fleet leader: the other two samples of 3800 or more seconds EFPL had 17 cracked blades between them. (There are 59 blades in the engine.) Next, we have abandoned the $2x$ rule and substituted equal time (1375). And finally, the 1375 is where a crack was discovered. We can say that no crack had been found below 1375, but the last time we looked and saw no cracks was 1100 seconds EFPL. We do not know when the crack formed between these times. For example, cracks may have been formed at 1150 seconds EFPL. (Approximately two-thirds of the blade sets tested in excess of 1375 seconds EFPL had cracks. Some recent experiments have, indeed, shown cracks as early as 1150 seconds.) It was important to keep the number high, for the shuttle had to fly its engines very close to their limit by the time the flight was over.

Finally, it is claimed that the criteria have not been abandoned, and that the system is safe, by giving up the FAA convention that there should be no cracks, and by considering only a completely fractured blade a failure. With this definition no engine has yet failed. The idea is that since there is sufficient time for a crack to grow to fracture, we can ensure that all is safe by inspecting all blades for cracks. If cracks are found, replace the blades, and if none are found, we have enough time for a safe mission. Thus, it is claimed, the crack problem is no longer a flight safety problem, but merely a maintenance problem.

This may in fact be true. But how well do we know that cracks always grow slowly enough so that no fracture can occur in a mission? Three engines have run for long time periods with a few cracked blades (about 3000 seconds EFPL), with no blade actually breaking off.

A fix for this cracking may have been found. By changing the blade shape, shot-peening the surface, and covering it with insulation to exclude thermal shock, the new blades have not cracked so far.

A similar story appears in the history of certification of the HPOTP, but we shall not give the details here.

In summary, it is evident that the flight readiness reviews and certification rules show a deterioration in regard to some of the problems of the space shuttle main engines that is closely analogous to the deterioration seen in the rules for the solid rocket boosters.

Avionics

By "avionics" is meant the computer system on the orbiter as well as its input sensors and output actuators. At first we will restrict ourselves to the computers proper, and not be concerned with the reliability of the input information from the sensors of temperature, pressure, et cetera; nor with whether the computer output is faithfully followed by the actuators of rocket firings, mechanical controls, displays to astronauts, et cetera.

The computing system is very elaborate, having over 250,000 lines of code. Among many other things it is responsible for the automatic control of the shuttle's entire ascent into orbit, and for the descent until the shuttle is well into the atmosphere (below Mach 1), once one button is pushed deciding the landing site desired. It would be possible to make the entire landing automatic. (The landing gear lowering signal is expressly left out of computer control, and must be provided by the pilot, ostensibly for safety reasons.) During orbital flight the computing system is used in the control of payloads, in the display of information to the astronauts, and in the exchange of information with the ground. It is evident that the safety of flight requires guaranteed accuracy of this elaborate system of computer hardware and software.

In brief, hardware reliability is ensured by having four essentially independent identical computer systems. Where possible, each sensor also has multiple copies—usually four—and each copy feeds all four of the computer lines. If the inputs from the sensors disagree, either a certain average or a majority selection is used as the effective input, depending on the circumstances. Since each computer sees all copies of the sensors, the inputs are the same, and because the algorithms used by each of the four computers are the same, the results in each computer should be identical at each step. From time to time they are compared, but because they might operate at slightly different speeds, a system of stopping and waiting at specified times is instituted before each comparison is

made. If one of the computers disagrees or is too late in having its answer ready, the three which do agree are assumed to
be correct and the errant computer is taken completely out
of the system. If, now, another computer fails, as judged by
the agreement of the other two, it is taken out of the system,
and the rest of the flight is canceled: descent to the landing
site is instituted, controlled by the two remaining computers.
It is seen that this is a redundant system since the failure of
only one computer does not affect the mission. Finally, as an
extra feature of safety, there is a fifth independent computer,
whose memory is loaded with only the programs for ascent
and descent, and which is capable of controlling the descent
if there is a failure of more than two of the computers of the
main line of four.

There is not enough room in the memory of the mainline
computers for all the programs of ascent, descent, and payload
programs in flight, so the memory is loaded by the astronauts
about four times from tapes.

Because of the enormous effort required to replace the
software for such an elaborate system and to check out a new
system, no change in the hardware has been made since the
shuttle transportation system began about fifteen years ago.
The actual hardware is obsolete—for example, the memories
are of the old ferrite-core type. It is becoming more difficult to
find manufacturers to supply such old-fashioned computers
that are reliable and of high enough quality. Modern computers are much more reliable, and they run much faster. This
simplifies circuits and allows more to be done. Today's computers would not require so much loading from tapes, for their
memories are much larger.

The software is checked very carefully in a bottom-up fashion. First, each new line of code is checked; then sections of code (modules) with special functions are verified. The scope is increased step by step until the new changes are incorporated into a complete system and checked. This complete output is considered the final product, newly released. But working completely independently is a verification group that takes an adversary attitude to the software development group and tests the software as if it were a customer of the delivered product. There is additional verification in using the new programs in simulators, et cetera. An error during this stage of verification testing is considered very serious, and its origin is studied very carefully to avoid such mistakes in the future. Such inexperienced errors have been found only about six times in all the programming and program changing (for new or altered payloads) that has been done. The principle followed is: all this verification is not an aspect of program safety; it is a test of that safety in a noncatastrophic verification. Flight safety is to be judged solely on how well the programs do in the verified tests. A failure here generates considerable concern.

To summarize, then, the computer software checking system is of highest quality. There appears to be no process of gradually fooling oneself while degrading standards, the process so characteristic of the solid rocket booster and space shuttle main engine safety systems. To be sure, there have been recent suggestions by management to curtail such elaborate and expensive tests as being unnecessary at this late date in shuttle history. Such suggestions must be resisted, for they do not appreciate the mutual subtle influences and sources of error generated by even small program changes in one part of a program on another. There are perpetual requests for program changes as new payloads and new demands and modifications are suggested by the users. Changes are expensive because they require extensive testing. The proper way to save money is to curtail the number of requested changes, not the quality of testing for each.

One might add that the elaborate system could be very much improved by modern hardware and programming techniques. Any outside competition would have all the advantages of starting over. Whether modern hardware is a good idea for NASA should be carefully considered now.

Finally, returning to the sensors and actuators of the avionics system, we find that the attitude toward system failure and reliability is not nearly as good as for the computer system. For example, a difficulty was found with certain temperature sensors sometimes failing. Yet eighteen months later the same sensors were still being used, still sometimes failing, until a launch had to be scrubbed because two of them failed at the same time. Even on a succeeding flight this unreliable sensor was used again. And reaction control systems, the rocket jets used for reorienting and control in flight, still are somewhat unreliable. There is considerable redundancy, but also a long history of failures, none of which has yet been extensive enough to seriously affect a flight. The action of the jets is checked by sensors: if a jet fails to fire, the computers choose another jet to fire. But they are not designed to fail, and the problem should be solved.

Conclusions

If a reasonable launch schedule is to be maintained, engineering often cannot be done fast enough to keep up with the expectations of the originally conservative certification criteria designed to guarantee a very safe vehicle. In such situations, safety criteria are altered subtly—and with often apparently logical arguments—so that flights can still be certified in time. The shuttle therefore flies in a relatively unsafe condition, with a chance of failure on the order of a percent. (It is difficult to be more accurate.)

Official management, on the other hand, claims to believe the probability of failure is a thousand times less. One reason for this may be an attempt to assure the government of NASA's perfection and success in order to ensure the supply of funds. The other may be that they sincerely believe it to be true, demonstrating an almost incredible lack of communication between the managers and their working engineers.

In any event, this has had very unfortunate consequences, the most serious of which is to encourage ordinary citizens to fly in such a dangerous machine—as if it had attained the safety of an ordinary airliner. The astronauts, like test pilots, should know their risks, and we honor them for their courage. Who can doubt that McAuliffe* was equally a person of great courage, who was closer to an awareness of the true risks than NASA management would have us believe?

Let us make recommendations to ensure that NASA officials deal in a world of reality, understanding technological weaknesses and imperfections well enough to be actively trying to eliminate them. They must live in a world of reality in comparing the costs and utility of the shuttle to other methods of

---

* Christa McAuliffe, a schoolteacher, was to have been the first ordinary citizen in space—a symbol of the nation's commitment to education, and of the shuttle's safety.

entering space. And they must be realistic in making contracts and in estimating the costs and difficulties of each project. Only realistic flight schedules should be proposed—schedules that have a reasonable chance of being met. If in this way the government would not support NASA, then so be it. NASA owes it to the citizens from whom it asks support to be frank, honest, and informative, so that these citizens can make the wisest decisions for the use of their limited resources.

For a successful technology, reality must take precedence over public relations, for Nature cannot be fooled.

Epilogue

PREFACE

When I was younger, I thought science would make good things for everybody. It was obviously useful; it was good. During the war I worked on the atomic bomb. This result of science was obviously a very serious matter: it represented the destruction of people.

After the war I was very worried about the bomb. I didn't know what the future was going to look like, and I certainly wasn't anywhere near sure that we would last until now. Therefore one question was—is there some evil involved in science?

Put another way—what is the value of the science I had dedicated myself to—the thing I loved—when I saw what terrible things it could do? It was a question I had to answer.

"The Value of Science" is a kind of report, if you will, on many of the thoughts that came to me when I tried to answer that question.

Richard Feynman

THE VALUE OF SCIENCE*

From time to time people suggest to me that scientists ought to give more consideration to social problems— especially that they should be more responsible in considering the impact of science on society. It seems to be generally believed that if the scientists would only look at these very difficult social problems and not spend so much time fooling with less vital scientific ones, great success would come of it.

It seems to me that we *do* think about these problems from time to time, but we don't put a full-time effort into them— the reasons being that we know we don't have any magic formula for solving social problems, that social problems are very much harder than scientific ones, and that we usually don't get anywhere when we do think about them.

I believe that a scientist looking at nonscientific problems is just as dumb as the next guy—and when he talks about a

* A public address given at the 1955 autumn meeting of the National Academy of Sciences.

nonscientific matter, he sounds as naive as anyone untrained in the matter. Since the question of the value of science is *not* a scientific subject, this talk is dedicated to proving my point—by example.

The first way in which science is of value is familiar to everyone. It is that scientific knowledge enables us to do all kinds of things and to make all kinds of things. Of course if we make *good* things, it is not only to the credit of science; it is also to the credit of the moral choice which led us to good work. Scientific knowledge is an enabling power to do either good or bad—but it does not carry instructions on how to use it. Such power has evident value—even though the power may be negated by what one does with it.

I learned a way of expressing this common human problem on a trip to Honolulu. In a Buddhist temple there, the man in charge explained a little bit about the Buddhist religion for tourists, and then ended his talk by telling them he had something to say to them that they would *never* forget—and I have never forgotten it. It was a proverb of the Buddhist religion:

To every man is given the key to the gates of heaven;
the same key opens the gates of hell.

What then, is the value of the key to heaven? It is true that if we lack clear instructions that enable us to determine which is the gate to heaven and which the gate to hell, the key may be a dangerous object to use.

But the key obviously has value: how can we enter heaven without it?

Instructions would be of no value without the key. So it is evident that, in spite of the fact that it could produce enormous horror in the world, science is of value because it *can* produce *something.*

Another value of science is the fun called intellectual enjoyment which some people get from reading and learning and thinking about it, and which others get from working in it. This is an important point, one which is not considered enough by those who tell us it is our social responsibility to reflect on the impact of science on society.

Is this mere personal enjoyment of value to society as a whole? No! But it is also a responsibility to consider the aim of society itself. Is it to arrange matters so that people can enjoy things? If so, then the enjoyment of science is as important as anything else.

But I would like *not* to underestimate the value of the world view which is the result of scientific effort. We have been led to imagine all sorts of things infinitely more marvelous than the imaginings of poets and dreamers of the past. It shows that the imagination of nature is far, far greater than the imagination of man. For instance, how much more remarkable it is for us all to be stuck—half of us upside down—by a mysterious attraction to a spinning ball, which has been swinging in space for billions of years, than to be carried on the back of an elephant supported on a tortoise swimming in a bottomless sea.

I have thought about these things so many times alone that I hope you will excuse me if I remind you of this type of thought that I am sure many of you have had, which no one could ever have had in the past because people then didn't have the information we have about the world today.

For instance, I stand at the seashore, alone, and start to think.

There are the rushing waves
mountains of molecules
each stupidly minding its own business
trillions apart
yet forming white surf in unison.

Ages on ages
before any eyes could see
year after year
thunderously pounding the shore as now.
For whom, for what?
On a dead planet
with no life to entertain.

Never at rest
tortured by energy
wasted prodigiously by the sun
poured into space.
A mite makes the sea roar.

Deep in the sea
all molecules repeat
the patterns of one another
till complex new ones are formed.
They make others like themselves
and a new dance starts.

Growing in size and complexity
living things
masses of atoms

DNA, protein
dancing a pattern ever more intricate.

Out of the cradle
onto dry land
here it is
standing:
atoms with consciousness;
matter with curiosity.

Stands at the sea,
wonders at wondering: I
a universe of atoms,
an atom in the universe.

The same thrill, the same awe and mystery, comes again and again when we look at any question deeply enough. With more knowledge comes a deeper, more wonderful mystery, luring one on to penetrate deeper still. Never concerned that the answer may prove disappointing, with pleasure and confidence we turn over each new stone to find unimagined strangeness leading on to more wonderful questions and mysteries—certainly a grand adventure!

It is true that few unscientific people have this particular type of religious experience. Our poets do not write about it; our artists do not try to portray this remarkable thing. I don't know why. Is no one inspired by our present picture of the universe? This value of science remains unsung by singers: you are reduced to hearing not a song or poem, but an evening lecture about it. This is not yet a scientific age.

Perhaps one of the reasons for this silence is that you have to know how to read the music. For instance, the scientific article may say, "The radioactive phosphorus content of the cerebrum of the rat decreases to one-half in a period of two weeks." Now what does that mean?

It means that phosphorus that is in the brain of a rat—and also in mine, and yours—is not the same phosphorus as it was two weeks ago. It means the atoms that are in the brain are being replaced: the ones that were there before have gone away.

So what is this mind of ours: what are these atoms with consciousness? Last week's potatoes! They now can *remember* what was going on in my mind a year ago—a mind which has long ago been replaced.

To note that the thing I call my individuality is only a pattern or dance, *that* is what it means when one discovers how long it takes for the atoms of the brain to be replaced by other atoms. The atoms come into my brain, dance a dance, and then go out—there are always new atoms, but always doing the same dance, remembering what the dance was yesterday.

When we read about this in the newspaper, it says "Scientists say this discovery may have importance in the search for a cure for cancer." The paper is only interested in the use of the idea, not the idea itself. Hardly anyone can understand the importance of an idea, it is so remarkable. Except that, possibly, some children catch on. And when a child catches on to an idea like that, we have a scientist. It is too late* for them to get the spirit when they are in our universities, so we must attempt to explain these ideas to children.

I would now like to turn to a third value that science has.

* I would now say, "It is late—although not too late—for them to get the spirit . . ."

It is a little less direct, but not much. The scientist has a lot of experience with ignorance and doubt and uncertainty, and this experience is of very great importance, I think. When a scientist doesn't know the answer to a problem, he is ignorant. When he has a hunch as to what the result is, he is uncertain. And when he is pretty darn sure of what the result is going to be, he is still in some doubt. We have found it of paramount importance that in order to progress we must recognize our ignorance and leave room for doubt. Scientific knowledge is a body of statements of varying degrees of certainty—some most unsure, some nearly sure, but none *absolutely* certain.

Now, we scientists are used to this, and we take it for granted that it is perfectly consistent to be unsure, that it is possible to live and *not* know. But I don't know whether everyone realizes this is true. Our freedom to doubt was born out of a struggle against authority in the early days of science. It was a very deep and strong struggle: permit us to question— to doubt—to not be sure. I think that it is important that we do not forget this struggle and thus perhaps lose what we have gained. Herein lies a responsibility to society.

We are all sad when we think of the wondrous potentialities human beings seem to have, as contrasted with their small accomplishments. Again and again people have thought that we could do much better. Those of the past saw in the nightmare of their times a dream for the future. We, of *their* future, see that their dreams, in certain ways surpassed, have in many ways remained dreams. The hopes for the future today are, in good share, those of yesterday.

It was once thought that the possibilities people had were not developed because most of the people were ignorant. With universal education, could all men be Voltaires? Bad can be taught at least as efficiently as good. Education is a strong force, but for either good or evil.

Communications between nations must promote understanding—so went another dream. But the machines of communication can be manipulated. What is communicated can be truth or lie. Communication is a strong force, but also for either good or evil.

The applied sciences should free men of material problems at least. Medicine controls diseases. And the record here seems all to the good. Yet there are some patiently working today to create great plagues and poisons for use in warfare tomorrow.

Nearly everyone dislikes war. Our dream today is peace. In peace, man can develop best the enormous possibilities he seems to have. But maybe future men will find that peace, too, can be good and bad. Perhaps peaceful men will drink out of boredom. Then perhaps drink will become the great problem which seems to keep man from getting all he thinks he should out of his abilities.

Clearly, peace is a great force—as are sobriety, material power, communication, education, honesty, and the ideals of many dreamers. We have more of these forces to control than did the ancients. And maybe we are doing a little better than most of them could do. But what we ought to be able to do seems gigantic compared with our confused accomplishments.

Why is this? Why can't we conquer ourselves?

Because we find that even great forces and abilities do not seem to carry with them clear instructions on how to use them. As an example, the great accumulation of understanding as to how the physical world behaves only convinces one that this behavior seems to have a kind of meaninglessness. The sciences do not directly teach good and bad.

Through all ages of our past, people have tried to fathom the meaning of life. They have realized that if some direction or meaning could be given to our actions, great human forces would be unleashed. So, very many answers have been given to the question of the meaning of it all. But the answers have been of all different sorts, and the proponents of one answer have looked with horror at the actions of the believers in another— horror, because from a disagreeing point of view all the great potentialities of humanity are channeled into a false and confining blind alley. In fact, it is from the history of the enormous monstrosities created by false belief that philosophers have realized the apparently infinite and wondrous capacities of human beings. The dream is to find the open channel.

What, then, is the meaning of it all? What can we say to dispel the mystery of existence?

If we take everything into account—not only what the ancients knew, but all of what we know today that they didn't know—then I think we must frankly admit that *we do not know*.

But, in admitting this, we have probably found the open channel.

This is not a new idea; this is the idea of the age of reason. This is the philosophy that guided the men who made the democracy that we live under. The idea that no one really knew how to run a government led to the idea that we should arrange a system by which new ideas could be developed, tried out, and tossed out if necessary, with more new ideas brought in—a trial-and-error system. This method was a result of the fact that science was already showing itself to be a successful venture at the end of the eighteenth century. Even then it was clear to socially minded people that the openness of possibilities was an opportunity, and that doubt and discussion were essential to progress into the unknown. If we want to solve a problem that we have never solved before, we must leave the door to the unknown ajar.

We are at the very beginning of time for the human race. It is not unreasonable that we grapple with problems. But there are tens of thousands of years in the future. Our responsibility is to do what we can, learn what we can, improve the solutions, and pass them on. It is our responsibility to leave the people of the future a free hand. In the impetuous youth of humanity, we can make grave errors that can stunt our growth for a long time. This we will do if we say we have the answers now, so young and ignorant as we are. If we suppress all discussion, all criticism, proclaiming "This is the answer, my friends; man is saved!" we will doom humanity for a long time to the chains of authority, confined to the limits of our present imagination. It has been done so many times before.

It is our responsibility as scientists, knowing the great progress which comes from a satisfactory philosophy of ignorance, the great progress which is the fruit of freedom of thought, to proclaim the value of this freedom; to teach how doubt is not to be feared but welcomed and discussed; and to demand this freedom as our duty to all coming generations.

Index

HEAR RICHARD FEYNMAN

It's heartening to know that one hundred years after his birth, Richard Feyman's "adventures of a curious character" are still being read—on paper, no less!

Since these stories were meant to be heard, you can hear some of them in Feynman's own voice (assuming the Internet still exists in its present form when you read this) by visiting Feynman.com.